PocketGuide to
Communication
Disorders

Hegde's PocketGuide to Communication Disorders

M. N. Hegde, Ph.D.
Department of Communicative Sciences and Disorders
California State University–Fresno

THOMSON

DELMAR LEARNING

Australia   Canada   Mexico   Singapore   Spain   United Kingdom   United States

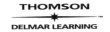

THOMSON

DELMAR LEARNING

Hegde's PocketGuide to
Communication Disorders
by M. N. Hegde

Vice President, Health Care Business Unit:
William Brottmiller

Director of Learning Solutions:
Matthew Kane

Senior Acquisitions Editor:
Sherry Dickinson

Senior Product Manager:
Juliet Steiner

Editorial Assistant:
Angela Doolin

Marketing Director:
Jennifer McAvey

Marketing Manager:
Chris Manion

Marketing Coordinator:
Vanessa Carlson

Production Director:
Carolyn Miller

Content Project Manager:
Katie Wachtl

Senior Art Director:
Jack Pendleton

Library of Congress
Cataloging-in-Publication Data
Hegde, M. N. (Mahabalagiri N.), 1941–
Hegde's PocketGuide to communication disorders / M. N. Hegde.
p. ; cm.
Includes bibliographical references.
ISBN 978-1-4180-5210-2
1. Communicative disorders—Handbooks, manuals, etc. I. Title.
II. Title: Hegde's pocket guide to communication disorders. III. Title:
PocketGuide to communication disorders. [DNLM: 1. Communication Disorders—Handbooks.
WL 39 H462hp 2008]
RC423.H3827 2008
616.85'5—dc22
2007016111

NOTICE TO THE READER

Publisher does not warrant or guarantee any of the products described herein or perform any independent analysis in connection with any of the product information contained herein. Publisher does not assume, and expressly disclaims, any obligation to obtain and include information other than that provided to it by the manufacturer.

The reader is expressly warned to consider and adopt all safety precautions that might be indicated by the activities described herein and to avoid all potential hazards. By following the instructions contained herein, the reader willingly assumes all risks in connection with such instructions.

The publisher makes no representations or warranties of any kind, including but not limited to, the warranties of fitness for particular purpose or merchantability, nor are any such representations implied with respect to the material set forth herein, and the publisher takes no responsibility with respect to such material. The publisher shall not be liable for any special, consequential, or exemplary damages resulting, in whole or part, from the reader's use of, or reliance upon, this material.

Major Entries

About the Author

M. N. (Giri) Hegde, Ph.D., is Professor of Communication Sciences and Disorders at California State University–Fresno. He holds a Master's degree in experimental psychology from the University of Mysore, India; a post-Master's diploma in Medical (Clinical) Psychology from Bangalore University, India; and a doctoral degree in Speech-Language Pathology from Southern Illinois University at Carbondale, Illinois.

Dr. Hegde is a specialist in fluency disorders, language disorders, research methods, and treatment procedures in communicative disorders. He has published many research articles on language and fluency disorders. He has made numerous presentations to national and international audiences on both basic and applied topics in communicative disorders and experimental and applied behavior analysis. With his deep, as well as wide scholarship, Dr. Hegde has authored several highly regarded and widely used scientific and professional books, including: *Treatment Procedures in Communicative Disorders, Clinical Research in Communicative Disorders, Introduction to Communicative Disorders, A Coursebook on Aphasia and Other Neurogenic Language Disorders, Language Disorders in Children: An Evidence-Based Approach to Assessment and Treatment* (with Christine Maul), *Clinical Methods and Practicum in Speech-Language Pathology* (with Deborah Davis), *Treatment Protocols for Stuttering,* the two-volume *Treatment Protocols for Language Disorders in Children, A Coursebook on Scientific and Professional Writing in Speech-Language Pathology, An Advanced Review of Speech-Language Pathology* (with Celeste Roseberry-McKibbin), and *Assessment and Treatment of Articulation and Phonological Disorders in Children* (with Adriana Peña-Brooks). He also has served on the editorial boards of several scientific and professional journals and continues to serve as an editorial consultant to the *American Journal of Speech-Language Pathology* and the *Journal of Fluency Disorders.*

Dr. Hegde is the recipient of various honors including: the Outstanding Professor Award from California State University–Fresno; CSU–Fresno Provost's Recognition for Outstanding Scholarship and Publication; Distinguished Alumnus Award from the Southern Illinois University Department of Communication Sciences and Disorders; and Outstanding Professional Achievement Award from District 5 of California Speech-Language-Hearing Association. Dr. Hegde is a Fellow of the American Speech-Language-Hearing Association.

Preface

This PocketGuide to Communication Disorders has been designed as a companion volume to the third editions of *Hegde's PocketGuide to Assessment in Speech-Language Pathology* and *Hegde's PocketGuide to Treatment in Speech-Language Pathology*. These three PocketGuides combine the most desirable features of a specialized dictionary of terms, clinical resource books, and textbooks. The Pocket-Guides are meant to be quick reference books like a dictionary because the entries are alphabetized, but they offer more than a dictionary because they contain extensive information on the disorders, their assessment, or treatment. The PocketGuides offer more than most resource books by alphabetically organizing detailed and specific information. Unlike textbooks that address only one disorder each, these PocketGuides are organized such that in-depth information can be quickly retrieved on most disorders of communication.

This new PocketGuide was created to offer systematic information on communication disorders themselves, so that the other guides could be more fully devoted to either assessment or treatment. The ever-expanding research base in communication disorders and related medical conditions made it necessary to create a new guide that is exclusively concerned with the disorders. This new guide made it possible to expand the assessment and treatment guides to include new information.

How the PocketGuide is Organized

This PocketGuide on communication disorders is organized like the previous two guides. It summarizes the available research and clinical information on disorders of communication, epidemiology and ethnocultural factors, symptomatology, onset and development, etiological factors, and major theoretical concepts. Whenever appropriate, neurophysiological and neuropathological factors related to a communication disorder also are described.

Each major disorder of communication is an alphabetized entry in the guide. Within each major entry, types or varieties of that disorder are alphabetically described. For example, under the main entry Aphasia, the specific types of aphasia are described (e.g., Broca's Aphasia, Wernicke's Aphasia). Under the main entry Fluency Disorders, the reader will find entries for Cluttering, Neurogenic Stuttering, and Stuttering.

Entries in the guide are not limited to major disorders. Neurophysiological diseases or disorders of relevance and various clinical and related concepts are also defined and described.

How to Use this PocketGuide

The guide may be used much like a dictionary. A clinician who wants to find out information about a specific communication disorder will access it by its main alphabetical entry. The table of contents will quickly direct the clinician to the major entries in the book; most of these are names of various disorders. Under each main entry, the clinician will find information within a standard format as described. The clinician also may be referred to related concepts and disorders that are cross-referenced. All cross-referenced entries are underlined. Thus, throughout the guide, an underlined term means that the reader can find more about it in its own main alphabetical entry.

Serious attempts have been made to include most reliable information on communication disorders. However, the author is aware that not every symptom and not every theoretical concept have been included in this guide. To support evidence-based practice, information generally supported by empirical research has been given priority, although controversial concepts are noted as well.

Acknowledgments

I would like to thank several anonymous reviewers for their thoughtful and detailed comments which have been invaluable in finalizing this book. I would also like to thank Francine Pomaville, my colleague and friend at California State University–Fresno, who reviewed and offered excellent comments on laryngectomy. Finally, I am thankful to Juliet Steiner, Senior Product Manager at Thomson Delmar Learning, for her excellent, friendly, and sustained support to complete this book.

A

Abductor Spasmodic Dysphonia. A type of voice disorder; also known as *phonation breaks, intermittent abductory dysphonia*, and *abductor spasms*; thought to be functional in origin, although it may be considered a type of Spasmodic Dysphonia, in which case it may be a suspected neurological disorder (laryngeal dystonia); the most significant feature of the disorder is sudden, intermittent, and fleeting cessation of voice (aphonia) because of vocal fold abduction; howevere, the voice may be normal except for such phonation breaks; the voice may remain normal for only a few seconds or days altogether; excessive effort (hyperfunction) in producing voice and speech is also part of this problem; because of such excessive laryngeal muscle tension associated with abrupt abductions and phonation breaks, some clinicians continue to describe this problem as *spastic dysphonia*.

Colton, R. H., Casper, J. K., & Leonard, R. (2006). *Understanding voice problems* (3rd ed.). Philadelphia, PA: Lippincott Williams and Wilkins.

Boone, D. R., McFarlane, S. C., & Von Berg, S. L. (2005). *The voice and voice therapy* (7th ed.). Boston, MA: Allyn and Bacon.

Abulia. Extreme lack of motivation, found in some psychiatric and neurological disorders; not an independent disease entity, but a symptom of some disease conditions; the client with abulia is disinterested in any kind of activity, including speaking; an extreme form of abulia is called akinetic Mutism, in which the client is alert, does not have neuromotor disorders related to speech, but still lacks motivation to speak; in some cases, associated with severe frontal lobe damage; see also Psychiatric Problems Associated with Communication Disorders.

Acquired Immune Deficiency Syndrome (AIDS). A syndrome caused by human immunodeficiency virus; pathology includes destruction of white blood cells that reduce cell-mediated immunity; although there is no cure for the disease, several drugs have checked the progression of the disease and have increased clients' survival rate and duration; one of the causes of dementia, known as the AIDS Dementia Complex.

Acrocephaly. A cranial abnormality resulting in high-domed skull; part of certain genetic syndromes including Waardenburg syndrome (see Syndromes Associated With Communication Disorders).

Adaptation Effect. Progressive decrease in the frequency of stuttering when a printed passage is orally read repeatedly; maximum decrease often on the second reading; decrease is progressively less on subsequent readings; little or no decrease after the fifth reading; reduced or eliminated by rest pause between readings; shows no transfer across passages; marked effect suggests relatively weak stimulus control of stuttering; contrasts with Consistency Effect.

Adjacency Effect. Occurrence of new stuttering on previously fluently read words because they are adjacent to words that were stuttered in prior oral readings of the same passage; methodologically, studied by blotting out the previously stuttered words and asking the client to read the passage aloud; some of the words printed before, after, above, and below the blotted words may be stuttered on repeated readings even though they were initially read fluently; shows that stuttering is under stimulus control.

Agenesis. Absence of an organ due to genetic defect.

Agnosia. A group of disorders in which recognition of sensory stimuli is impaired to varying extents; not due to impaired sense organs but to central nervous system dysfunction; the clients can see, hear, or feel stimuli or objects but are unable to grasp the meaning of stimuli and objects they come in contact with; although pure agnosia is rare, some clients with cerebral pathology may give the impression of agnosia when difficulty recognizing stimuli may be due to impaired intellect (as in dementia), disturbed sensory discrimination, or simple comprehension deficit; to diagnose agnosia, it should not be a function of intellectual deterioration or dementia; once recognized, the clients will be able to name the stimulus; a client who cannot recognize an object presented visually may recognize it in some other modality (e.g., tactile or auditory); there are several types of agnosia and the following are the major types:

- Auditory agnosia: Difficulty recognizing the meaning of auditory stimuli including language; clients have normal peripheral hearing as assessed by pure tone audiometry; bilateral damage to the auditory association areas is the typical cerebral pathology; the clients:
  o Can hear sounds and respond to them, but cannot understand their meaning
  o May visually recognize objects, but cannot match the object with its sound characteristics
- Auditory verbal agnosia: Difficulty understanding the meaning of spoken words, though the clients can hear them; also known as *pure word deafness*; a rare form of agnosia; bilateral temporal lobe lesions that isolate Wernicke's area from the other parts of the brain are thought to cause this form of agnosia; the clients:
  o May have significant problems understanding the meaning of what others say
  o May recognize nonverbal sounds
  o May recognize printed or written words
  o May have intact spontaneous speech, reading, and writing
- Prosopagnosia: Difficulty recognizing familiar faces; found in clients with right hemisphere syndrome; the client
  o May fail to recognize the faces of family members, friends, and other familiar persons
  o May recognize the face when the person speaks to the client
- Tactile agnosia: Difficulty recognizing or discriminating objects through touch when the client is blindfolded and does not hear the sounds that are associated with them (if any); lesion in the parietal lobe that isolates the somatosensory cortex from other parts of the brain is the most common cause of tactile agnosia; the clients:
  o Report normal sensation through touch, but cannot name the objects they touch or hold in their hand while they cannot see them
  o May correctly name the objects when they see them or hear the characteristic sounds
- Visual agnosia: Difficulty recognizing or discriminating visual stimuli; a rare form of agnosia; bilateral occipital lobe lesions, posterior parietal lobe lesions,

or damaged fibers that connect the visual cortex to other brain regions may cause visual agnosia; the clients:

o Cannot name what they see
o May have no difficulty naming the objects when they hear their characteristic sounds
o May name the objects when they touch them

Agrammatism. Language production with omitted grammatic elements or features; deficient grammar; telegraphic speech; limited sentence length and variety; a characteristic of nonfluent forms Aphasia, especially Broca's Aphasia.

Agraphia. Writing disorders due to recent brain pathology; agraphia is loss of previously acquired writing skills; in children, developmental writing problems are typically associated with learning disorders and are not classified as agraphia; in adults, agraphia is associated with aphasia, dementia, and other neurological disorders; the foot of the second frontal gyrus was suggested as the area that controls writing (Exner's area) and is damaged in agraphia, although this suggestion has remained controversial; some experts believe that several areas in the left hemisphere may be involved in writing; speech-language pathologists assess and treat writing problems in the context of aphasia and other language disorders; see Aphasia; major types of agraphia and their neuropathological bases are as follows:

- Left hemisphere lesions: These lesions produce structural and syntactic writing problems; the writing:
  o Tends to contain morphologic and syntactic errors
  o May include neologistic constructions, reflecting the verbal expressions of clients with aphasia
- Right hemisphere lesions: These lesions may affect the spatial aspects of writing; these problems are a part of the right hemisphere syndrome; the client:
  o May fail to give margins and adequate spaces in between words and sentences
  o May neglect the left side of the page in writing
- Apraxic agraphia: These are writing problems associated with Apraxia; focal brain lesions in the parietal lobe is the suspected cause; problems include:
  o Disorders of letter formation, numerous spelling errors, and repeated words
  o In severe cases, each letter of the alphabet may be only a scribble, although the client could name each letter correctly
  o Writing only in capital letters; all forms of writing (spontaneous, copying, writing to dictation) may be equally affected
- Motor agraphia: Writing problems due to impaired neuromotor control; upper and lower motor neuron pathology may affect the muscles of the hand and thus lead to motor agraphia; clients may:
  o Write with very small letters or the size of the letters may progressively decrease (hypokinetic agraphia or micrographia)
  o Write in a highly disorganized manner or may find it impossible to write because of tremors, tics, chorea, and dystonia (hyperkinetic agraphia)
- Pure agraphia: An isolated writing disorder in the context of normal language functions, including normal auditory comprehension; hence, not a part of aphasia; technically pure agraphia should not include alexia, although a few

cases of pure agraphia with alexia has been reported; a controversial diagnostic category because some doubt its existence; suggested neuroanatomic sites of lesions include the premotor cortex (Exner's area) and the superior parietal lobe; the client:

o May not write anything although there is no motor involvement

o May produce spontaneous writing full of errors but automatic writing and copying may be normal or nearly so

Benson, D. E., & Ardila, A. (1996). *Aphasia: A clinical perspective.* New York: Oxford University Press.

AIDS Dementia Complex. Dementia associated with acquired immune deficiency syndrome; resembles subcortical dementia in the beginning and cortical dementia in the advanced stages; one of several infection-induced forms of dementia; also known as *human immunodeficiency virus encephalopathy*; currently, the most frequently reported form of dementia.

Epidemiology and Ethnocultural Variables

- Most of the statistics reported here are from various sources, including the Center for Disease Control which periodically publishes information on the prevalence and incidence of various diseases (http://www. cdc.gov); the reader should check this web site for the latest information because the information is constantly changing and available sources my offer inconsistent information

- Estimates of the prevalence of AIDS in the U.S. population vary from about 25 to 39 per 100,000 people; estimates of the number of people living in the U.S. with the AIDS infection vary from a low of 350,000 to a high of 950,000 people

- Prevalence rates vary across the different states; the highest (232 cases per 100,000) is reported for the District of Columbia, contrasted with the lowest of 1.5 in Wyoming

- Throughout the 1990s, about 40,000 people in the U.S. were infected annually

- Infection rates vary among homosexual and heterosexual people; men who have sex with men have the highest rate of infection

- Generally, more men than women are infected annually

- A majority of women (up to 78%) who are HIV-infected belong to minority groups

- A majority of children infected with AIDS are African American

- Groups with limited access to health care have a disproportionately high prevalence of AIDS; lack of early detection and medical intervention are thought to be the cause of this disparity

- In the year 2001, the incidence rate of AIDS in African Americans was nine times the rate for whites

- The rate of infection is higher for African American women than for white women

- Hispanic males who have sex with males are infected at a rate that is twice the rate found for white men with similar sexual behavior

- Death rate due to AIDS is higher among less educated and lower income groups than among college educated and higher income groups

- AIDS is the fifth leading cause of death among people who are in the age range of 25 to 45 years
- There has been a decline in the incidence of HIV infection in the United States and European countries although the decline is uneven among different ethnocultural groups and in different parts of the world; the decline has been less impressive among African Americans; whereas there was a 24% decline among Native Americans and Native Alaskans, the decline was only 8% for African Americans
- Infection continues at a high rate in some Asian and African countries
- Worldwide prevalence of HIV infection is estimated at 30 million or more people

Onset and Early Symptoms
- Prominent early symptoms include the following:
  - Forgetfulness, slow thinking, and generally slow response time
  - Apathy, diminished sex drive, and loss of interest in work
  - Social withdrawal and depression
  - Attention deficits relative to speaking and writing
  - Disorientation to time and space
  - Frequent and severe headaches
  - Progressive deterioration in balance and weakness in legs
  - Deterioration in handwriting
  - Reduced verbal output

Progression and Advanced Characteristics
- Serious and general cognitive deterioration including:
  - Severe memory impairment
  - Severely impaired concentration
  - Confusion and indifference
  - Hallucinations and delusions
  - Disorientation to time, place, and person
- Severe neurological symptoms including:
  - Further deterioration in motor skills and performance
  - More serious balance problems (ataxia)
  - Neuromotor disorders including hypertonia, myoclonus, seizures, tremors, facial nerve paralysis, and rigidity of the muscles
- Incontinence
- Opportunistic infections (organisms that can infect only when a client's immune system is weak)
- Slow progression in the beginning but rapid physical and cognitive decline in the advanced stage
- Mutism in the final stage of the disease
- Diagnosis of dementia may precede the diagnosis of full-blown AIDS in some cases

Etiologic Factors
- Human immunodeficiency virus
- Depletion of white blood cells
- Impaired immune system

- Neural degeneration in subcortical white matter and the basal ganglia
- Degeneration of cortical layers in the advanced stage of the disease

Theories

- Various sources, including the Web sites of the National Institutes of Health and the Center for Disease Control discuss several theories of AIDS, including the following:
  o HIV infection that weakens the immune symptoms is the cause of AIDS
  o HIV may be a mutated form of Simian Immunodeficiency Virus found in chimpanzees
  o Contaminated needle use by drug abusers as well as health care professionals is a suggested means of spreading the disease
  o Main mechanisms of transmission of the infection include sexual contact where one partner is already infected, birth of babies to infected mothers, drug abuse through injection, and receiving infected blood
  o Loss of T-helper cells (bearing CD4 markers on the surface) that compromise the immune system
  o Invasion of various opportunistic infections that often lead to death
  o Some popular theories discount the idea that HIV infection causes AIDS, but such theories are not scientifically supported
  o Body's response to HIV may partly be due to a genetic defect; a new gene named *Nef* that normally lowers the body's immune response to infection may lose this function in clients with AIDS; consequently, the immune system overworks and weakens to a point where the AIDS infection begins to damage the body
  o There also are various versions of *conspiracy theories* of AIDS which suggest that U.S. scientists or the U.S. military may have created the HIV virus as a means of biological warfare, but the mainstream scientists do not subscribe to this view

Center for Disease Control (2002). Update: Aids—United States, 2000. *MMWR Weekly, 51*(27), 592–595. http://www.cdc.gov/mmwr/preview/mmwrhtml/mm5127a2.htm. Accessed June 18, 2006.

Clark, C. M., & Trojanowski, J. Q. (2000). *Neurodegenerative dementias.* New York: McGraw-Hill.

Larsen, C. (1998). *HIV and communication disorders.* Clifton Park, NY: Thomson Delmar Learning.

Lubinski, R. (Ed) (1991). *Dementia and communication.* Philadelphia, PA: B.C. Decker.

National Institutes of Health (n.d.). http://www.nih.gov

Ripich, D. N. (1991). *Handbook of geriatric communication disorders.* Austin, TX: Pro-Ed.

Akinesia.   Absent or reduced voluntary movement; a symptom of several neurological diseases including Parkinson's disease and supranuclear palsy.

Alexia.   A general term that describes reading problems in adults; the problems are of recent origin and due to neuropathological conditions; in children, such problems are often associated with learning disabilities and are called *dyslexia*;

in adults, alexia is typically found in clients with neurological disorders of recent onset; not due to peripheral visual problems; speech-language pathologists assess and treat reading problems because of their frequent association with neurodegenerative diseases that cause communication deficits, including Aphasia; several varieties of alexia have been described including the following:

Alexia with Agraphia. This includes reading and writing problems due to recent cerebral pathology; often found in clients with aphasia; also called parietal-temporal alexia; the severity of reading and writing problems are roughly equal; reading nonalphabetic symbols, such as musical notations and mathematical formulae, also are affected; see Agraphia for associated writing problems; due to lesions in the angular gyrus and the dominant parietal and temporal lobes; lesions may be caused by strokes, tumors, metastatic tumors, trauma, and gunshot wounds; includes reading and writing problems associated with Wernicke's Aphasia and Broca's Aphasia (see Aphasia: Specific Types); characteristics include:

- Reading difficulties that reflect problems of oral expression
- Reading comprehension deficits that are more serious in clients with Wernicke's aphasia; generally related to the degree of auditory comprehension of spoken language; clients may be unable to comprehend words that are spelled out for them
- Better reading of concrete nouns than abstract words by clients with Broca's aphasia
- Better comprehension of read material by Broca's clients than by Wernicke's clients
- Writing problems that parallel an individual client's reading problems; letter combinations in writing may be nonsensical
- Letter and word copying skills may be better than spontaneous writing skills

Alexia without Agraphia. Reading difficulties that are due to recent neuropathological conditions; with relatively intact writing skills; also known as *occipital alexia* and *pure alexia*; causes include various neuropathologies associated with Aphasia and, more specifically, a disassociation between occipital association cortex (damage to the visual cortex) and the dominant angular gyrus; occlusion of the posterior cerebral artery, malformations of the arteries, and tumors cause this neural damage; the characteristics include:

- Variety of reading problems as in alexia with agraphia; clients may be unable to read normally because of lost word recognition skill, although they may read letter-by-letter in a laborious manner because of intact or regained letter and number recognition; the clients may recognize words spelled out for them or spell words when asked to; they may write nearly normally, although their writing skill may show slow deterioration; clients cannot read what they write
- Right visual field deficits (right hemianopia) in some clients who are right-handed; left hemianopia in left-handed individuals
- A marked difficulty in naming colors; found in some but not all clients; clients cannot point to a named color; they still can correctly answer questions

about colors (e.g., *What color is the sky?*) or correctly use the color names in their spontaneous speech

Deep Dyslexia. A reading disorder characterized by a variety of semantic reading errors; errors are in some way related to the meaning of the printed word the client tries to read; etiology is not well understood, although involvement of right hemisphere has been suggested; the characteristics include:
- General semantic errors (e.g., misreading the printed word *close* as *shut*, and printed *tall* as *long*)
- Derivational errors (e.g., misreading printed word *wise* as *wisdom*, and *entertain* as *entertainment*; deletion of suffixes as in misreading the printed word *hardest* as *hard*or, *walking* as *walk*)
- Errors based on visual similarity of printed words and misreading (e.g., misreading the printed word *crocus* as *crocodile*, *crowd* as *crown*)
- Misreading of grammatical function words (e.g., misreading the printed word *the* as *yes*)
- Inability to read nonsense syllables or misreading them as meaningful words (e.g., responding with *I don't know* for the printed syllable *wux*, or misreading *dup* as *dump*)

Frontal Alexia. A reading disorder associated with frontal brain lesions; the most frequently observed site of lesion is the posterior portion of the inferior frontal gyrus; cerebrovascular accidents, tumors, or trauma may cause the lesion; frontal alexia may be a part of Broca's aphasia, although not all clients with this type of aphasia have frontal alexia; also called the *third alexia* or *anterior alexia*; the characteristics include:
- Significant and marked reading problems; most clients can read only individual words; clients may flatly refuse to read; clients tend to avoid reading
- Greater difficulty with abstract nouns and function words than with concrete nouns
- Comprehension of only what is read; relatively better reading comprehension of content words; increased difficulty in comprehending the meaning of relational words (e.g., adjectives, conjunctions, and prepositions)
- Difficulty in comprehending words spelled aloud
Omission of printed morphological elements in reading (e.g., present progressive *ing* or plural inflections)
- Absence of letter-by-letter reading (the client uses the whole word approach to reading)
- Difficulty in deriving meaning of sentences from their syntactic structures
- Better comprehension of spoken language than printed material the clients read

Alternating Motion Rates (AMRs). Also known as *diadochokinetic rates*, AMRs are a measure of the speed and regularity with which repetitive movements of the articulatory structures are made; slower AMRs suggest impaired functional and structural integrity of the lips, jaw, and tongue; significantly slower AMRs are typically associated with Dysarthria; see also Sequential Motion Rates (SMRs); see the companion volume, *Hegde's PocketGuide to Assessment in Speech-Language Pathology* (3rd ed.), for assessment procedures.

Alzheimer's Disease (AD). A degenerative neurological disease characterized by deterioration in behavior, intellectual skills (cognition), memory, language, general communication, and personality; a significant health problem associated with aging; AD is responsible for 50% of dementias; first described in 1906 by the German neuropsychiatrist Alois Alzheimer.

Epidemiology and Ethnocultural Variables

- An estimated 2% to 3% of clients under 75 years of age, and 6% of those between 75 and 84 years, and nearly 15% of those 85 or older may have AD
- Onset during the 40s has been reported, but infrequent
- More common in women than men, due to women's longevity, which puts them in older age groups with greater risk
- A family history of Down syndrome is a known risk factor; AD is more common in families with individuals who have Down syndrome; brain morphologic changes associated with AD also are often found in older individuals with Down syndrome
- The familial incidence of AD is higher than that in the general population; the prevalence rate among the first-degree relatives of clients with AD is about 50%
- Without effective treatment, the incidence of Alzheimer's disease is estimated to quadruple by year 2047; in the 1990s, 2.3 million people were affected in the United States; the incidence is expected to be 8.64 million people by the year 2047
- Some data suggest that AD may be more common in whites than in African Americans, Asian Americans, or Hispanic Americans; limited data suggest that AD may be uncommon in African people living in Africa; the disease is said to be nonexistent in Nigerians
- Generally, Vascular Dementia is more common than other types; in Americans of European descent, dementia associated with AD is more common than vascular dementia
- Cultural and social factors may affect the reported incidence data; in certain cultural groups, early signs of dementia may be thought of as the inevitable result of the aging process
- Ethnocultural variables that influence access to health care also may affect the reported incidence of AD and dementias; more nonwhite elderly than white elderly may receive care at home and may not use health care facilities, resulting in a possible underestimation of dementia in nonwhite populations

Onset/Early Symptoms

- Onset is typically gradual
- AD begins with mild symptoms that gradually intensify; additional symptoms appear as the disease progresses
- Subtle memory problems are the earliest and most frequently noted symptoms of AD; both recent and remote memory may be impaired; early symptoms may be ignored or noticed only by family members
- Marked difficulty in learning and retaining new material

- Subtle behavior or personality changes that my be compensated; avoiding certain tasks (e.g., cooking or reading); self-neglect; asking others to do what he or she has being doing
- Mild psychiatric symptoms, including irritability, hostility, apathy, suspiciousness, depression, frustration, and disorientation and confusion limited to new surroundings; frequent mood changes in some individuals; the client may be indifferent to his or her problems; symptoms may intensify over the years
- Language and communication problems
  o Anomia; mild naming problems are among the earliest problems of AD; difficulty generating a list of nouns starting with a specific letter of the alphabet
  o Paraphasic but generally fluent and effortless speech; paraphasia possibly due to anomia the client is aware of
  o Problems in language comprehension; often undetected difficulty understanding abstract or implied meanings
  o Impaired picture description
  o Difficulty maintaining a topic of conversation
  o No associated articulation, voice, or prosodic problems; intact syntactic skills; unimpaired gestural behaviors; normal oral reading and writing skills
- Impaired inferential ability; difficulty understanding implied meanings of what others say
- Impaired construction and other visual-spatial orientation; difficulty copying three-dimensional drawings, constructing block designs, or locating such personal belongings as car keys or shoes
- Poor reasoning and judgment; inappropriate social and personal behaviors; may forget to pay bills or pay them more than once; these may be the early signs that alert family members to more serious problems that follow

Progression/Advanced Symptoms

- Gradual intensification of initial symptoms and appearance of additional problems as the diseases progresses
- Serious and obvious memory problems for both recent and remote events
- Generalized intellectual (cognitive) deterioration
  o Severe problems in managing daily activities
  o Impaired cooking, shopping, and personal grooming skills
  o Impaired self-help skills
  o Inability to take care of personal and family finances
- Progression of behavioral deterioration and appearance of aberrant behaviors
  o Indifference, poor social judgment, and lack of emotional responses
  o Making false accusations (due to paranoia)
  o Delusion of persecution; belief that family members or health care providers are conspiring against himself or herself
  o Acting on one's own delusions (e.g., trying to protect himself or herself from harm others are falsely believed to be planning on inflicting)
  o Stealing or hiding things
  o Rummaging through other persons' rooms or belongings
  o Urinating or masturbating in public places

- o Expressing inappropriate humor, incongruous laughter, or catastrophic emotional reactions at trivial incidents
- o Restlessness, agitation, and hyperactivity
- o Purposeless pacing, ritualistic or meaningless handling of objects; picking things
- o Loss of initiative; unmotivated
- o Violence and emotional lability in some clients
- o Delusions and misidentification (especially associated with cerebral white matter damage)
- o Global deterioration in intellectual functioning
- o Disorganized behavior
- Severe visuospatial problems; in the more advanced stages, such routine skills as dressing, eating, walking, and bathing may be impaired
- Profound disorientation; getting lost in one's own home or other familiar surroundings; wandering off; eventual loss of all sense of orientation to time, place, and person
- Acalculia; intensified difficulty dealing with mathematical and arithmetic operations
- Agnosia; failure to identify objects; frequent misidentification of objects (e.g., trying to use a spoon as a knife); eventually, failure to recognize family members
- Language and communication problems
  - o Phonemic paraphasia (sound substitution in words as in *Lamerica* for *America* or sound addition as in *Amelrican* for *American*)
  - o Circumlocution and failure to use correct pronouns
  - o Jargon and empty speech
  - o Incoherent speech, evidence of disorganized thinking
  - o Impaired comprehension of spoken speech
  - o Disturbed conversational skills; difficulty initiating or maintaining conversation
  - o Impaired reading skills; difficulty comprehending what is read
  - o Impaired writing skills; poor letter formation
  - o Echolalia (repeating what is heard), palilalia (repeating one's own productions), and logoclonia (repeating the final syllable of words)
  - o Neglect of social-verbal conventions (forgetting to greet or bid farewell)
  - o Confused and meaningless speech in the final stages
  - o A superimposed dysarthria because of neurological complications in the final stages
  - o Mutism or repetition of nonlanguage sounds in the final stages
- Rigidity and spasticity; unstable gait and frequent falls, forcing the client to be sitting or lying down most of the time; a bewildered facial expression
- Ideomotor apraxia (difficulty performing an action on command though it is correctly performed spontaneously) in some cases, especially in later stages
- Ideational apraxia (difficulty demonstrating such routine acts as filling a glass with water)
- Seizures, re-appearance of grasping and sucking reflexes, loss of weight
- Swallowing difficulties; aspiration pneumonia

- Periodic incontinence; loss of control of urinary and fecal function in the advanced stage of AD
- Diurnal rhythm disturbances (inappropriate sleep-wake cycles) in some clients
- Death often due to aspiration pneumonia, heart failure, or infection

Etiologic Factors

- Genetic factors; several chromosomal abnormalities have been noted in clients with AD and include:
  - Familial AD is suspected to have an autosomal dominant inheritance, although family history of AD is positive in only 4% to 8% of clients
  - Not all members of monozygotic twin pairs develop AD, thus suggesting the influence of environmental variables
  - Early-onset familial cases may have mutations affecting the gene for amyloid precursor protein on chromosome 21; mutations on chromosome 14 may be involved in other familial cases; the protein involved is called *presenilin 1.*
  - Late-onset dementia of the Alzheimer type may be associated with abnormalities on chromosome 19, affecting apolipoprotein E (ApoE), which metabolizes and transports fats in the body and has three gene variants, ApoE2, ApoE3, and ApoE4; among these, the presence of ApoE4 poses an increased risk for dementia of the Alzheimer's type whereas the presence of ApoE2 may be protective; other chromosomes that may be involved in late onset dementia and Alzheimer's disease include chromosome 12, chromosome 3 (called the *K variant*), chromosome 17 (containing another protein called microtubule-associated protein tau), and chromosome 10 (D10S1423)
  - Other genetic abnormalities include mutations in mitochondria (structures in the cytoplasm of cells responsible for cell metabolism), although it is not clear whether such mutations are inherited or occur anew in each case or generation
  - Trisomy 21, which causes Down syndrome, also is associated with an increased risk of Alzheimer's disease; trisomy 21 is a genetic abnormality of three free copies of chromosome 21, resulting in Alzheimer's disease that manifests in the fourth decade of life
- Disturbed immune functions, noted in some clients; not clear whether this is a cause or a consequence of AD
- Viral infections have been suggested but the evidence is questionable
- Additional risk factors for AD include:
  - Old age, which is associated with an increase in free radicals (reactive oxygen species) that damage cells
  - Family history of AD or dementia of the Alzheimer type (DAT), although this does not account for a majority of individuals with AD
  - History of head trauma (20 or more years before the onset of AD), which is important, but makes only a minor contribution to the development of AD
  - Limited education and intellectual activity, although the evidence is not uniform
  - Reduced cerebral blood flow, due to a variety of causes, including vascular diseases

o Strokes, although in some individuals, AD and strokes may be independent of each other
o Epilepsy, which causes senile plaque development at relatively younger age levels
o Inflammation of the brain, suggesting an environmental cause
- Some factors thought to decrease the risk of Alzheimer's disease include:
o Estrogen replacement therapy in women
o Apolipoprotein E2
o Nerve growth factors
o Antioxidants
o Sustained intellectual activity
o Cholesterol-lowering drugs and activities
o Regular and sustained physical activity
o Control of factors that lead to vascular diseases (e.g., hypertension)
o Anti-inflammatory drugs (e.g., aspirin)
o Higher education and life-long intellectual pursuits, although the evidence is not uniform

Neuropathology of AD

- Definitive evidence of neuropathology of AD can be obtained only through autopsy; no conclusive laboratory findings help make a diagnosis of AD or dementia associated with AD
- Routine blood, urine, and cerebrospinal fluid examinations, though showing certain abnormalities, do not offer definitive evidence of AD
- Even cerebral atrophy found at gross examination may not distinguish AD from the normal aging effects; only microscopic examinations reveal neuronal atrophy unique to AD
- Brain imaging techniques may not produce strong evidence for an unequivocal diagnosis of AD, although they may offer supportive evidence; used in conjunction with other diagnostic procedures, imaging with positron emission tomography may be more useful than other imaging techniques in making an early diagnosis of AD
- Neurofibrillary tangles, neuritic plaques, and neuronal loss are the three dominant structural neuropathologies associated with AD and dementia associated with AD; these structural changes lead to neurochemical changes
- Neurofibrillary tangles are thickened, twisted, and tangled neurofibrils (filamentous structures in the nerve cell's body, dendrites, and axons); in clients with AD, these neurofibrils form unusual loops and triangles; the tangles are most often found in the pyramidal neurons of the cortex, the hippocampus, and the amygdala; also found in other neurological diseases (e.g., postencephalitic Parkinson's disease and progressive supranuclear palsy), older persons with Down's syndrome without dementia, and apparently healthy older individuals; it is the excessive formation of neurofibrillary tangles that lead to pathological changes that cause AD
- Neuritic (senile) plaques are minute areas of cortical and subcortical tissue degeneration, especially in the cerebral cortex and hippocampus (a structure deep within the brain presumably concerned with memory); also may

be seen in the corpus striatum, amygdala, and thalamus; plaques affect synaptic connections and thus impair neuronal transmission of messages; also found in clients with Down syndrome, clients with Creutzfeldt-Jakob disease, lead encephalopathy, and apparently healthy older persons, suggesting that similar to neurofibrillary tangles, neuritic plaques also are normal within tolerable limits; by their eighth decade, nearly 75% of otherwise healthy individuals may have some degree of neuritic plaques

- Neuronal loss in the cerebral hemispheres, especially in the temporal and parietal lobes, of clients with Alzheimer's disease results in shrinkage of the brain by about 10%; the ventricles of the brain enlarge as the brain tissue is atrophied or shrunk; neuronal loss in the hippocampus and surrounding areas may begin years before the onset of intellectual decline, especially in clients with high risk for AD; loss is spread to other structures

- Neurochemical changes that characterize the brains of clients with AD include a severe depletion of various brain chemicals that facilitate neural transmission, including acetylcholine, somatostatin, vasopressin, and β-endorphin; this depletion may be due to selective neuronal death; many cognitive deficits may be due to a depletion of neurotransmitters

- Neurochemical changes include not only depletion of desirable neurochemicals, but also an accumulation of the *β-amyloid protein* in the brain, suggesting a potential metabolic impairment in clients with Alzheimer's disease

- Neural damage may extend to such deeper brain structures as the nucleus basalis of Meynert, which produce such neurotransmitters as acetylcholine (ACh); white matter changes in Alzheimer's disease may be responsible for such psychiatric symptoms as delusions and misidentification

- Other possible neuropathologies include diffused slowing of the brain electrical activity as evident on electroencephalograms (EEGs), decreased dendritic branches, reduced cerebral blood flow, and reduced cortical glucose metabolism as measured by positron emission tomography

Theories of AD

- Infection, such as the one found in scrapie, has been hypothesized as a potential cause of AD; scrapie is a disease that affects sheep; the hypothesis needs more evidence than is currently available

- Various kinds of toxicity of the brain has been suggested as a cause of neuronal changes associated with AD; note that aluminum toxicity, which was frequently mentioned in the past, has been questioned or even discounted

- Hypothesis of vascular pathologies, in contrast to the typical hypothesis of neurodegenerative hypothesis, has also been proposed, because of the association of hypertension and AD and the presence of ischemic white matter rarefaction (atrophy)

- Hyperinsulinemia has also been a suggested causative factor

- Genetic transmission is currently the most frequently mentioned theory of AD; supported by greater Familial Incidence, higher Concordance Rate for monozygotic twins than for ordinary siblings, and AD's association with Down syndrome; needs additional substantiation; no specific mode of genetic transmission has been discovered

American Psychiatric Association (1994). *Diagnostic and statistical manual of mental disorders* (4th ed.). Washington, DC: Author.

Clark, C. M., & Trojanowski, J. Q. (2000). *Neurodegenerative dementias.* New York: McGraw-Hill.

Brookshire, R. H. (2003). *An introduction to neurogenic communication disorders* (5th ed.). St. Louis, MO: Mosby Year Book.

Cummings, J. L., & Benson, D. F. (1983). *Dementia: A clinical approach.* Boston, MA: Butterworth.

Forbes-McKay, K. E., & Venneri, A. (2005). Detecting subtle spontaneous language decline in early Alzheimer's disease with a picture book description. *Neurological Sciences, 26*(4), 243–254.

Hegde, M. N. (2006). *A coursebook on aphasia and other neurogenic language disorders* (3rd ed.). Clifton Park, NY: Thomson Delmar Learning.

Jaques, A., & Jackson, G. A. (2000). *Understanding dementia* (3rd ed.). New York: Churchill Livingstone.

Munoz, D. G., & Feldman, H. (2000). Causes of Alzheimer's disease. *Canadian Medical Association Journal, 162*(11), 65–72.

Simon, R. P., Aminoff, M. J., & Greenberg, D. A. (1999). *Clinical neurology* (4th ed.). Stamford, CT: Appleton & Lange.

Weiner, M. F. (1996). *The dementias: diagnosis, management, and research* (2nd ed.). Washington, DC: American Psychiatric Press.

Amnesic Aphasia. The same as Anomic Aphasia.

Amyloid Angiopathy (Cerebral). Vascular disease in which amyloid (fatty) substance accumulates in the small and medium vessels of the brain causing microinfarcts; a pathology associated with Alzheimer's Disease.

Amyotrophic Lateral Sclerosis (ALS). A progressive neurological disease that affects both the upper and lower motor neurons; more common in men than in women, ALS affect 1% to 5% of the population worldwide; the peak incidence rate is reached in the age group of 60 to 70 years; a majority of clients die of pneumonia and respiratory failures within 5 years of onset; associated with Flaccid Dysarthria, Spastic Dysarthria, or Mixed Dysarthria; characteristics include:
- Degeneration of motor neurons in the precentral and postcentral cortex, corticospinal tracts, motor nuclei of the cranial nerves, and parts of the spinal cord
- Varied motor and speech symptoms depending on the site of neuronal loss; limb weakness and hypotonia in cases of spinal nerve damage; facial and oral weakness, dysphagia, flaccid dysarthria, and tongue atrophy in cases of cranial nerve damage; limb weakness and spasticity in cases of corticospinal tract damage; facial and oral weakness, dysphagia, and spastic dysarthria in cases of corticobulbar tract damage

Anarthria. Speechlessness or mutism due to severe impairment of the neuromuscular mechanism of speech; it is the most severe form of Dysarthria; in most cases, anarthria is associated with mixed spastic-flaccid, spastic-ataxic, and spastic-hypokinetic dysarthrias; typical neuropathology involves bilateral damage to the direct and indirect activation pathways; clients have a desire to communicate, hence, not a form of typical mutism in which the desire is lost; in the absence of language problems and intellectual disabilities, the client is unable to speak because of a loss of control over the speech mechanism; muteness is relative in most cases, not absolute; the clients may be functionally mute, but may have some speech that is inadequate to meet the personal and social needs; brainstem strokes, multiple bilateral strokes, amyotrophic lateral sclerosis, encephalopathy, and multiple sclerosis combined with multiple strokes are often associated with anarthria in dysarthric clients.

Aneurysm. A form of arterial disease; a balloon-like swelling of a weakened and thinned-out portion of an artery that eventually ruptures resulting in hemorrhage; cerebral aneurysm is a cause of hemorrhagic strokes; common aneurysm sites include the basal ganglia, base of the brain, vertebral arteries, the basilar artery, anterior and middle cerebral arteries, and the Circle of Willis.

Angelman Syndrome. See Syndromes Associated With Communication Disorders.

Anoxia. Lack of oxygen; a condition of blood that may cause damage to body tissue, including brain tissue; a cause of brain lesions associated with aphasia and other communication problems.

Anomia. Difficulty in naming people, places, or things; the client may suggest the word in other ways, including gestures, descriptions, and writing, but cannot say it; anomia is a major symptom of aphasia; also found in Dementia, Right Hemisphere Syndrome, and Traumatic Brain Injury; Anomic Aphasia is a separate syndrome with naming difficulties as its main characteristic, although the current opinion is that it is the end point of most types of aphasia; see Aphasia.

Major Symptoms and Types of Anomia
- *Delayed response;* presumably due to the slow activation of the naming process
- *Limited anomia;* disconnection anomias; such category-specific problems as difficulty naming animals or vegetables
- *Paraphasias;* unintended word or sound substitutions; see Aphasia
- *Perseveration;* persistence of speech errors; repeating the same error response
- *Self-corrected-errors;* relatively fast or slow self-correction of errors; self-correction is partially or fully successful
- *Semantic anomia;* failure to recognize the words not produced
- *Unrelated words;* word retrieval problems resulting in irrelevant responses
- *Word production anomia;* anomia due mainly to motor problems
- *Word selection anomia;* clients can describe, gesture, write, and draw to suggest a word they cannot say, and can correctly recognize the name when given

Etiologic Factors and Neuropathology
- Lesions in cortical and subcortical regions are suspected
- Angular gyrus in the parietal lobe of the left hemisphere, along with the left posterior superior temporoparietal region, have been suggested
- Subcortical structures including the insula-putamen also are suspected

Basso, A. (2003). *Aphasia and its therapy*. New York: Oxford University Press.

Davis, G. A. (2000). *Aphasiology: Disorders and clinical practice*. Needham Heights, MA: Allyn and Bacon.

Hegde, M. N. (2006). *A coursebook on aphasia and other neurogenic language disorders* (3rd ed.). Clifton Park, NY: Thomson Delmar Learning.

Nadeau, S. E., Gonzalez Rothi, L., & Crosson, B. (2000). *Aphasia and language: Theory to practice*. New York: Guilford Press.

Anomic Aphasia. A syndrome of aphasia; main characteristic is persistent and severe naming or word finding difficulties, although it might be the final stage of most clients who have recovered from their major aphasic symptoms but are now left with naming problems; see Aphasia: Specific Types.

Anterior Isolation Syndrome. The same as Transcortical Motor Aphasia; see Aphasia: Specific Types.

Aphasia. A language disorder caused by brain injury in which all aspects of language comprehension and production are impaired to varying degrees; loss of previously acquired language in adults versus a failure to learn (acquire) language in early childhood; is of recent origin, typically due to a known adverse neurological event; some aspects of language may be more impaired than other aspects, suggesting the possibility of classifying aphasia on the basis of dominant symptoms; controversially classified into different types (e.g., Broca's Aphasia, Global Aphasia, Primary Progressive Aphasia, Subcortical Aphasia, Transcortical Motor Aphasia, Transcortical Sensory Aphasia, and Wernicke's Aphasia); more pronounced language impairments; negligible or no general cognitive impairment, although some experts attribute language impairment to impaired cognitive processes that underlie language; impaired social participation and social role fulfillment as a hallmark of impaired communication skills; presence or absence of neurological symptoms, depending on the site of cerebral lesion; the most common cause is a stroke or cerebrovascular accident that deprives oxygen and causes lesions in the brain; most immediate causes of strokes and aphasia have many chained events behind them, each a cause of the next effect (e.g., oxygen deprivation to brain tissue, which is due to an arterial occlusion, which in turn is due to cholesterol build up, which again may be due to poor eating habits, genetic predisposition, or a combination of the two).

Epidemiology and Ethnocultural Variables

- Epidemiology of aphasia is a function of various diseases that result in aphasia; how the factors that result in aphasia are distributed in the general population will determine the pattern of incidence or prevalence of aphasia and related disorders
- Factors that lead to strokes, the leading cause of aphasia, are unevenly distributed in the general population:
  - Strokes, also known as *cerebrovascular accidents* or *"brain attacks,"* are the third leading cause of death in the United States (after heart disease and cancer); for every 100,000 persons in the country, 56 deaths may occurr due to stroke; a death due to strokes occurs every 3 minutes; strokes cause about 12% of total mortality

- o A stroke occurs every 45 seconds; about 700,000 cases of strokes are reported each year; roughly 47% are males and 53% are females; the difference is due mainly to the longevity of females
- o Death rates due to strokes are higher for women than for men (a ratio of 3:2)
- o More than 300,000 people who have a stroke also may have permanent disability; stroke clients are a large number of clients admitted to nursing homes
- o Strokes and aphasia are an expensive health care problem; in the year 2005, the estimated healthcare cost was approximately $57 billion
- o Incidence of strokes increases rapidly after age 65; about two-thirds of all strokes occur in people age 65 and older; 12% of men and 11.5% of women age 75 and older have a stroke; some have multiple strokes
- o Ischemic strokes (that limit or interrupt blood supply to the brain) are more common than hemorrhagic strokes (bleeding in the brain due to ruptured blood vessels)
- Types of aphasia that result from various causes are differentially distributed in the population
  - o Broca's aphasia is more common in younger clients than in older clients
  - o Wernicke's aphasia is more common in older clients than in younger clients
  - o Wernicke's aphasia is more common in women than in men
  - o Global aphasia is more common in women than in men
- Prevalence of aphasia and the diseases that cause it are distributed differently in different ethnocultural segments of society
  - o Stroke incidence is higher in African Americans than in whites; age-adjusted stroke incidence rate per 100,000 persons is 167 for white males and 138 for white females; the same rate is 323 for African American males and 260 for African American females
  - o Age of onset of strokes is generally younger in African American women than in white women
  - o For people of all ethnocultural backgrounds combined, women who have had strokes outnumber men who have had them
  - o Death rates due to strokes differ among different ethnocultural groups; according to recent statistics, the stroke death rate per 100,000 individuals was 54 for white men, 53 for white women, and 82 for African American men, and 72 for African American women; the rate was 40 for all Hispanics, 40 for American Indians/Alaska Natives, and 52 for Asians/Pacific Islanders
  - o Limited survey results suggest a higher incidence of 168 strokes per 100,000 Mexican Americans compared to 136 strokes per 100,000 non-Hispanic whites
  - o Incidence of ischemic strokes, transient attacks, and extracerebral strokes are more common in whites than in other ethnocultural groups; hemorrhagic strokes are more common in Native Americans than in whites
  - o South Asians living in the United States have a higher incidence of strokes and heart disease than the general U.S. population
  - o Hispanics and African Americans tend to have strokes at earlier age levels than do whites

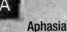
- o Fewer Hispanics than whites die of strokes after age 65, possibly due to a lower blood pressure documented in the former group
- o High blood pressure, smoking, untreated high cholesterol levels, obesity, poor diet, and lack of exercise are the main reasons for strokes in African Americans
- o High blood pressure, smoking, lack of exercise, alcohol consumption, diabetes, and malnutrition are the risk factors for Native Americans and Alaskan Natives
- o Lack of exercise, obesity, poor eating habits, alcohol consumption, smoking, and high blood pressure are the risk factors for Hispanics
- o Lack of exercise, smoking, obesity, high-sodium diet, high cholesterol diet, alcohol consumption, high blood pressure, and diabetes are the risk factors for Asian Americans and Pacific Islanders.
- o First strokes in African Americans have more serious consequences than the same strokes in whites
- o Compared to other groups, African Americans need more time to recover from strokes, and generally recover to a lesser extent
- o The extent of disability due to strokes is highest for African American females and lowest for white males
- Prevalence of aphasia and the diseases that cause it are low in children, but children have strokes
  - o Although comprehensive statistics are unavailable, California hospitals treated 2,278 children with strokes in a period of 10 years
  - o Strokes strike 28% more boys than girls
  - o Ischemic strokes are more common than hemorrhagic strokes (the same is true for adults)
  - o Infants up to 1 year are more likely to have ischemic strokes and teenagers are more likely to have subarachnoid hemorrhagic strokes
  - o Children with head trauma are more likely to have strokes than those without it; head trauma incidence is higher in boys than in girls
  - o Children with Sickle Cell Disease are more likely to have strokes than those without the disease
  - o African American children, possibly because of their proneness to sickle cell disease, have a higher risk of strokes than all other groups; Asian and white children have roughly the same risk; Hispanic children have the lowest risk

Classification of Aphasia

- There are arguments for and against classifying aphasia
- Aphasia in many clients cannot be strictly classified into a specific type
- Some types of aphasia evolve into other types over a period of time
- Many symptoms are common across the different types
- Additional clinical conditions (such as the presence of dysarthria) create clinical impressions of different forms of aphasia, although a dual diagnosis (e.g., aphasia and dysarthria) may be appropriate
- Many clinicians find some general classification system useful, and some popular diagnostic tests of aphasia classify it into types
- A basic classification is that of *fluent* and *nonfluent* aphasias

- Generally, more posterior lesions in the brain are associated with fluent aphasia and more anterior lesions are associated with nonfluent aphasia
- *Broca's aphasia, transcortical motor aphasia, mixed transcortical aphasia, and global aphasia* are the four main types of nonfluent aphasia; *Wernicke's aphasia, conduction aphasia, transcortical sensory aphasia,* and *anomic aphasia* are the four major forms of fluent aphasia
- Other classifications include primary progressive aphasia, subcortical aphasia, and various atypical syndromes that are described as Alexia, Agraphia, and Agnosia.
- Following this general description of aphasia, the different types are described in alphabetical entries under Aphasia: Specific Types

Onset and Early Symptoms of Stroke

- Acute onset (sudden), except for primary progressive aphasia
- Headaches at the time of onset, especially with anterior cerebral ischemia
- Altered consciousness, especially with posterior Ischemia
- Stupor and coma (especially with hemorrhage in the pons region)
- Episodes of vomiting; more common with hemorrhagic strokes
- Convulsions, along with other symptoms, especially with hemorrhagic strokes that affect subcortical white matter
- Hemiparesis or hemiplegia, depending on the site of the brain lesion
- Blurred vision at the onset of stroke; other sensory impairments such as reduced sensation on one side of the body
- Confusion and loss of memory
- Sudden respiratory problems; difficulty breathing
- Dizziness, difficulty standing or walking, suddenly fall; more common with cerebellar damage
- Interrupted or otherwise impaired speech; may be severe impairments; more common in clients who have anterior ischemia
- Difficulty comprehending what others say
- Symptoms lasting at least 24 hours to be classified as a full-fledged stroke
- Symptoms that last less than 24 hours and are less severe are *transient ischemic attacks (TIA)*; less pronounced symptoms at the time of onset; the typical cause is ischemia, not hemorrhage; may not be associated with vomiting, seizures, stupor, and coma that accompany full-fledged strokes

Stabilization/Subsequent Symptoms

- In the absence of repeated strokes and other illnesses, good recovery from physical symptoms; physical condition improves and stabilizes; variable rate of recovery
- Spontaneous recovery of communication skills but emergence of a constellation of communication problems
- Auditory comprehension deficits that vary in severity from mild to severe; moderate to severe in certain global aphasia, isolation aphasia, Wernicke's aphasia, and transcortical sensory aphasia; mild or no significant auditory comprehension problems in Broca's aphasia, transcortical motor aphasia, conduction aphasia, and anomic aphasia; problems may include:
  o Auditory Agnosia (impaired recognition of sounds)

- o Auditory verbal Agnosia, also known as word deafness (impaired recognition of words)
- o Word comprehension deficits
- o Isolated sentence comprehension deficits
- o Varying degrees of complex discourse comprehension deficits
- Speech fluency problems to varying degrees; more severe in nonfluent types of aphasia than in fluent types; production of five or more words without dysfluencies indicates acceptable fluency; problems may include:
  - o Impaired word fluency (production of many words in succession as a response to a single word given as stimuli)
  - o Impaired fluency in phrase or sentence production (speech filled with pauses, repetitions, and other forms of dysfluencies)
  - o Reduced speaking rate (e.g., *very slow rate:* 0 to 50 words per minute (wpm); *slow rate:* 51 to 90 wpm; *normal rate:* 90 or more wpm)
  - o Impaired rhythm, intonation, or melodic line of speech
  - o Impaired facility in producing phonemes and syllables
  - o Reduced variety of grammatical forms and types
- Difficulty repeating modeled speech; variable across different types of aphasia; somewhat severe and more frequent repetition errors in Wernicke's aphasia, possibly due to auditory comprehension deficits; some difficulty repeating modeled speech in Broca's aphasia, mainly because of production problems; relatively unimpaired repetition in transcortical sensory aphasia; repetition skills, along with other symptoms, may help support diagnosis of certain types of aphasia; problems include:
  - o Impaired repetition of single words
  - o Impaired repetition of phrases and sentences
- Persistent naming problem when confronted with physical stimuli (Anomia); a core problem of aphasia; may be a residual problem in clients with good recovery of language skills; anomia is a specific symptom of aphasia whereas Anomic Aphasia is a syndrome by itself; naming problems include:
  - o Impaired confrontation naming of objects and pictures (naming in response to "What is this?")
  - o Impaired naming in response to descriptions or definitions of objects (e.g., asking, *What is this? It is a tool for writing* to evoke *pen*)
  - o Impaired sentence completion (e.g., *You write with a . . .* to evoke *pen*)
- Word finding problems in discourse and spontaneous speech, measured through picture description and discourse analysis; causes a cluster of symptoms called Paraphasia, which is unintended word substitutions when the right word eludes the client; like anomia, paraphasia is another hallmark of aphasia; a client with this problem tends to:
  - o Substitute such general terms as *this, that, thing,* and *stuff* for specific terms
  - o Substitute words that belong to a class, but not produce the specific words (e.g., *flower* for all kinds of specific flowers)
  - o Produce Semantic Paraphasia in which the client substitutes a word that is related in meaning (e.g., substituting the word *son* for *daughter*)

- Exhibit <u>Random Paraphasia</u>, in which the intended and substituted words have no apparent connection (e.g., substituting the word *window* for *banana*)
- Show <u>Phonemic Paraphasia</u> in which one phoneme in the intended word is substituted for another phoneme (e.g., saying *loman* for *woman*); an unnecessary phoneme is added to a word (e.g., saying *wolman* for *woman*); also known as <u>Literal Paraphasia</u>
- Produce <u>Neologistic Paraphasia</u>, also known as <u>Jargon</u>, in which the substituted words are an entire creation of the client; usually meaningless to the listeners
- Increased frequency of dysfluencies (e.g., repetitions or pauses) because of word finding problems; more pronounced in nonfluent aphasias
- Reduced rate of speech due to word finding problems
- Grammatical deficiencies (<u>Agrammatism</u>); aggravated in nonfluent forms of aphasias; includes an overuse of content words (nouns, verbs, adjectives) and exclusion of grammatical morphemes; clients tend to:
  - Omit such function words as articles, prepositions, and pronouns
  - Omit such grammatical morphemes as the regular plural, auxiliary verbs, and past tense inflections
  - Speak in a telegraphic manner
  - Speak mostly in terms of nouns, main verbs, and adjectives
- Impaired use and understanding of gestures (a controversial deficit)
- Various kinds of reading problems (<u>Alexia</u>), and include:
  - Lack of recognition of printed words
  - Dysfluent, effortful, and slow reading
  - Word-by-word reading of sentences
  - Substitution and omission of words
- Difficulty comprehending read material; more serious in Wernicke's aphasia
- Writing problems (<u>Agraphia</u>); some due to the necessity of having to use the nonpreferred left hand because of paresis or paralysis of the preferred right hand; problems include:
  - Poor letter formation due to paresis of the dominant hand
  - Poor word formation
  - Poor script writing
  - Reversed, confused, or substituted letters, resulting in neologistic writing (more common in Wernicke's aphasia)
  - Writing nonsensical syllables
  - Repeated but unsuccessful attempts at self-correction
  - Perseverative writing errors
  - Omission of grammatical forms (unusual in Wernicke's aphasia, common in Broca's)
  - Syntactic deficiencies (short phrases, inadequate sentence structures, confused syntax, especially in Wernicke's aphasia)
  - Omission or substitution of words
  - Wrong word order in sentences
  - Frequent misspelling

o Omission or misuse of punctuation marks
o Disorganized writing (poor spacing between letters)
o Sparse writing (especially common in clients with Broca's aphasia)
o Totally illegible writing (especially in global aphasia)
- Differential bilingual deficits; aphasia may differentially affect the language skills of a bilingual person
  o Better performance in the native language in some clients
  o Faster recovery of expressive skills in the native language in some clients
  o Better performance in the most frequently used language in other clients
  o Sudden recovery of few or more expressions of infrequently used or forgotten native language in some clients
- Potential pragmatic communication problems; need research substantiation of pragmatic problems; possibly, the problems include:
  o Poor communication in spite of apparently better language skills, especially in clients with Wernicke's aphasia
  o Potential problems in topic initiation, topic maintenance, and turn taking in discourse
- Potential impairments in automatic speech and singing; not found in most clients with aphasia; musical impairment suggestive of right-hemisphere pathology; possibly, the problems include:
  o Impaired automatic speech (e.g., recitation of days of the week, number sequence)
  o Impaired ordinary musical skills (e.g., failure to hum a song, sing overlearned poems or nursery rhymes)

Etiologic Factors

- Etiologic factors that result in aphasia are a chain of events; generally, a stroke is the most proximal (immediate) cause of aphasia; a stoke will result in a sudden onset of aphasia, but strokes have causes that may be at work for years; vascular disorders that cause strokes develop over many years; traumatic brain injury earlier in life may increase the probability of a stroke much later in life
- In general, damage to the language structures of the brain is the main and proximal cause of aphasia
- Many factors cause damage to the language areas of the brain; hence, aphasia has multiple causes
- Vascular disorders cause Cerebrovascular Accidents (Strokes) and include:
  o Thrombosis, a vascular disease in which a collection of blood material (a *blood clot*) restricts or completely blocks the blood flow through a blood vessel; brain tissue thus deprived of blood supply is damaged because of lack of oxygen; thrombosis causes roughly two-thirds of all ischemic strokes; *thrombi* (plural of *thrombus*) are formed because of a slowly developing disease process known as Atherosclerosis in which the arteries are narrowed and hardened from an accumulation of lipids, calcium deposits, and fibrous material that result in *atherosclerotic plaques*
  o Embolism, another arterial disease in which a moving fragment of arterial debris blocks blood flow in small arteries through which it cannot pass;

an *embolus* is typically formed elsewhere and found in a distant place, whereas the thrombus is found in its place of origin; blockage of blood flow causes an ischemic stroke

- o Aneurysm, another cause of hemorrhagic strokes, is a balloon-like swelling of a weakened and thinned-out portion of an arterial wall; the balloon eventually bursts and spills blood into the surrounding areas, resulting in brain hemorrhage
- Strokes are of two major types:
  - o *Ischemic*: Death of neural tissue due to reduced or interrupted blood supply, caused by a Thrombosis, often associated with Atherosclerosis (arteriosclerosis) or Embolism
  - o *Hemorrhagic*: Ruptured cerebral blood vessel causing Cerebral Hemorrhage
- Traumatic Brain Injury, a risk factor for strokes and aphasia; automobile accidents, gunshot wounds, and blows to the head, among others, are causes of traumatic brain injury, which may be either
  - o Penetrating (open head): The skull is fractured or lacerated and the meninges are torn; either the penetrating object or the fragments of fractured skull may cause injury to the brain tissue
  - o Nonpenetrating (closed head): The meninges are intact though the skull may be fractured or intact; brain is damaged by the impact, although there is no penetration of foreign objects
- Brain Tumors (intracranial neoplasms), which cause aphasia less frequently than strokes; classified as Grade I, II, III, or IV, tumors may be
  - o Primary: Tumors originally grown in the brain; often found in the cerebrum and the cerebellum
  - o Metastatic: Tumors grown elsewhere in the body but migrated into the brain; migrated tumor cells then begin to grow in the brain; also called *secondary intracranial tumors*
  - o Meningiomas: Tumors grown within the meninges; also called extracerebral tumors
- Toxicity of the brain, including:
  - o Prescription drug overdose and drug interactions
  - o Heavy metal toxicity from lead and mercury
  - o Drug abuse, including chronic use of cocaine, amphetamines, and heroin are risk factors for stroke, especially in younger adults; cocaine hydrochloride abuse is associated more often with hemorrhagic strokes than ischemic strokes; alkaloid cocaine (crack cocaine) abuse is associated with ischemic strokes, although hemorrhagic strokes also are possibilities; amphetamines tend to cause ischemic strokes
- Infections that attack brain tissue, including:
  - o Bacterial meningitis that affects the meninges and the cerebrospinal fluid, resulting in fever, headache, lethargy, drowsiness, and possibly coma
  - o Brain abscess, caused by bacteria, fungus, or parasites migrating into the brain from sinuses, middle ear, or the mastoid
- Viral infections that cause brain injury, including:
  - o Mumps, measles, or untreated syphilis may eventually lead to impaired language problems of the kind found in aphasia

- Equine encephalitis and rabies also are associated with aphasic symptoms in a few cases
- HIV infection and AIDS; may result in aphasia or dementia; in the final stages, dementia dominates
- Herpes simplex encephalitis, a brain infection that causes headache, confusion, fever, and coma and affects parts of the temporal and frontal lobes of the brain; recovering clients may have symptoms of aphasia; generalized dementia may follow and overshadow aphasia
- Postulated *prion* infection associated with the Creutzfeldt-Jakob Disease that causes aphasic symptoms and, more notably, dementia
- Metabolic disorders affecting brain functions, including:
  - Hypoglycemia and thyroid disorders
- Nutritional disorders affecting brain function, including:
  - Thiamin deficiency

Neuropathology of Aphasia

- Cerebral cell death due to the listed etiologic factors is the main neuropathology associated with aphasia; either ischemia or hemorrhage results in cerebral cell death; a common term for cerebral cell death is *lesions*
- Hypometabolism (reduced metabolic rate) is a result of various kinds of neuropathology associated with aphasia in almost all clients (regardless of lesion sites)
- Regions of the brain where lesions occur affect the total symptom complex, suggesting different types of aphasia and cerebral localization of functions
- Lesions in the posterior-inferior (third) frontal gyrus of the left hemisphere, served by the upper division of the middle cerebral artery, are involved in producing the predominantly nonfluent type of aphasia (Broca's Aphasia); portions of frontal, temporal, and parietal lobes also may be involved
- Lesions in the superior frontal lobes are associated with Transcortical Motor Aphasia (TMA); supplemental motor areas, areas supplied by the anterior cerebral artery, and the anterior branch of the middle cerebral artery may also be affected in TMA
- Hypoxia or Anoxia of various regions of the brain, resulting in cell death, is associated with Mixed Transcortical Aphasia (MTA); cardiac arrests, cerebral edema, and multiple embolic strokes also may result in lesions that cause MTA
- Lesions of the entire perisylvian region is associated with Global Aphasia, a most severe form of aphasia; lesions may be found in both Broca's and Wernicke's areas; regions supplied by the middle cerebral artery are often involved
- Lesions in the posterior portion of the superior temporal gyrus in the left hemisphere, also known as Wernicke's area, causes Wernicke's Aphasia; the lesion may extend to the second temporal gyrus, the surrounding parietal region, the angular gyrus, and the supramarginal gyrus; lesions in subcortical regions that impair connection to the temporal cortex may also be associated with Wernicke's aphasia; the site of lesions associated with
- Wernicke's area is supplied by the posterior branch of the left middle cerebral artery

- Lesions in the temporoparietal region, especially in the posterior portions of the middle temporal gyrus, are typically is associated with Transcortical Sensory Aphasia (TSA); in some cases, lesions may extend to the lateral aspects of the occipital lobe, the angular gyrus, and the visual and auditory association cortex; generally, the lesions that cause TSA are the watershed areas of the middle cerebral artery
- Lesions in the left parietal lobe, supramarginal gyrus, inferior parietal gyrus, and the lower portion of the postcentral sulcus may be associated with Conduction Aphasia
- Lesions in the basal ganglia and the thalamus may be associated with Subcortical Aphasia

Theories of Aphasia

- Theories of aphasia address the underlying factors that initially lead to problems (e.g., hypercholesterolemia or high blood pressure), the nature of neuropathology, and the mechanisms by which pathological conditions produce their effects
- Explanations include both environmental and genetic factors
- Genetic predisposition to certain vascular diseases; a significant number of South Asians, for example, lack a genetic mechanism that regulates the natural cholesterol production by the liver, causing the liver to overproduce cholesterol
- Various environmental factors affect disease prevalence in different ethno-cultural groups; for instance, higher prevalence of strokes, disability arising from them, and mortality rates in certain minority groups in the United States may partly be a function of limited access to health care, inferior quality of care received, and absence of treatment and follow-up due to lack of health insurance; inadequate resources for transportation to medical facilities and inability to pay for aphasia treatment compound the problems
- Some of the early theories that are still debated concern the relationship between brain and behavior, including verbal behavior and the relationship between language and cognition; localizationist versus holistic theories contrast in explaining how the human brain handles language skills
- Localizationists, who are also associationists, propose that specific areas of the brain specialize in specific functions; it is this view of brain-language relationship that gives rise to such diagnostic categories as Broca's aphasia and Wernicke's aphasia with somewhat contrasting symptoms
- Holists contend that the brain is a network of integrated structures and, as such, it handles language (or any other function), as a single, integrated unit; lesions in a particular area of the brain cannot affect an isolated function attributed to it because the language areas are embedded in a neural network of connections; although certain symptoms may dominate a clinical picture in a client, various other, subtle symptoms, often unobserved, invalidate a strict localizationist view
- Subsequent to the discoveries of Broca and Wernicke, the localizationist view has been more generally understood and advocated than the alternative views, although this in itself is no justification of the localization theories;

criticisms of strict localization theories of language functions continue and, based on neuroimaging studies of language activation, some contend that language activation is rarely limited to the left hemisphere

- Two kinds of theories have been proposed to explain the relation between cognition, language, and aphasia; one set of theories suggests that language and cognition are different functions and that aphasia is a disturbance of only language, not cognition; other theories propose that cognition is impaired to varying extents in clients with aphasia and that pure disassociation between linguistic elements is rare in aphasia; critics continue to counter that various aspects of memory, attention, linguistic information processing—all parts of cognition—are impaired in clients with aphasia
- The resource theory of aphasia presents a different view of deficits; essentially, the theory states that clients with aphasia have diminished resources to process language input, all clients—including the healthy have only limited attentional and other resources and because of the lesions, clients with aphasia have further compromised resources that explain their deficits
- No single theory of aphasia, or the relationship between language and the brain, is universally accepted

Basso, A. (2003). *Aphasia and its therapy*. New York: Oxford University Press.

Benson, D. E., & Ardila, A. (1996). *Aphasia: A clinical perspective*. New York: Oxford University Press.

Brookshire, R. H. (2003). *An introduction to neurogenic communication disorders* (6th ed.). St. Louis, MO: Mosby Year Book.

Catani, M., & ffytche, D. (2005). The rises and falls of disconnection syndromes. *Brain, 128*(10), 2224–2239.

Chapey, R. (Ed.) (2001). *Language intervention strategies in adult aphasia* (4th. ed.) Baltimore, MD: Lippincott Williams & Wilkins.

Darley, F. (1982). *Aphasia*. Philadelphia, PA: W. B. Saunders.

Davis, G. A. (2000). *Aphasiology: Disorders and clinical practice*. Needham Heights, MA: Allyn and Bacon.

Demonte, J., Guillaume, T., & Cardebat, D. (2005). Renewal of the neurophysiology of language: Functional Neuroimaging. *Physiological Review, 85*, 49–95.

Hegde, M. N. (2006). *A coursebook on aphasia and other neurogenic language disorders* (3rd ed.). Clifton Park, NY: Thomson Delmar Learning.

Helm-Estabrooks, N., & Albert, M. L. (2004). *Manual of aphasia therapy* (2nd ed.). Austin, TX: Pro-Ed.

LaPointe, L. L. (Ed.) (2005). *Aphasia and related neurogenic language disorders* (2nd ed.). New York: Thieme Medical Publishers.

Nadeau, S. E., Gonzalez Rothi, L., & Crosson, B. (2000). *Aphasia and language: Theory to practice*. New York: Guilford Press.

Payne, J. C. (1997). *Adult neurogenic language disorders: Assessment and treatment*. Clifton Park, NY: Thomson Delmar Learning.

Sarno, M. T. (Ed.) (1998). *Acquired aphasia* (3rd ed.). New York: Academic Press.

Aphasia: Specific Types. Aphasia is classified into specific types; the classification is based on the view that certain parts of the left hemisphere specialize in
different kinds of verbal behaviors (e.g., listening, talking, language formulation,
grammar, meaning, and so forth); there are significant arguments against aphasia
classification; many clients cannot be strictly categorized into specific types;
although major and obvious symptoms may suggest specific types, subtle symptoms,
carefully observed, may blur the distinctions; clients with one kind of aphasia may
evolve into another kind; suggested sites of lesions for each type are sometimes
neither necessary nor sufficient to produce the specific kind of aphasia; nonetheless, aphasia literature continues to describe the following major types of aphasia:

Anomic Aphasia. Traditionally considered a separate type of fluent aphasia,
with persistent and severe naming problems as its dominant characteristic;
also known as Amnesic Aphasia; pure anomic aphasia may be rare, hence
controversial; some doubt its existence; chronic clients with a history of other
kinds of aphasia may remain as anomic aphasic individuals; most now consider
anomic aphasia as an endpoint of *most other types of aphasia* (except
perhaps global aphasia).

Major Symptoms
- Marked naming problems, almost debilitating in conversation, exceed-
  ing all other communication problems in severity
- Verbal paraphasia; frequent word substitutions, resulting in empty speech
- Good repetition of modeled speech
- Relatively better auditory comprehension; can follow conversation
  although some subtle problems may be evident
- Fluent speech, although naming problems cause pauses and repetitions
- Acceptable articulation of speech sounds
- Acceptable prosody of speech
- Production of near-normal syntactic and morphologic features of language
- Unimpaired pointing of stimuli the client cannot name
- Normal or near-normal reading and writing skills, including good compre-
  hension of read material

Etiologic Factors and Neuropathology
- Lesions sites are controversial for anomic aphasia as a syndrome; may
  not be identifiable in some clients; focal lesions in the angular gyrus or
  the second temporal gyrus are often mentioned
- The same etiologic factors described for other types of aphasia if considered an endpoint of all types of aphasia; as such, would include vascular
  disorders, brain tumors, infections, closed head injury, and others listed
  under Aphasia

Broca's Aphasia. A type of nonfluent aphasia, named after the nineteenth-
century French physician Paul Broca; less commonly referred to as *expressive aphasia, motor aphasia*, and *verbal aphasia*; a somewhat controversial
diagnostic category because injury limited to Broca's area may produce
apraxia of speech along with transient mutism, not aphasia; injury to Broca's
area may produce transcortical motor aphasia; injury to Broca's area, though
the basis for the diagnostic category, is neither necessary nor sufficient to

produce aphasia; injury to other areas, and generally more extensive damage than originally thought, may be involved in Broca's aphasia.

Major Symptoms

- Obvious neurological symptoms including right-sided hemiparesis, hemiplegia, and initial confinement to a wheelchair; later, the use of a walker or a cane
- Nonfluent and slow speech; word output may be limited to less than 50 words per minute; uneven flow; long and frequent pauses in speech; speech is filled with other types of dysfluencies, including interjected sounds, revisions, sound or syllable prolongations, and repetitions
- Excessive speaking effort; speech associated with struggles, facial grimaces, and hand gestures
- Limited phrase length; telegraphic speech
- Brief answers to questions, too little speech to meet the social demands
- Missing grammatical elements (agrammatic speech); speech often limited to content words (nouns and verbs); missing articles, conjunctions, auxiliary verbs, copulas, prepositions, and inflections
- Impaired repetition of words and sentences when clinician models them; grammatical features especially difficult to imitate
- Marked naming problems, especially with naming something or someone when asked to (*confrontation naming*: response to "What is this?")
- Lack of intonation; abnormal prosodic features; monotonous speech
- Limited syntax, short sentences
- Better auditory comprehension, although mild to moderate deficits are common
- Associated Dysarthria and Apraxia of Speech; these are motor speech disorders, and not diagnostic of aphasia; hence, they are co-existing problems
- Poor oral reading skills and writing problems including poor formation of letters, spelling errors, and letter omissions; oral reading and writing may resemble the problems found in oral communication (e.g., missing grammatical elements)
- Depression and emotional reactivity; exhibiting catastrophic response, some clients may weep and refuse to participate in assessment activities

Etiologic Factors and Neuropathology

- Controversially, the lesion or lesions are in the posterior-inferior third frontal gyrus of the left hemisphere, known as Broca's area or Brodmann's area 44; area supplied by the upper division of the middle cerebral artery
- Areas beyond Broca's may be involved
- Deep cortical damage (extending below Broca's area) is necessary to produce Broca's aphasia
- Portions of temporal and parietal lobes may be involved
- Wernicke's area may be affected
- Symptoms of Broca's aphasia may occur without damage to Broca's area
- Though injury to Broca's area is evident, the type of aphasia may be different; it may be Transcortical Motor Aphasia

Conduction Aphasia. A type of fluent aphasia; somewhat rare, no more than 10% of clients with aphasia may have it; first postulated by Wernicke; also known as *central aphasia, efferent conduction aphasia,* and *repetition aphasia*; a controversial type; similar to Wernicke's aphasia, except for better auditory comprehension; impaired repetition and good fluency are its hallmarks.

Major Symptoms

- Paresis of the right side of the face and right upper extremity in some; others may have no neurological symptoms
- Persistent oral and limb apraxia in some; others may recover from motor symptoms
- Marked impairment in repetition skills, the most important distinguishing feature of conduction aphasia; not attributable to poor auditory comprehension of spoken speech; spontaneous production of what cannot be repeated
- Normal or near normal auditory comprehension of spoken speech; any difficulty may be limited to grammatically more complex language
- Fluent but paraphasic speech; phonemic paraphasia is more common than semantic or neologistic paraphasia; reduced fluency compared to Wernicke's aphasia; hesitations and self-corrections interrupt fluency
- Moderate to mild auditory comprehension deficits
- Adequate articulation and prosody, although phoneme substitutions and deletions are common
- Near-normal syntactic and morphologic features
- Severe to mild naming problems; greater problems with content words than function words, resulting in empty speech
- Recognition and awareness of errors; frequent and failed attempts at self-correction
- Variable but not too severe reading problems; paraphasic reading; occasional failure to read
- Writing problems characterized by spelling errors, letter omissions, reversals, and substitutions
- Buccofacial apraxia; failure to follow commands to make buccofacial movements

Etiologic Factors and Neuropathology

- Etiological factors and neuroanatomic bases are highly controversial
- Site of lesions include the supramarginal gyrus, inferior parietal gyrus, the lower part of the postcentral sulcus, and the superior temporal lobe
- Regions between Broca's and Wernicke's area (arcuate fasciculus) may be damaged
- The left temporal lobe and the auditory association areas also may be involved

Crossed Aphasia. Aphasia in right-handed clients with right hemisphere injury; a somewhat rare occurrence; it is assumed that in clients with crossed aphasia, the cerebral dominance for language is in the left hemisphere; aphasia is *uncrossed* if the right-handed individual has a clearly established right-dominance for language; aphasia is *crossed* only when right brain injury causes it in a client with normal language dominance (left); the syndrome is poorly understood and the lesions and language dominance in clients with crossed aphasia have been a subject of speculation.

Major Symptoms

- Nonfluent and agrammatic speech
- Minimal naming and auditory comprehension problems
- Symptoms of Broca's aphasia in some cases; symptoms of Wernicke's, transcortical, or conduction aphasia
- Features inconsistent with the main type of crossed aphasia; for instance, intact reading skills in Broca's crossed aphasia; only minimal auditory comprehension deficits in Wernicke's crossed aphasia
- Varied language comprehension skills
- Varied repetition skills
- May include symptoms consistent with right hemisphere damage (e.g., left-sided neglect and difficulties in drawing)

Etiologic Factors and Neuropathology

- Most of the suggested etiologic factors and neuropathology is speculative and contradictory
- Right-hemisphere damage in right-handed individuals distinguish crossed aphasia from other syndromes of aphasia caused by damage to the left hemisphere
- Some have speculated that the lesion or lesions may be in both hemispheres or the lesion in the left hemisphere may not have been documented
- Others have speculated that individuals with crossed aphasia have diffuse language representation in their brains
- Right hemisphere lesion effects may spread to the left hemisphere

Global Aphasia. The most severe form of aphasia; a nonfluent aphasia characterized by severe deficits in comprehension and production of language as well as nonverbal communication; caused by extensive brain damage; 30% to 50% of all clients with aphasia may have this type; other kinds of aphasia may appear to be global if assessed in the acute stage.

Major Symptoms

- Obvious neurological symptoms; right hemiparesis or hemiplegia is likely to be present
- Hemineglect (neglect of one side of the body)
- Globally and seriously impaired communication skills
- Verbal expressions limited to a few recognizable or unrecognizable words, exclamations, or stereotypic expressions
- Repetition of consonant-vowel combinations (e.g., do-do-do) or constant repetition of short phrases (verbal perseveration)
- Severely reduced speech fluency
- Severely impaired naming and repetition skills
- Extreme difficulty in auditory comprehension
- Impaired gestural skills

- Impaired reading and writing
- Verbal and nonverbal apraxia

Etiologic Factors and Neuropathology

- Lesions in the frontal, temporal, and parietal lobes; may involve the entire perisylvian region
- Broca's and Wernicke's areas may both be involved
- Lesions may extend to the white matter of the brain
- Basal ganglia, the internal capsule, and the thalamus may be affected
- Lesions may be limited to the anterior region, the posterior region, or subcortical structures
- The most commonly affected areas are supplied by the middle cerebral artery

Isolation Aphasia. A rare type of nonfluent aphasia in which the perisylvian speech and language areas are isolated; resembles global aphasia.

Major Symptoms

- Severely impaired fluency
- Severely impaired auditory comprehension
- Marked naming difficulties
- Moderate to mild problems in repetition
- Symptoms similar to global aphasia except for better preserved repetition skills

Etiologic Factors and Neuropathology

- Lesions surrounding the perisylvian area
- Isolation of the speech-language areas from other areas of the brain

Primary Progressive Aphasia (PPA). Also classified as *progressive dysarthria* or *progressive anarthria,* primary progressive aphasia is not a classic form of aphasia because it is progressive (neurodegenerative) and its end point is dementia; some believe it may be *apraxia of speech with dysarthria;* classic aphasic syndromes are not progressive and do not terminate in dementia; unlike classic syndromes whose onsets are sudden, PPA has an insidious onset; more men than women may be affected, but when affected, women tend to have more serious symptoms; PPA is a part of the larger frontotemporal dementia, which includes Pick's disease and dementia due to Pick's disease; because the initial symptoms are aphasic-like language problems, it is called *progressive aphasia;* the onset is typically in the fifth decade of life (earlier than most classic forms of aphasia); clients are aphasic with no symptoms of dementia for about 2 years postonset, although some may remain aphasic much longer whereas others may show signs of dementia sooner; both fluent and nonfluent forms of PPA have been identified, although all clients, regardless of the initial form, become nonfluent and mute; some clients cannot be classified into fluent or the nonfluent variety; in a few individuals, the disease may be genetic; symptoms and neuropathology are integrated in the following description.

Major Symptoms and Their Neuropathology

- Nonfluent primary progressive aphasia
  o Clinically similar to Broca's aphasia

- No history of strokes or tumors associated with the classic aphasia syndromes
- Word finding and naming difficulties, although not as severe as those in the fluent variety of PPA
- Language comprehension deficits
- Reduced phrase length
- Agrammatic, effortful, and halting speech, though sometimes mentioned, may not be a significant factor (a feature that distinguishes the nonfluent PPA from Broca's aphasia)
- Reduced fluency, perhaps due to dysarthria because of the absence of significant agrammatism
- Repetition deficits
- Greater impairment in letter fluency (generating a list of words that start with a particular phoneme) than category fluency (generating a list of words that belong to a category such as *animals*)
- Minimal difficulty in comprehending the meanings of single words (contrasts with fluent PPA)
- Difficulty understanding the meaning of phrases
- Language deficits most prominent even as other symptoms emerge in the progression of the disease
- Presence of acalculia and ideomotor apraxia
- Dysarthria in a majority of clients (helps distinguish the nonfluent from the fluent PPA)
- No signs of dementia or cognitive deficits during the first 2 years postonset; absence of memory problems, visuospatial problems, visual recognition deficits, sensory motor problems, apathy, and disinhibition
- Lesions in the left inferior frontal region may be more common than in the fluent variety; however, lesions for the nonfluent and fluent varieties may not be distinct
- Atrophy and reduced metabolic activity in the anterior insula (as in Broca's aphasia)

- Fluent primary progressive aphasia
  - The fluent form of primary progressive aphasia has also been called *semantic dementia*
  - Resembles Wernicke's aphasia
  - May be more common in women
  - Normal fluency, absence of agrammatic speech
  - Paraphasia, even during confrontation naming tasks
  - Repetition deficits
  - Impaired category and letter fluency
  - Significant auditor comprehension deficits
  - Failure to comprehend the meaning of single words as the disease progresses, a feature that contrasts with the nonfluent variety, which is why this is also called *semantic dementia*, a potentially confusing term
  - Despite difficulty understanding single word meaning, some may understand the meaning of phrases

- o Dysarthria is uncommon (helps distinguish the fluent from the nonfluent PPA)
- o As in the nonfluent variety, no signs of dementia or cognitive deficits during the first 2 years postonset, though the signs may appear sooner or later
- o Nonfluent speech and eventual mutism
- o Lesions in the left temporal lobe may be more common than in the nonfluent variety; however, lesion sites for the two varieties may not be distinct; progressive atrophy of temporal lobe tissue as the disease progresses into dementia
- See the following journal articles because PPA is not adequately covered in many sources cited at the end of the main entry

Clark, D. G., Charuvastra, A., Miller, B. L., Shapira, J. S., & Mendez, M. F. (2005). Fluent versus nonfluent primary progressive aphasia: A comparison of clinical and functional neuroimaging features. *Brain and Language, 94*, 54–60.

Mesulam, M. M. (2001). Primary progressive aphasia. *Annals of Neurology, 49*, 425–432.

Soliveri, P., Piacentini, S., Carella, F., Testa, D., Ciano, C., & Girotti, F. (2003). Progressive dysarthria: Definition and clinical follow-up. *Neurological Science, 24*, 211–212.

Subcortical Aphasias.   Several newer syndromes of aphasia due to damage of left subcortical regions, contrasted with better known syndromes that are caused by damage to left cortical regions of the brain; more clinical research needed to understand these communication deficits and neuropathology; some doubt that lesions limited to subcortical structures cause aphasia; cortical damage may still be present in clients supposed to have subcortical aphasia; damaged subcortical structures may or may not be involved in language; effects of subcortical lesions may spread to cortical lesions because of tissue swelling (edema) and reduced cortical metabolism; to produce aphasia, subcortical damage must be extensive; symptoms depend on the different subcortical structures involved; therefore, symptoms and neuropathology are integrated in the following description.

Major Symptoms and Their Neuropathology

- Lesions of the anterior limb of the internal capsule and putamen cause
  - o Severe dysarthria
  - o Severe writing problems
  - o Mild to moderate problems in word repetition, naming, reading, and auditory comprehension
  - o Normal or near-normal syntax and phrase length
  - o Right hemiplegia
- Lesions of the left posterior limb of the internal capsule and putamen cause
  - o Severe problems in auditory comprehension and naming
  - o Near-normal fluency and syntax with mild articulation problems, if any
  - o Right hemiplegia

- Subcortical anterior and posterior lesions affecting internal capsule, putamen, and thalamus cause
  - Global aphasia, severely affecting all language functions
  - Severe dysarthria
  - Severe auditory comprehension problems
  - Serious reading and writing problems
- Thalamic lesions or hemorrhages cause
  - Hemiplegia, hemisensory loss, right-visual field problems, and possibly coma
  - Initial mutism from which the clients recover
  - Difficulty initiating spontaneous speech
  - Sparse, fluctuating, perseverative, neologistic, and echolalic speech
  - Severe naming problems
  - Relatively intact repetition, reading, and comprehension skills
  - Symptoms generally similar to transcortical motor aphasia

Transcortical Motor Aphasia.   A type of nonfluent aphasia; also known as *dynamic aphasia* and *anterior isolation syndrome*; resembles Broca's aphasia with intact repetition skills; compared and contrasted with <u>Transcortical Sensory Aphasia</u>, which resembles Wernicke's aphasia with good repetition skills.

Major Symptoms

- Motor disorders, including rigidity of upper extremes, <u>Akinesia</u> (lack of movement or limited movement), <u>Bradykinesia</u> (slowness of movement), <u>Hemiparesis</u> (legs more involved than the arms), and buccofacial apraxia in a few individuals
- Muteness in the acute stage, possibly due to akinesia
- <u>Echolalia</u> and perseverative speech following recovery from the acute stage
- Intact repetition; can repeat long and complex sentences, in spite of not being able to produce them spontaneously; a diagnostic feature
- Lack of spontaneous speech; limited speech output only when strongly urged to speak; difficulty initiating speech although attempts at initiating speech by such motor prompts as clapping, vigorous head nodding, or hand waving
- Naming problems resulting in paraphasic speech
- Agrammatic telegraphic speech as in Broca's aphasia; good understanding of grammaticality; will correct ungrammatical sentences
- Generally fluent speech with good articulation, in spite of difficulty generating a word list
- Generally intact serial speech (count numbers or recite days and months)
- Better auditory comprehension for simple conversation than for complex speech
- Reading problems; both reading aloud and reading comprehension may be affected
- Writing problems; generally disinterested in writing; need to be coaxed to write; the writing may be sparse, characterized by spelling errors and large and ill-formed letters

Etiologic Factors and Neuropathology

- Lesions are typically located outside Broca's area; usually either above or below that area
- Anterior superior frontal lobe is often affected
- Supplemental motor areas may be involved; it is speculated that the lesion or lesions may disconnect this area from Broca's area
- Lesions affect the association pathways that connect perisylvian regions with other brain regions
- Lesions also may be found in the deep white matter below the supplementary motor area
- The areas affected are supplied by the anterior cerebral artery and the anterior branch of the middle cerebral artery; the watershed area of the brain that receives marginal blood supply also may be effected

Transcortical Sensory Aphasia (TSA). A type of fluent aphasia; also known as *posterior isolation syndrome* and *Wernicke's aphasia type II*; similar to Wernicke's aphasia except that repetition skills are impaired in Wernicke's aphasia and intact in TSA; compared and contrasted with transcortical motor aphasia (TMA); TSA is a fluent counterpart of the nonfluent TMA; a form of aphasia commonly associated with Alzheimer's disease, although with Alzheimer's disease, the condition is progressive; TSA also may be associated with the Gertsmann syndrome, a neurological disease with finger agnosia, agraphia, confusion of laterality, and acalculia.

Major Symptoms

- Hemiparesis at onset; no significant physical symptoms after the initial recovery period
- Neglect of one side of the body
- Intact repetition (contrasted with Wernicke's aphasia); can repeat long and complex sentences
- Echolalia, which is not a significant feature of Wernicke's aphasia
- Auditory comprehension deficits as in Wernicke's aphasia
- Moderate to severe naming difficulties
- Generally fluent but empty (paraphasic) speech; adequate phrase length, syntax, and prosody; similar to the fluent speech of Wernicke's aphasia
- Generally good syntactic skills as in Wernicke's aphasia
- Once initiated, normal automatic speech
- Poor reading comprehension; the clients may read aloud with word substitutions
- Writing problems that parallel spoken language problems

Etiologic Factors and Neuropathology

- Lesion in the temporoparietal region is the most frequent cause of TSA
- Lateral aspects of the occipital lobe may be involved in some cases
- Damage to the posterior portion of the middle temporal gyrus is typical
- Angular gyrus and visual and auditory association cortex may be involved
- The areas affected are in the watershed areas of the middle cerebral artery

Wernicke's Aphasia. A type of fluent aphasia characterized by somewhat excessively fluent verbal expressions and reduced auditory comprehension of spoken speech; a less controversial syndrome than nonfluent Broca's aphasia, with which it contrasts; Carl Wernicke, the nineteenth-century German neuropsychiatrist, first described the syndrome and called it *sensory aphasia*; also called *receptive aphasia*; less commonly referred to as *word deafness, syntactic aphasia*, and *central aphasia.*

Major Symptoms

- Absence of paresis or paralysis (contrasted with Broca's aphasia); no motor symptoms
- Signs of confusion, because of somewhat meaningless hyperfluency
- Absence of insight into disability; lack of appreciation of one's own communication problems
- Lack of frustration in spite of failed attempts at communication
- Presence of psychiatric symptoms; paranoid, homicidal, suicidal, or depressed; may accuse others of speaking in a code they do not understand (possibly due to severe auditory comprehension deficits); depression is associated with strokes (not unique to Wernicke's aphasia)
- Normal or even excessive fluency; rapid rate and incessant and effortless speech (in contrast to those with Broca's aphasia); may need signals to stop talking; a distinguishing feature
- Relatively normal (or longer) phrases, articulation, and grammar; may have excessive use of grammatical morphemes; sentences may be pseudo-grammatical
- Normal prosodic features with good patterns of intonation even as they speak in meaningless sentences
- Mild to severe naming difficulties and severe word finding problems that cause paraphasia, neologism, jargon, and circumlocution that may result in partially or totally meaningless speech; the speech may be filled with such general terms as *this, that stuff*, and *thing*
- Copious but empty (meaningless) speech production
- Severe auditory comprehension deficits, another dominant and distinguishing feature; may be severe for names and longer sentences; significant difficulty in distinguishing words that are phonemically minimally different (e.g., *pat* and *bat*)
- Impaired repetition, the degree of impairment commensurate with the degree of auditory comprehension deficit
- Impaired conversational skills, possibly due to the auditory comprehension deficits that are worse in such adverse conditions as background noise; topic initiation, turn taking, and staying on a single topic may all be impaired to more or less extent depending on the severity of speech comprehension deficits
- Poor reading comprehension; failure to recognize the meaning of printed words; failure to recognize the letters of the alphabet
- Free, copious, and effortless but also meaningless writing that parallels language production

Etiologic Factors and Neuropathology

- In most cases, the lesion is found in the posterior portion of the superior temporal gyrus in the left hemisphere (Wernicke's area)
- Lesion may extend to the second temporal gyrus, the surrounding parietal region, the angular gyrus, and the supramarginal gyrus
- Subcortical damage that disconnects the temporal cortex
- Areas of cortical lesions supplied by the posterior branches of the left middle cerebral artery
- Damage to Wernicke's area may not always produce symptoms consistent with the syndrome although when such symptoms are present, the damage almost always is in the dominant superior temporal gyrus, whether extended to other areas or not

Basso, A. (2003). *Aphasia and its therapy*. New York: Oxford University Press.

Benson, D. E., & Ardila, A. (1996). *Aphasia: A clinical perspective*. New York: Oxford University Press.

Brookshire, R. H. (2003). *An introduction to neurogenic communication disorders* (6th ed.). St. Louis, MO: Mosby Year Book.

Catani, M., & ffytche, D. (2005). The rises and falls of disconnection syndromes. *Brain, 128*(10), 2224–2239.

Chapey, R. (Ed.) (2001). *Language intervention strategies in adult aphasia* (4th. ed.) Baltimore, MD: Lippincott Williams & Wilkins.

Darley, F. (1982). *Aphasia*. Philadelphia, PA: W. B. Saunders.

Davis, G. A. (2000). *Aphasiology: Disorders and clinical practice*. Needham Heights, MA: Allyn and Bacon.

Demonte, J., Guillaume, T., & Cardebat, D. (2005). Renewal of the neurophysiology of language: Functional Neuroimaging. *Physiological Review, 85*, 49–95.

Hegde, M. N. (2006). *A coursebook on aphasia and other neurogenic language disorders* (3rd ed.). Clifton Park, NY: Thomson Delmar Learning.

Helm-Estabrooks, N., & Albert, M. L. (2004). *Manual of aphasia therapy* (2nd ed.). Austin, TX: Pro-Ed.

LaPointe, L. L. (Ed.) (2005). *Aphasia and related neurogenic language disorders* (2nd ed.). New York: Thieme Medical Publishers.

Nadeau, S. E., Gonzalez-Rothi, L., & Crosson, B. (2000). *Aphasia and language: Theory to practice*. New York: Guilford Press.

Payne, J. C. (1997). *Adult neurogenic language disorders: Assessment and treatment*. Clifton Park, NY: Thomson Delmar Learning.

Sarno, M. T. (Ed.) (1998). *Acquired aphasia* (3rd ed.). New York: Academic Press.

Aphonia.   Loss of voice; may be complete and continuous or intermittent (voice breaks); may be due to vocal fold paralysis or a response to stressful situations (psychiatric or "psychogenic"); see Voice Disorders and Psychiatric Problems Associated with Communication Disorders

Aplasia. Underdevelopment of an organ or tissue. See also Agenesis and Hypoplasia.

Apraxia. Disordered volitional movement in the absence of muscle weakness, paralysis, fatigue, sensory impairment, comprehension problems, or failure to understand verbal or gestural commands; a motor sequencing disorder; theorized as a motor planning disorder; in the absence of peripheral neuromuscular disorders, the client is thought to have impaired motor programming and motor integration capacity in the brain; a basic apraxic condition may be associated with speech production, resulting in Apraxia of Speech (AOS) in Adults; there are varieties of apraxia; the major forms include:

- Apraxia of speech: Impaired voluntary movements involved in speech production although the muscles involved in speech production are normal; see Apraxia of Speech (AOS) in Adults
- Childhood apraxia of speech: Difficulty sequencing speech movements for articulating speech sounds; controversial diagnostic category because of lack of documented neuropathology associated with apraxia of speech in adults; see Childhood Apraxia of Speech
- Constructional apraxia: Difficulty constructing or replicating spatial designs such as block designs; associated with various kinds of cerebral pathologies and trauma; the client may be:
  o Unable to draw pictures (e.g., a house, a clock, a human face)
  o Unable to replicate or copy block designs or match designs
- Limb apraxia: Impaired volitional movements of the arms and legs; although the muscular strength is adequate or unaffected, clients are unable to move their limbs when a command is given; when asked to do, the client may be:
  o Unable to wave good-bye
  o Unable to pick up an object
- Oral (nonverbal) apraxia: Difficulty performing nonspeech movements with the oral structures when requested; also known as *buccofacial apraxia, facial apraxia, orofacial apraxia,* or *lingual apraxia*; the client may be:
  o Unable to perform acts with the oral articulators when requested
  o Unable to lick lips, whistle, clear throat, protrude tongue, and so forth when requested
  o No difficulty performing the impaired activities spontaneously

Apraxia of Speech (AOS) in Adults. A neurogenic speech disorder with documented neuropathology in the left cerebral hemisphere including such areas as Broca's and supplementary motor; primarily an articulatory sequencing disorder characterized by problems in positioning and sequentially moving muscles for the volitional production of speech; unimpaired reflexes and automatic acts; associated with prosodic problems; not caused by muscle weakness or slowness; presumed to be a disorder of motor programming for speech; also called *aphemia, afferent motor aphasia, anarthria, apraxic dysarthria, cortical dysarthria, oral verbal apraxia, primary verbal apraxia,* and *pure motor aphasia*; frequently, Aphasia may be a co-existing disorder; less often, Dysarthria of unilateral upper motor neuron type may coexist; may be an independent problem (speech programming deficit) in some clients with aphasia; in its pure form, may not affect language skills; frequently, but not always, associated with nonverbal oral apraxia; some individuals may present apraxia of speech as the only symptom of a neurological disease.

Epidemiology and Ethnocultural Variables

- AOS exists both as an isolated symptom (a primary diagnosis) and as a coexisting condition associated with other neurological disorders or diseases
- In its pure form, AOS occurs less frequently than as a coexisting problem with other neurogenic communication deficits; severe AOS may occur more frequently than milder AOS; also, severe AOS tends to coexist with other disorders (most often, aphasia and dysarthria)
- Information on the incidence and prevalence of apraxia of speech in adults and its distribution across different ethnocultural populations is limited
- Apraxia of speech may be found in 8% or more of all clients diagnosed with a motor speech disorder

Nonverbal and Neurological Symptoms

- AOS is associated with nonverbal oral apraxia (NVOA); this is difficulty in voluntary movements of the oral and laryngeal structures when asked to imitate, although reflexive and more spontaneous movements are unaffected
- Lesions in the frontal or parietal lobes
- Neurological symptoms are not remarkable unless there is coexisting dysarthria; the neurological symptoms include weak facial and tongue muscles, and the resulting speech production problems are attributed to dysarthria and are not considered in diagnosing AOS
- Impaired oral sensation may or may not be present in AOS; when they do exist, they are not considered a critical diagnostic feature of AOS
- In the absence of dysarthria, swallowing, chewing, and gag reflex are normal in clients with AOS
- Many clients with AOS also have nonverbal oral apraxia (NVOA), which may be independent of AOS; clients with NVOA:
  - Are unable to perform oral motor acts when asked to
  - Cannot imitate actions modeled for them
  - Find it difficult to cough, click tongue, smack the lips, blow, or whistle when instructed to do so; clients nonetheless may try but with awkward movements, groping gestures, many false starts, and trials-and-errors; some clients may also repeat the command as they try to perform the act with repeated failures
  - Are aware of their difficulties and react emotionally to failures or awkward attempts; may be upset or frustrated; some are perplexed; almost all are embarrassed
  - May reflexively or spontaneously perform the acts they fail to execute on command or as imitation

- Right hemiparesis and sensory deficits may be present
- Limb apraxia may be present; not an invariable symptom

Verbal (Speech) Symptoms

- General characteristics
  - Because of awareness of speech problems, clients may be surprised, frustrated, or embarrassed by their mistakes
  - Volitional sequencing of movements required for speech most notably affected; automatic speech is usually less affected than spontaneous or volitional speech
  - The speech errors were initially thought to be highly variable (different kinds of errors on repeated attempts of the same word); this characteristic has lately been questioned; more recently, location of errors within words or utterances and error types have been found to be somewhat consistent
  - Use of such compensatory strategies as slower rate of speech to better articulate speech sounds
  - Multiple and varied stress points within the same production, causing increased difficulty; similarly, longer words and phrases also cause increased articulatory problems
  - Even those with severe AOS and limited speech intelligibility may count numbers or sing a song (semiautomatic skills)
- Articulatory, acoustic, and speech physiologic problems
  - The most basic feature of AOS is the multiple substitutions, distortions, and omissions of speech sounds
  - Substitution errors, especially on consonants, may exceed all other kinds of errors; however, most of the substitutions may also be classified as distortions; if so, the distortions are the most frequent articulatory errors found in AOS
  - The greatest number of substitutions involve place-related productions and include manner, voicing, and oral/nasal distinction errors
  - Replacement of a phoneme that occurs earlier in the word with one that occurs later in the same word in *anticipatory substitutions* (e.g., *lelo* for *yellow*)
  - Substitution of a later sound with an earlier sound in the word in *postpositioning errors* (e.g., *dred* for *dress*)
  - *Metathetic errors* in which the sound positions are switched (e.g., *tefalone* for *telephone*)
  - Consonant substitutions that may actually complicate, not simplify, intended productions
  - Distorted or substituted productions that are generally closer to the intended sound productions
  - Addition of sounds to a word, but the added sounds also may be distorted
  - Fewer errors on bilabial and lingual-alveolar consonants but greater on affricates and fricatives than on other sound classes and on consonant clusters than on singletons
  - Generally fewer errors on vowels than on consonants

- o Because of distortions, lost distinction between voiced and voiceless speech sounds
- o Increased frequency of errors with increasingly complex productions (e.g., longer words and phrases)
- o Delayed speech initiation
- o Trial-and-error articulatory groping and struggle associated with repeated speech attempts
- o A higher frequency of errors on infrequently occurring sounds than on more frequently occurring words
- o Easier automatic productions than volitional/purposive productions
- o Nonsense syllables more difficult to produce than meaningful words
- o Repeated attempts at self-correction
- o Errors in imitation, which are comparable to those in spontaneous speech
- o Limited speech production associated with the most severe form of AOS; mutism, called *apraxia of phonation* in this case, may be relatively permanent; if not mute, clients may produce only a few meaningful syllables or repetitively utter a few meaningless syllables; even automatic speech (including singing and counting) and imitative speech may be severely impaired; because of such extremely limited speech repertoire, the errors they make are predictable (less variable)
- Prosodic problems
  - o Dysprosody or prosodic problems, a hallmark of AOS, is a function of several variables, including rate, stress, intensity, and frequency abnormalities
  - o Reduced rate of speech, a reliable symptom of AOS, is probably not a compensatory strategy because most clients cannot modify their speech rate when requested; they find it especially difficult to increase their speech rate even though at times they can produce speech at a faster rate
  - o Production of words and even syllables with noticeable silent pauses between them; such silent pauses also contribute to an overall reduction in speech output for given units of speaking time; syllable productions with pauses in between has prompted a speculation that the impaired motor programming cannot handle such larger units as words and phrases; speech is thought to be programmed at the syllable level
  - o Increased duration of consonants and vowels in syllables, words, and phrases; may be another factor that contributes to a slower rate of speech; they may stretch the vowel duration; also may produce syllables with the same duration regardless of normal durational variations
  - o Even stress on syllables, resulting in monotonous speech
  - o Limited intonation variations; fundamental frequency may not naturally vary and may not show the typical decline toward the end of longer utterances
  - o Lack of the normal loudness variations; restricted range of loudness variation may contribute to the monotonous speech
  - o Limited pitch variations and limited range within which such variations take place

o Characteristics of a foreign accent; see Foreign Accent Syndrome
o Highly variable voice onset time (VOT)
o Overlapping VOT values for voiced and voiceless stops, leading to a blurring of distinction between the voiced and voiceless speech sounds; a failure to achieve complete vocal tract closure while producing stop sounds may result in leakage of air giving speech a noisy quality and resulting in distorted speech sounds
o Inconsistent or delayed coarticulation of speech sounds
o Abnormal variations in lower lip and jaw movement velocity as shown by kinematic studies; longer duration of movements and unnecessary changes in velocity of movement; highly variable movement of articulators
o Discoordination between amplitude and velocity of jaw, lip, tongue, and velar movements
• Fluency problems
o A high frequency of silent pauses, marked difficulty in initiating speech
o Repetition of words and syllables, possibly due to false starts and frequent attempts at correcting articulatory errors
o Prolongation of speech sounds, although the sound prolongations, unlike those of people who stutter, may be distorted

Auditory Processing Deficits (APDs)
• Normal or near-normal auditory skills
• APDs may be present if clients also have a coexisting aphasia; APDs, if present, do not explain the speech problems; the presence of APDs may exacerbate AOS

Etiologic Factors and Neuropathology of AOS
• Generally, injury or damage to brain structures in the dominant hemisphere (the left hemisphere in most cases) involved in motor speech planning and programming; injury that produces focal damage (contrasted with diffuse damage) likely to be associated with apraxia
• The most frequent cause is a stroke; vascular lesions (resulting in strokes) that specifically affect speech planning and programming structures and pathways; single left hemisphere stroke causes apraxia in about 40% of cases; multiple strokes in about 8%; frontal and parietal lesions are more often associated with AOS than other lesions elsewhere; occasionally, temporal lobe lesions may also be involved with lesions in the frontal and parietal lesions, but rarely alone
• Left hemisphere trauma due to external forces; surgical trauma to the left hemisphere in the process of tumor removal, aneurysm repair, and hemorrhage evacuation in about 15% of cases
• Tumors in the left hemisphere in about 4% of cases; in some cases of tumor, apraxia of speech may be the only initial symptom of the disease
• Undetermined etiology in about 4% of cases; although these clients may present clear signs of AOS, there may be no clear evidence of neuropathology
• Seizure disorders and multiple causes in a small number of individuals

- Inflammation, brain toxicity, metabolic disorders, and multiple sclerosis do not often produce AOS
- Corticobasal degeneration, Creutzfeldt-Jakob Disease (CID), Primary Progressive Aphasia, and Alzheimer's Disease may be associated with AOS; more than a quarter of all cases of AOS may be associated with a neurodegenerative disease; in some individuals, AOS may be the only initial sign of a progressive neurological disease

Theories of Apraxia of Speech

- The most widely discussed explanation of AOS is the motor planning, motor programming, or speech motor control hypothesis (Duffy, 2005; McNeil, Doyle, & Wambaugh, 2000)
- Most of the conceptual, linguistic, and motor planning and programming is hypothesized to take place in the hemisphere that is dominant for language (i.e., the left hemisphere in most individuals)
- Unless there is coexisting aphasia, AOS does not involve language conceptualization or linguistic planning deficits
- Motor planning and programming deficits underlie AOS; the message to be expressed is well conceptualized and formed; what is impaired in apraxia is the motor planning that is needed as an intermediate stage between language formulation and speech production; if the deficits are purely in the production realm, the disorder would be dysarthria; if the deficits are purely at the level of conceptualization and formulation of messages, the disorder would be aphasia; being neither, AOS involves a failure to program speech movements after the message has been conceptualized and before speech movements are executed
- Motor speech planning and programming functions are hypothesized to exist in the brain; motor planning is the highest level of cortical motor functioning; this planning unit receives the phonological representation of the planned message; to realize this message, the motor planning unit generates a motor plan that includes the necessary motor goals; generation of such a motor plan may be considered *preprogramming* of motor acts; plans include general strategies and goals, but not specific procedures of speech production
- The cortical structures involved do not have to generate motor plans for every instance of speech; with increased experience in speaking, motor plans for various speech events are stored as engrams that are later efficiently evoked
- Once a goal-oriented motor plan is generated for an act of speech, motor programming function, supposedly a lower level cortical function, is set into motion; motor programs specify how the procedures or manners in which the plan may be realized; programming specifies the spatial and temporal aspects of the plan; motor programs may specify commands for movement; sensory feedback from articulators may help modify the program as the speech is in progress (on-line modifications)
- The motor plan, once assembled, may be held in a buffer for a brief duration until the articulators are ready to move; the plan is then downloaded to

the articulators that unpack the downloaded commands, resulting in speech production; if the downloaded motor plan has wrong goals, inappropriate spatial targets, or is otherwise defective, the articulators may not produce speech normally even though they are structurally capable of normal movement; the result is AOS

- Various cortical and subcortical areas, including the motor cortex, supplementary motor area, basal ganglia, cerebellum, and frontolimbic systems are involved in motor planning and programming for speech; the somatosensory cortex and supramarginal gyrus may help integrate sensory information necessary for speech motor planning and programming
- In addition to cortical and subcortical structures, learning and experience play an important role in motor planning and programming; it is the repeated experiences in speaking that help store motor plans that may be evoked when necessary
- Lesions in one or more cortical and subcortical structures involved in motor planning and programming for speech may cause AOS
- The limitation of this explanation of apraxia is that the motor planning and programming units, buffer zones, and downloading of plans to articulators are mostly hypothetical; like many speech production models, these theories are modeled after the workings of computers; almost all evidence offered in support of the theories is indirect; the existence of planning or programming units have not been convincingly demonstrated; speech motor planning or programming model, like other models of speech production, are based on rational assumptions that parallel observed symptoms, but not on direct experimental evidence

Bhatnagar, S. C. (2002). *Neuroscience for the study of communication disorders* (2nd ed.). Baltimore, MD: Lippincott Williams & Wilkins.

Brookshire, R. H. (2003). *An introduction to neurogenic communication disorders* (6th ed.). St. Louis, MO: Mosby Year Book.

Croot, K. (2002). Diagnosis of AOS: Definition and criteria. *Seminars in Speech and Language, 23*(4), 267–279.

Darley, F. L., Aronson, A. E., & Brown, J. R. (1975). *Motor speech disorders*. Philadelphia, PA: W. H. Saunders.

Deger, K., & Wolfram, Z. (2002). Speech motor programming in apraxia of speech. *Journal of Phonetics, 30,* 321–335.

Duffy, J. R. (2005). *Motor speech disorders: Substrates, differential diagnosis, and management* (2nd ed.). St. Louis, MO: Elsevier Mosby.

Freed, D. (2000). *Motor speech disorders*. Clifton Park, NY: Thomson Delmar Learning.

Love, R. J., & Webb, W. G. (2001). *Neurology for the speech-language pathologist* (4th ed.). Boston, MA: Butterworth-Heinemann.

McClain, M., & Foundas, A. (2004). Apraxia. *Current Neurology and Neuroscience Reports, 4*(6), 471–476.

McNeil, M. R., Doyle, P. J., & Wambaugh, J. (2000). Apraxia of speech: A treatable disorder of motor planning and programming. In S. E. Nadeau,

L. J. Gonzalez-Rothi, & B. Crosson (Eds.), *Aphasia and language: Theory to practice* (pp. 221–266). New York: Guilford.

Ogar, J., Slama, H., Dronkers, N., Amici, S., & Gorno-Tempini, M. L. (2005). Apraxia of speech: An overview. *Neurocase: Case Studies in Neuropsychology, Neuropsychiatry, and Behavioral Neurology, 11*(6), 427–432.

Ogar, J., Willock, S., Baldo, J., Wilkins, D., Ludy, C., & Donkers, N. (2006). Clinical and anatomical correlates of apraxia of speech. *Brain and Language, 87,* 343–350.

Peña-Brooks, A., & Hegde, M. N. (2007). *Assessment and treatment of articulation and phonological disorders in children* (2nd ed.). Austin, TX: Pro-Ed.

Apraxia of Speech in Children.   See Childhood Apraxia of Speech, currently the preferred term.

Aprosodia or Dysprosody.   Prosodic disturbances; technically, aprosodia is the lack of prosodic features in speech whereas dysprosody means impaired prosody of speech; both result in monotonous, robot-like speech; Apraxia of Speech, Dysarthria, and Right Hemisphere Syndrome are often associated with prosodic impairment; people who have received the slow speech treatment to control their stuttering also may have prosodic impairments; in most individuals, dysprosody may be associated with slower rate and lack of pitch and loudness variations; in other cases, it may be associated with excessive or unpredictable variations in rate and loudness.

Arteriosclerosis.   Disease of the arteries in which the walls of the arteries thicken and lose elasticity; has several varieties including cerebral arteriosclerosis (a major cause of strokes and thus aphasia), and coronary arteriosclerosis (disease of the arteries of the heart); see Atherosclerosis.

Arthropathy.   Disease of joints; a symptom in some genetic syndromes including Stickler syndrome (see Syndromes Associated With Communication Disorders).

Articulation and Phonological Disorders.   Disorders of speech characterized by difficulty in producing speech sounds accurately; difficulty in producing single or a few sounds with no pattern or derivable rule is an articulation disorder; multiple errors that can be grouped on some principle and thus form patterns and severely affect intelligibility are Phonological Disorders; some consider both terms as referring to a group of speech disorders that are not due to structural deviations or neuromotor control problems; the same as *functional articulation disorders*; a common diagnostic category especially in school-age children; frequently associated with language disorders; articulation disorders due to documented central or peripheral nervous system pathology are known as Dysarthrias; articulation problems that are due to central nervous system pathology causing motor programming problems in the absence of weakness or paralysis of the speech muscles are described as Apraxia of Speech; although children with functional articulation disorders may have subtle neuromotor problems, and such speech disorders may persist into adulthood, much of the information presented in this section pertains to children's articulation disorders that cannot be explained on the basis of clear and convincing evidence of organic deficits.

Epidemiology and Ethnocultural Variables

- Prevalence has been difficult to estimate because of lack of systematic studies
- Nearly 10% of the population is estimated to have a disorder of communication; a majority of them, perhaps 50% to 80% have an articulation and phonological (Ar-Ph) disorder
- Clinicians in public schools serve a large number of children with Ar-Ph disorders; up to 97% of school-based clinicians serve children with these disorders
- Speech delay may be found in approximately 15% to 16% of 3-year-olds; however, some 75% of them achieve normal articulation by age 6
- Prevalence rate of Ar-Ph disorders in 6-year-old children is estimated to be 3.8%
- More boys than girls have Ar-Ph disorders
- Compared to the general prevalence, there is a higher prevalence of Ar-Ph disorders associated with developmental and intellectual impairments, neurological involvement (e.g., cerebral palsy), and hearing impairment
- Infants and toddlers who have repeated middle ear infections are at risk of speech delay and speech production problems
- Approximately 40% to 80% of children with Ar-Ph disorders also may have a coexisting language disorder
- Most children with Ar-Ph disorders have normal intellectual, sensory, and neurological status, although they may have auditory processing difficulties or subtle neuromotor problems
- Moderate to severe Ar-Ph disorder, if not remediated, may negatively affect a child's reading and writing skills
- Children with persistent and severe Ar-Ph disorders are likely to experience difficulties in socialization
- Some children with persistent and severe Ar-Ph disorders may exhibit behavior disorders
- Socioeconomic status of parents is not strongly correlated with Ar-Ph disorders in their children
- Familial incidence of Ar-Ph disorders may be higher than that in the general population; in about 35% to 40% of cases, a positive family history of speech disorders may be evident; no such influence is evident in 55% to 60%
- Parents with poor articulation tend to have children with similar skills
- Systematic data on ethnocultural variables and Ar-Ph disorders in minority groups are limited; when compared to white children, African American children may make more errors on standard English, but those errors do not constitute articulation disorders; their speech production patterns are a part of African American English
- There is no evidence that children with multicultural or bilingual family status are prone to Ar-Ph disorders; bilingual children may produce different phonological patterns (not disorders) that are influenced by their primary language; they may have an Ar-Ph disorder in their primary language, secondary language, or both, that is not a product of their bilingual status

Description of Articulatory Errors

- Traditionally, articulatory errors were described without an analysis of patterns found in the errors; individual sound errors were considered and classified; the most common classification included omissions, substitutions, distortions, and additions; the main concern in the traditional analysis is the correct or incorrect motoric production of individual sounds; individual error analysis with no consideration of patterns is still valid in the case of children who misarticulate a few speech sounds.

- Omissions or Deletions
  - Absence of a required sound in a word; one of the more common errors of articulation
  - Initial and final sounds in a word may be omitted more often than the medial sounds in words (e.g., *æt* for *cat* or *cæ* for *cat*)
  - Deletion of a sound in a sound cluster (e.g., *stike* for *strike*)

- Substitutions
  - Sound replacements
  - An incorrect sound is produced instead of a right sound (e.g., *dat* for *cat* or *bawoon* for *balloon*)

- Distortions
  - Inaccurate sound productions
  - Sounds distorted may be perceived as the target sound
  - Distortions of sibilants are more common than distortion of other classes of sounds

- Additions
  - Intrusion of a sound that does not belong to the target word; often an unstressed vowel
  - Characterized as *epenthesis* in phonological process analysis; (e.g., *səpoon* for *spoon*)

- Devoicing
  - Production of voiced sounds without vocal fold vibrations or with limited vibrations
  - Sounds thus produced are devoiced (e.g., *tum* for *gum*)

- Lisps
  - Frontal lisps: Production of sibilant consonants with tongue tip placed too anteriorly (far forward, against the teeth or between the teeth); distorted /s/ and /z/ sounds in different word positions, often in the initial positions
  - Lateral lisps: Production of sibilant sounds (which include /s/, /z/, /ʃ/, /ʒ/, /tʃ/ and /dʒ/, with air flowing over the sides of the tongue)

- Nasalization
  - Inappropriate nasal resonance in the production of oral sounds, especially oral stops (/p/, /t/, /k/, /b/, d/, and /g/)
  - Most oral sounds except for /m/, / n/, and /ŋ/ may be vulnerable

- Pharyngeal fricative
  - Fricatives produced in the pharyngeal area
  - Consonants produced by lingual-pharyngeal contacts often found in clients with cleft palate

- Initial position error
  - Error in the production of initial sounds in words
  - Common type of articulation error, may be a deletion or a substitution
- Medial position error
  - Error in the production of a middle sound of a word
  - Less frequent than errors in the initial and final word positions
- Final position error
  - Error in the production of a final sound of a word
  - A common type of error, may be a deletion of a sound or a substitution
- Intervocalic error
  - Error in producing a consonant that is preceded and succeeded by a vowel
  - Error in the medial position of words

Phonological Error Patterns or Processes

- A process is a pattern of errors, instead of a collection of unrelated individual sound errors; patterns are based on certain linguistic rules of sound production and sound combinations that apply to languages; errors are considered related (not independent) to other errors within a process; a process is a way of organizing errors into groups (patterns) that are understood in terms of underlying linguistic rules of operation
- There are varied descriptions of phonological processes, which are patterns of sound productions normal up to a chronological age and disorders beyond that point; some patterns are more common than others; some have greater effect on intelligibility than others; major phonological processes are described in alphabetical order
- Assimilation processes: Phonological patterns in which one sound in a word leads to a change in another sound in the same word; assimilative errors are similar to substitution errors; in assimilation, influence of one sound on another is the main source of error; such an influence is not a factor in simple substitutions
  - Alveolar assimilation: Production of an alveolar in place of a velar
    - *dot* for *goat*
    - *tot* for *coat*
  - Devoicing: Production of a voiceless consonant in place of a voiced consonant
    - *back* for *bag*
    - *sip* for *zip*
  - Diminutization: Addition of [i] or a consonant and [i]
    - *eggi* for *egg*
    - *nodi* for *no*
  - Epenthesis: Insertion of a vowel (an error of addition); often between two consonants in a consonantal cluster
    - *bə lu* for *blue*
    - *sə mile* for *smile*
  - Labial assimilation: Production of a labial consonant in place of a nonlabial consonant in a word that contains another labial
    - *beab* for *bead*
    - *bop* for *top*

- o Metathesis: Production of sounds in a word in their reversed order
  - *peek* for *keep*
  - *likstip* for *lipstick*
- o Nasal assimilation: Production of a nasal consonant in place of an oral consonant in a word that contains a nasal
  - *nam* for *lamb*
  - *nun* for *fun*
- o Prevocalic voicing (voicing assimilation): Voiced production of voiceless consonants when they precede a vowel (prevocalic position)
  - *bea* for *pea*
  - *Dom* for *Tom*
- o Reduplication (doubling): Repetition of a syllable within a word
  - *wawa* for *water*
  - *kaka* for *cat*
- o Velar assimilation: Production of a velar consonant in place of a nonvelar in a word that contains a velar
  - *keak* for *teak*
  - *guck* for *duck*
- Substitution processes (Simplification processes): Similar to *substitutions* in the traditional analysis, involve replacement of one sound for another sound
  - Apicalization: Production of an apical (tongue tip) consonant in place of a labial consonant
  - *dee* for *bee*
  - *tee* for *pea*
- o Backing: Production of more posteriorly placed consonants instead of more anteriorly placed consonants (velar consonants in place of alveolar consonants)
  - *boak* for *boat*
  - *hoop* for *soup*
- o Affrication: Production of an affricate in place of a fricative or stop
  - *chun* for *sun*
  - *chu* for *shoe*
- o Deaffrication: Production of a fricative in place of an affricate
  - *pez* for *page*
  - *ship* for *chip*
- o Denasalization: Production of an oral sound with a similar place of articulation (homorganic sound) in place of a nasal
  - *by* for *my*
  - *dame* for *name*
- o Depalatalization: Production of an alveolar fricative in place of a palatal fricative or affricate
  - *su* for *shoe*
  - *wats* for *watch* (diacritic ∪ under ts)
  - Final consonant devoicing: Production of an unvoiced final consonant in place of a voiced final consonant
  - *bet* for *bed*
  - *bik* for *big*

- o Fronting: Production of more anteriorly placed consonants in place of more posteriorly placed consonants (e.g., alveolar consonants instead of velar consonants)
  - *tee* for *key*
  - *su* for *shoe*
- o Gliding: Production of a glide (w, j) in place of a liquid (l, r)
  - *pwey* for *play*
  - *yewo* for *yellow*
- o Glottal replacement: Production of a glottal stop (ʔ) in place of other consonants
  - *tuʔ* for *tooth*
  - *buʔ* for *boot*
- o Labialization: Production of a labial consonant in place of a lingual consonant
  - *fum* for *thumb*
  - *vase* for *days*
- o Stopping: Production of stop consonants in place of other sounds (often fricatives)
  - *teat* for *seat*
  - *doup* for *soup*
- o Vocalization (vowelization): Production of vowels in place of liquids or nasals
  - *fawo* for *flower*
  - *dippo* for *zipper*
- • Deletion processes (Structure processes): Elimination of certain sounds in syllables and words; similar to *deletions* in the traditional analysis.
  - o Cluster reduction or cluster simplification: Omission (deletion) of one or more consonants in a cluster of consonants
    - *bes* for *best*
    - *seep* for *sleep*
  - o Consonant deletion: Omission of an intervocalic consonant
    - *mai* for *mommy*
    - *dai* for *Dotty*
  - o Initial consonant deletion: Omission of word-initial consonants
    - *at* for *pot*
    - *oop* for *soup*
  - o Final consonant deletion: Omission of a consonant at the end of a word or syllable
    - *kæ* for *cat*
    - *pu* for *pool*
  - o Unstressed (weak) syllable deletion: Omission of a syllable, usually an unstressed syllable
    - *nana* for *banana*
    - *tephone* for *telephone*

Factors Related to Articulation and Phonological Disorders

- • No specific cause or causes explain Ar-Ph disorders
- • Several factors are correlated with Ar-Ph disorders; such factors are not necessarily the causes of the disorders

- There are differences between those who do and those who do not have Ar-Ph disorders on specific variables; such differences also do not suggest causation
- Age
  Most children have near-normal speech skills by the time they are 4 or 5 years old
  Articulatory performance improves until children are about 8 years old
- Gender
  o Girls may be slightly ahead of boys in phonological acquisition
  o More boys than girls have Ar-Ph disorders, although no satisfactory explanation for this difference is available
- Socioeconomic status
  o A slightly greater number of children from lower socioeconomic groups have Ar-Ph disorders than those from higher socioeconomic groups
  o Nonetheless, socioeconomic status is not considered a significant variable
- Familial and genetic factors
  o As noted earlier, familial and genetic factors may influence speech production; there is a family history of articulation disorders in 35% to 40% of cases; no specific genetic abnormality in children with routine Ar-Ph disorders has been isolated
  o Older and only children have slightly better articulatory skills than children whose siblings are only slightly older, but birth order and sibling status are not considered important in the development of articulation or its disorders
- Personality and emotional disorders
  o Children with Ar-Ph disorders are not distinguished by unique personality or emotional disorders
  o Parents or other family members are not distinguished by unique personality or emotional factors
- Intelligence
  o Within normal limits, intelligence is not associated with Ar-Ph disorders because most children with these disorders have normal intelligence
  o Children with intellectual disabilities tend to exhibit Ar-Ph disorders; the greater the degree of impairment, the higher the number of errors and error severity
  o Children with intellectual disabilities do not exhibit a unique pattern of misarticulations; for the most part, their errors resemble those of younger children with normal intelligence
- Academic performance
  o Ar-Ph disorders are usually independent of academic performance
  o Children with severe Ar-Ph disorders and significant language delay have A high risk for poor academic performance including reading and spelling problems; these problems are related to limited language skills
- Structural variations in the speech production mechanism
  o Generally, variations within the normal range in the oral speech production mechanism are not a factor in Ar-Ph disorders
  o Extreme deviations are more likely to be associated with Ar-Ph disorders; extreme degrees of malocclusions, velopharyngeal incompetence, and tongue deformities may be positively correlated with Ar-Ph disorders

- Some individuals with notable deviations may still learn to produce the speech sounds correctly by adopting successful compensatory strategies
- So-called functional articulation disorders may be found in the absence of structural anomalies
- Oral sensory factors
  - The relationship between oral sensory perception and articulation skills is not clear; the limited evidence is contradictory
  - Research on oral tactile sensitivity and oral form recognition has failed to produce convincing evidence that oral sensory impairment causes Ar-Ph disorders
- Hearing loss
  - Hearing loss is associated with Ar-Ph disorders
  - Significant degree of loss at all ages is related to articulation disorders (may not be classified as phonological disorders)
  - Even mild loss during the period of speech sound acquisition (of the kind associated with otitis media) may slow down speech sound acquisition
  - Many children with Ar-Ph disorders have normal hearing; thus hearing loss does not explain their disorder
- Motor skills
  - Children with Ar-Ph disorders do not necessarily have deficits in general motor skills
  - Although some children with Ar-Ph disorders may score slightly below average on diadochokinetic tests, other children may perform as well as, or even better than, the average rates on such tests
- Tongue thrust
  - Anterior tongue resting position during swallow may be associated with lisping
  - Distortions of /z/ and /l/ and interdentalization of /t/, /d/, /n/, and /l/ have been noted in children with tongue thrust
  - Tongue thrust is not a significant factor in a most children with Ar-Ph disorders
- Auditory speech sound discrimination skills
  - Ar-Ph disorders may be associated with speech sound discrimination problems
  - Whether such auditory discrimination problems are due to their Ar-Ph disorders or vice versa is unclear
  - Generally, auditory discrimination problems play a minor, if any, role in most children with Ar-Ph disorders
- Language skills
  - Speech and language disorders may coexist in approximately 50% of preschool children
  - Some 40% to 80% of children with Ar-Ph disorders have language disorders and roughly the same number of children with specific language impairment have Ar-Ph problems
  - A smaller percentage of children with Ar-Ph disorders (10% to 40%) also may have language comprehension problems

54

- o Children with significant Ar-Ph disorders may use less complex language, shorter utterances, and incomplete sentences
- o Both the number and severity of Ar-Ph disorders may increase when syntactic complexity is combined with syllabic complexity
- o Mild to moderate Ar-Ph disorders in many children may not be associated with significant language problems
- Phonological awareness
  - o Children with Ar-Ph disorders may have deficiencies in <u>Phonological Awareness</u>
  - o Children with Ar-Ph disorders may have difficulty in analyzing the phoneme components of syllables and words; may have difficulty with such skills as rhyming, sound segmentation, syllable identification, sound blending, and alliteration

Theories of Articulation and Phonological Disorders

- No specific cause or causes explain articulation and phonological (Ar-Ph) disorders
- There are factors that may coexist, and hence be correlated, with Ar-Ph disorders; such correlations do not suggest causation
- There are differences between those who do and those who do not have Ar-Ph disorders on specific variables; such differences, too, do not suggest causation
- Subtle neuromotor or sensory processing deficits that may exist in children with Ar-Ph disorders do not explain the disorders
- Deficiencies in phonological awareness may be a part or an effect of Ar-Ph disorders, not the cause of the disorders; treating phonological awareness may not automatically improve speech production skills
- Theories of articulation and phonological disorders address patterned phonological disorders, not isolated difficulties in speech sound production; most are linguistically based and seek to explain speech production in children who speak normally and those who speak with phonological errors
- The classic and basic theory (explanation) of phonological disorders, which is a liner explanation of phonological skills and errors, is that children make phonological errors because
  - o Speech production is a complex task that is difficult for some children
  - o Children simplify what they hear in the speech of adults around them and such simplifications are phonological processes
  - o Typically, as the child becomes more proficient in speech production, the processes fade
  - o But in some children, attempts to simplify phoneme productions and phoneme sequences persist, creating phonological disorders
- Fundamental assumptions of newer and current phonological theories are that all speakers, including children
  - o Have underlying *mental representations* of phonemes
  - o Children who produce speech sounds normally have correctly realized the underlying mental representation
  - o Those who make phonological errors have failed to realize an accurate mental representation of their sound system

- One of the newer nonlinear phonological theories, called the **naturalness and markedness** theory, explains certain phonological error patterns by stating that
  - Phonological errors are due to a tendency to move from the marked features to the natural (unmarked) features of a language
  - The features of languages are not evenly distributed across the languages of the world; some features occur more frequently and more commonly among the languages; other features are either unique to certain languages or found less commonly among languages; features that are found frequently and across many languages are called *natural*; those that are infrequent or unique are called *marked*
  - Some common phonological processes are due to a tendency to use more natural features because they are easier and less complex than marked features; final consonant deletion, for example, creates open syllables or the CV type, which is the most natural (unmarked) syllable type; similarly, the stopping of fricatives and affricates is also due to a tendency to move from the less natural (fricatives and affricates) to more natural (stops).
- **Optimality theory**, another nonlinear phonological theory, postulates that
  - Grammars (including phonological rules) are a set of conflicting constraints that are differently ranked across languages; rules ranked lower in a given language may be ranked higher in other languages
  - Speakers of each language obey rules ranked higher in their own language and ignore lower-ranked rules
  - All speakers have, in their innate grammar, universal and natural constraints (*rules* in older terminology) that are unmarked and more natural, but they also have to learn what is unique to their particular language (marked, less natural); a child with a phonological disorder may have an innate grammar in which constraints are ranked differently than in the adult grammar of that language; the result is a phonological disorder
  - Final consonant deletions by an English-speaking child, for example, is explained by pointing out that the markedness constraint CODA (which says, "no final consonants") outranks the faithfulness constraint MAX (which says, "no deletion"); in English grammar, which has many final consonants, MAX is ranked higher than CODA, so the normal adult productions include final consonants; a child or any other speaker of English who deletes final consonants obeys CODA ("no final consonants") and ignores MAX ("no deletions"), whereas those who include final consonants do the opposite—they obey MAX and ignore CODA
  - Children who reduce clusters to singletons have in their grammar (input representation) COMPLEX ("no clusters") ranked higher than MAX ("no deletion"); unfortunately, the language they speak has the opposite ranking: MAX is ranked higher than COMPLEX
  - Children exhibit *gliding* because in their grammar, *LIQUIDS ("no liquids") is ranked higher than IDENT [consonantal] ("don't change [consonantal])
  - Children who exhibit *stopping* (substitution of stops for fricatives as in [du] for [zoo]) obey the markedness constraint FRICATIVES ("no fricatives"); thus in each case, children's misarticulations are due to deviant

grammars that have a ranking of constraints different from those in adult grammars

- No theory is complete or generally accepted; most phonological theories are rationalist models that tend to be speculative

Barlow, J. A., & Gierut, J. A. (1999). Optimality theory in phonological acquisition. *Journal of Speech, Language, and Hearing Research, 42,* 1482–1498.

Bernhardt, B., & Stoel-Gammon, C. (1994). Nonlinear phonology: Introduction and clinical application. *Journal of Speech and Hearing Research, 37,* 123–143.

Bernthal, J. E., & Bankson, N. W. (2004). *Articulation and phonological disorders* (5th ed.). Boston, MA: Allyn and Bacon.

Clements, G. N. (1995). Constraints based approaches to phonology. *Proceedings of the XIIIth International Congress of Phonetic Sciences, 3,* 66–73.

Dekkers, J., van der Leeuw, F., & van der Weijer, J. (2000). *Optimality theory: Phonology, syntax, and acquisition.* Oxford, UK: Oxford University Press.

Goldsmith, J. A. (1990). *Autosegmental and metrical phonology.* Oxford, UK: Basil Blackwell.

Goldston, C. (1996). Direct optimality theory: Representation as pure markedness. *Language, 72,* 713–748.

Grunwell, P. (1997b). Natural phonology. In M.J. Ball & R.D. Kent (Eds.), *The new phonologies: Developments in clinical linguistics.* San Diego, CA: Singular Publishing Group.

Gussmann, E. (2002). *Phonology: Analysis and theory.* Cambridge, UK: Oxford University Press.

Lowe, R. J. (1994). *Phonology: Assessment and intervention applications in speech pathology.* Baltimore, MD: Williams & Wilkins.

Peña-Brooks, A., & Hegde, M. N. (2007). *Assessment and treatment of articulation and phonological disorders in children* (2nd ed.). Austin, TX: Pro-Ed.

Smit, A. B. (2004). *Articulation and phonology: Resource guide for school-age children and adults.* Clifton Park, NY: Thomson Delmar Learning.

Stoel-Gammon, C., & Dunn, C. (1985). *Normal and disordered phonology in children.* Austin, TX: Pro-Ed.

Williams, A. L. (2003). *Speech disorders: Resource guide for preschool children.* Clifton Park, NY: Thomson Delmar Learning.

Articulation and Phonological Disorders in African American Children.

Disorders of speech sound production in children who speak African American English (AAE); these children are more likely to speak both AAE and a variety of Standard American English (SAE); speech-language pathologists who assess and treat articulation disorders in African American children should be knowledgeable in the phonological, semantic, and syntactic aspects of AAE; if not, the clinician may make an inappropriate diagnosis of an articulation (or language) disorder in an African American child and may offer unjustified treatment; conversely, the clinician may miss a true articulation (or language) disorder in an African American child.

Articulation and Phonological Disorders in African American Children

Overview of African American English
- African American English is a product of the African American cultural heritage, like other languages and dialectal variations that are cultural products
- African American English shares many phonological features with SAE; however, it has a few unique phonological rules
- Varied AAE phonological rules are neither haphazard nor deviant; they are systematic; rules or patterns can be derived from AAE speech like they have been derived from SAE
- Not all African American children speak AAE; many African American children who speak AAE also speak SAE competently; the degree of proficiency may vary in both AAE and SAE in children who speak both languages
- An articulation disorder may be evident in one or both forms of English, but a disorder in SAE is not diagnosed without a reference to AAE; SAE production differences that are due to the influence of AAE are not an indication of an articulation disorder

Factors Related to Articulation and Phonological Disorders
- No unique factors that cause articulation and phonological disorders in African American children have been convincingly demonstrated
- Factors associated with articulation and phonological disorders in other children also may be associated with such disorders in African American children; see under <u>Articulation and Phonological Disorders</u> for a summary of associated factors

Articulatory Skills of African American Children
- Error patterns of African American children are the same as those of monolingual children (e.g., omissions, deletions, substitutions, additions, and specific phonological processes); see under <u>Articulation and Phonological Disorders</u> for a summary of common error patterns found in children who misarticulate speech sounds
- Phoneme inventory of children speaking AAE matches that of SAE; a majority of phonemes are used in the same way in both AAE and SAE; only some phonemes will be used differently, substituted for other phonemes, or omitted in certain contexts—all understood as regular and patterned according to rules derived from them
- The following phonological patterns are characteristic of AAE:
  - /l/ lessening or omission (e.g., *too'* for *tool; a'ways* for *always*)
  - /r/ lessening or omission (e.g., *doah* for *door; mudah* for *mother*)
  - /θ/ substitution for /f/ in word final or medial positions (e. g., *teef* for *teeth, nofin'* for *nothing*)
  - /t/ substitution for / θ/ in word initial positions (e.g., *tink* for *think*)
  - /d/ substitution for /ð/ in word initial and medial positions (e.g., *dis* for *this* and *broder* for *brother*)
  - /v/ substitution for /ð/ at word final positions (e.g., *smoov* for *smooth*)
  - Omission of consonants in clusters in word initial and final positions (e.g., *thow* for *throw* and *des'* for *desk*)
  - Consonant substitutions within clusters (e.g., *skrike* for *strike*)

- o Unique syllable stress patterns (e.g., *gui* tar for *guitar* and *Ju* ly for *July*)
- o Modification of verbs ending in /k/ (e.g., *li-id* for *liked* and *wah-tid* for *walked*)
- o Metathetic productions (e.g., *aks* for *ask*)
- o Devoicing of final voiced consonants (e.g., *bet* for *bed* and *ruk* for *rug*)
- o Deletion of final consonants (e.g., *ba'* for *bad* and *goo'* for *good*)
- o /i/ substitution for /e/ (e.g., *pin* for *pen* and *tin* for *ten*)
- o /b/ substitution for /v/ (e.g., *balentine* for *valentine* and *bes'* or *vest*)
- o Diphthong reduction or ungliding (e.g., *fahnd* for *find* and *ol* for *oil*)
- o /n/ substitution for /ŋ/ (e.g., *walkin'* for *walking* and *thin'* for *thing*)
- o Unstressed syllable deletion (e.g., *bout* for *about* and *member* for *remember*)

- Clinicians who assess and treat African American children may consult the following additional cited resources and the two companion volumes, *Hegde's PocketGuide to Assessment in Speech-Language Pathology* (3rd ed.) and *Hegde's PocketGuide to Treatment in Speech-Language Pathology* (3rd ed.).

Battle, D. E. (2002). *Communication disorders in multicultural populations* (3rd ed.). Boston, MA: Butterworth-Heinemann.

Genesee, F., Paradis, J., & Crago, M. B. (2004). *Dual language development and disorders*. Baltimore, MD: Paul H. Brookes.

Goldstein, B. A. (2004). *Bilingual language development and disorders in Spanish-English speakers*. Baltimore, MD: Paul H. Brookes.

Kamhi, A. G., Pollack, K. E., & Harris, J. L. (1996). *Communication development and disorders in African American children*. Baltimore, MD: Paul H. Brookes

Kayser, H. (1995). *Bilingual speech-language pathology: An Hispanic focus*. San Diego, CA: Singular Publishing Group.

Peña-Brooks, A., & Hegde, M. N. (2007). *Assessment and treatment of articulation and phonological disorders in children* (3rd ed.). Austin, TX: Pro-Ed.

Roseberry-McKibbin, C. (2002). *Multicultural students with special language needs* (2nd ed.). Oceanside, CA: Academic Communication Associates.

Articulation and Phonological Disorders in Bilingual Children. Disorders of speech sound production in children who speak two (or more) languages; the disorder may be evident in one or both the languages spoken by a large and varied group of children in the United States; clinicians who assess and treat articulation and phonological disorders (or any other communication disorder) in bilingual children should have a basic understanding of the primary language of the child; quite often, the primary language is other than English.

Overview of Bilingualism in the United States

- Bilingual children in the United States speak several other languages, often as their primary languages
- Children whose primary language is a variety of Spanish probably constitute the largest number of bilingual children in the country

- Children who speak an Asian language may constitute the second largest group of bilingual children
- Children who speak one of the Native American languages also are a considerable number, although this number has been dwindling over the past several decades
- Children of European background who speak a language other than English are increasing in number

Factors Related to Articulation and Phonological Disorders

- No unique factors that cause articulation and phonological disorders in bilingual children have been convincingly demonstrated
- Factors that are associated with articulation and phonological disorders in monolingual children also may be associated with such disorders in bilingual children; see under Articulation and Phonological Disorders for a summary of such factors
- Many error patterns found in bilingual children also will be similar to the patterns found in monolingual English-speaking children, although there will be unique characteristics; see under Articulation and Phonological Disorders for basic patterns of articulatory and phonological errors

Description of Articulatory Errors in Bilingual Children

- Error patterns of bilingual children are the same as those found in monolingual children (e.g., omissions, deletions, substitutions, additions, and specific phonological processes)
- The issue is not whether bilingual children exhibit unique patterns of errors; it is whether a given pattern of production is an articulation or a phonological disorder according to the rules of their first language
- See under Articulation and Phonological Disorders for a summary of common error patterns found in children who misarticulate speech sounds

Phonological Characteristics of Spanish-Influenced English

- Compared to English, Spanish has a simpler phonological system; Spanish phonological features that contrast with English features include the following:
  - English has 15 vowels, whereas Spanish has only 5 vowels: /i/, /e/, /u/, /o/, and /a/
  - The English consonants /v/, /θ/, /ð/, /z/, /dʒ/, and /ʒ/ are not in Spanish; the nasal /ŋ/ and the liquid /j/ also are absent in Spanish; while speaking English as a second language, some Spanish-speaking children may produce those consonants as allophonic variations of phonemes present in Spanish
  - The Spanish consonants /ŋ/, /ʎ/, /ɣ/, /χ/, /ř/, and /β/ are absent in English
  - Some Spanish consonants, though similar to certain consonants in English, may be produced differently; for example, the Spanish /s/ may be produced more frontally, giving the impression of a lisp
  - Spanish has only a few consonants in word final positions (only /s/, /n/, /r/, /l/, and /d/); consequently, other English consonants in final word positions may be omitted
  - Spanish vowels a, e, i, o, u may also be found in word final positions

o Spanish consonantal clusters are fewer and simpler; the /s/ cluster, most common in English, does not occur in Spanish; final clusters are rare in Spanish

o English /t/, /d/, and /n/ tend to be dentalized

o Final consonants may be devoiced (e.g, *dose* for *doze*)

o /b/ may be substituted for /v/ (e.g., *bery* for *very*)

o Weak or deaspirated stops, giving the impression of omission of stop sounds

o /ʧ/ may be substituted for /ʃ/ (e.g., *Chirley* for *Shirley*)

o /d/ or /z/ may be substituted for /ð/, which does not exist in Spanish (e.g., *dis* for *this* or *zat* for *that*)

o Schwa may be inserted before word-initial consonant clusters (*eskate* for *skate* or *espend* for *spend*)

o /r/ may be trapped (as in the English word *butter*) or trilled

o Word-initial /h/ may be silent (e.g., *old* for *hold* or *it* for *hit*)

o /y/ may be substituted for /ʤ/, an absent sound in Spanish (e.g., *yulie* for *Julie*)

Phonological Considerations of Asian Languages

- Asian languages belong to different language families; therefore, it is not possible to succinctly categorize the influence of "Asian languages" on English; much of the available information may apply to a specific Asian language

- China has more than 80 languages and countless dialectal variations; India has more than 20 major languages with numerous dialects of each; Asian languages belong to many language families including (1) Sino-Tibetan (e.g., Thai, Yao, Mandarin, Cantonese); (2) Indo-Aryan, Indo-European, or Indic (e.g., Hindi, Bengali, Marathi spoken in India); (3) Dravidian (e.g., Kannada, Tamil, Telugu, Malayalam spoken in India); (4) Astro-Asiatic (e.g., Khmer, Vietnamese, Hmong); (5) Tibeto-Burman (e.g., Tibetan and Burmese); (6) Malayo-Polynesian or Astronesian (e.g., Chamorro, Ilocano, Tagalog); (7) Papuan (e.g., New Guinean); and (8) Altaic (e.g., Japanese, Korean).

- Because of the diversity of Asian languages—they belong to different language families with diverse phonological properties—a general description of phonological characteristics of children who speak an Asian language is not practical, meaningful, or appropriate

- Many descriptions in the literature under the heading of *Asian* children or speakers apply mostly to the Chinese; some or most of the characteristics that apply to the Chinese language may not apply to other Asian languages

Phonological Considerations of Native American Languages

- Native American languages also belong to a variety of language families; therefore, it is not practical or meaningful to list the special phonological characteristics of Native American languages.

- Approximately 800 Native American languages are spoken in North, Central, and South America; the North American continent has at least 200 Native American languages

- The estimated number of Native American language families varies from a high of 60 to a low of 3. One classification of 8 language families include:

Algonquian, Iroquoian, Caddoan, Muskogean, Siouan, Penutian, Athabascan, and Uto-Aztecan.

- Many children of Native Americans do not speak their parents' language or have only extremely limited proficiency in it
- There are useful websites on American Indian or Native American culture and languages that offer information on certain languages and their properties; use these resources in understanding aspects of Native American languages (see, for example, http//www.indians.org/welker.americans.htm)
- Determine first whether a Native American child is a bilingual speaker; then follow the guidelines offered in this section
- To make an appropriate assessment of Native American children's phonological skills, clinicians need to develop a database of the phonological characteristics of Native American languages spoken in their service area

Bayles, K., & Harris, G. (1982). Evaluating speech and language skills in Papago Indian children. *Journal of American Indian Education, 21*(2), 11–20.

Genesee, F., Paradis, J., & Crago, M. B. (2004). *Dual language development and disorders*. Baltimore, MD: Paul H. Brookes.

Highwater, J. (1975). *Indian America*. New York: David McKay Company.

Peña-Brooks, A., & Hegde, M. N. (2007). *Assessment and treatment of articulation and phonological disorders in children* (2nd ed.). Austin, TX: Pro-Ed.

Robinson-Zanartu, C. (1996). Serving Native American children and families: Considering cultural variables. *Language, Speech, and Hearing Services in Schools, 27*, 373–384.

Roseberry-McKibbin, C. (2002). *Multicultural students with special language needs* (2nd ed.). Oceanside, CA: Academic Communication Associates.

U.S. Bureau of the Census. (2005). *Statistical abstract of the United States*. Washington, DC: U.S. Government Printing Office.

Welker, G. (1996). Native American languages. [Online]: Available FTP: www.indians.org/welker/americans.htm

Westby, C., & Vining, C. B. (2002). Living in harmony: Providing services to Native American children and families. In D. E. Battle (Ed.), *Communication disorders in multicultural populations* (3rd ed.) (pp. 136–178). Boston, MA: Butterworth-Heinemann.

Asperger's Disorder (Syndrome). An autism spectrum disorder; see under the main entry, Autism Spectrum Disorders.

Aspiration. Penetration of food and liquid into the airway, occurring at the level below the true vocal folds; a disorder of swallowing; food and liquid may enter the airway before swallow, during the pharyngeal phase of the swallow, after the swallow, or as a result of gastric reflux; causes aspiration pneumonia; see Dysphagia.

Aspiration Pneumonia. Lung infection due to aspiration, which is food and liquid penetration of the airway due to Dysphagia; inflammation of the walls of the smaller bronchial tubes; also called *broncho-* or *bronchial pneumonia*; causes breathing difficulties.

Assessment. A clinical procedure designed to find out whether a client has a disorder and if the client does have a disorder, to describe its characteristics, severity, potential causes, and treatment options; it includes several specific steps: (1) description and assessment of a client's existing and nonexisting communicative behaviors, background variables, and associated factors to evaluate or diagnose a communicative problem; (2) clinical measurement of a person's communicative behaviors; (3) evaluation of the communicative patterns of a client and his or her family; (4) assessment of the strengths, limitations, and needs of a client and his or her family; (5) prognosis for improvement with or without treatment; and (6) recommendation of treatment options for the client and family members; a clinical activity that precedes treatment, often continues throughout treatment, and is repeated before dismissal and during follow-up; see *Hegde's PocketGuide to Assessment in Speech-Language Pathology* (3rd ed.) for detailed assessment procedures; to complete an assessment, the clinician
- Obtains the case history
- Interviews the client (or caregivers of client)
- Conducts an orofacial examination
- Makes client-specific judgments on the use of standardized or nonstandardized measures; administers selected tests or other measurement instruments
- Uses measures appropriate to the client and his or her linguistic and ethnocultural background
- Screens hearing
- Obtains a speech-language sample
- Analyzes the results
- Draws conclusions; makes a diagnosis; suggests a prognosis; recommends treatment; disseminates information to the client, the family, and the referring professional

Assimilation Processes. A normal phonological pattern in children until age 3; one sound assumes the characteristics of another sound, typically another sound within the word; considered a phonological disorder if it persists beyond age 3; see Phonological Processes and Articulation and Phonological Disorders.

Assimilative Nasality. A disorder of resonance or a phonological process; undesirable nasal resonance on vowels that are adjacent to nasal consonants (a resonance disorder); a nonnasal sound being produced as a nasal sound because of an adjacent nasal sound in the same word (a phonological process called *nasal assimilation*).

Ataxia. A neurological disorder characterized by disturbed balance and movement due to injury to the cerebellum; neurological symptoms include impaired equilibrium and gait, unstable standing and walking, irregular steps while walking, difficulty maintaining balance leading to falls, overshooting or undershooting of objects while trying to reach them, slow initiation and execution of movements, irregular and poorly timed repetitive movements, hypotonia, and tremor associated with voluntary movements; associated with such diseases as Friedreich's ataxia, hereditary spinocerebellar ataxias, olivopontocerebellar atrophy, and such other neurological diseases; may also be caused by such other diseases as multiple sclerosis, vascular disorders, encephalitis, tumors, drug toxicity, and so forth.

Ataxic Dysarthria. A type of motor speech disorder associated with cerebellar damage and ataxia; see Dysarthria: Specific Types.

Atherosclerosis. A slowly developing vascular disorder in which the arteries are hardened and narrowed, leading eventually to the formation of thrombosis; prevents or severely restricts the blood flow to tissue; a frequent cause of ischemic strokes; also known as *arteriosclerosis*; accumulation of lipids and other forms of fat, calcium deposits, and fibrous materials cause the narrowing of arteries; causes of atherosclerosis include high blood pressure, high cholesterol, high triglycerides, diabetes, smoking, and use of oral contraceptives; genetic predisposition is suspected.

Athetosis. A neurological disorder characterized by slow, writhing, worm-like movements due to injury to the extrapyramidal motor pathways; movements may be more severe in the hands; a type of dyskinesia; see Cerebral Palsy for speech disorders associated with this type of neurological problem in children; acquired athetosis in adults if typically described as *dystonia*.

Atresia. Absence or closure of a normally open structure (e.g., closed external auditory canal); a congenital anomaly associated with many genetic syndromes.

Atrophy. Wasting away of tissues or organs; shrinking of cells in an organ or system; atrophy of muscles involved in speech or atrophy of neural tissue due to diseases and trauma are associated with communication disorders.

Auditory Agnosia. Impaired understanding or recognition of auditory stimuli; a central nervous system disorder; normal peripheral hearing; associated with certain adult neurological disorders; see Agnosia and Aphasia.

Auditory Comprehension Deficit. Difficulty in understanding spoken language; a problem found in a variety of communication disorders; symptom of dementia and aphasia, especially Wernicke's aphasia; also associated with intellectual disabilities and language disorders in children.

Auditory Verbal Agnosia. Difficulty comprehending the meaning of spoken words; the client can hear them; therefore, there is no peripheral hearing loss; a sign of central nervous system disorder; associated with some of the adult neurogenic communication disorders. See Aphasia.

Augmentative and Alternative Communication (AAC). Methods of communication that supplement oral communication or provide alternative means of communication for individuals with extremely limited oral communication skills or for individuals who have lost previously acquired communication skills due to disease, trauma, or surgical intervention (e.g., the removal of cancerous larynx); means of communication that partially or fully compensate for severe, oral-expressive communication deficits; involve a variety of methods to encode, transmit, and physically exhibit messages that individuals cannot vocally produce; always includes the residual vocal and verbal communication even if they are extremely limited; are always multimodal in that gestures, manual signs, vocal productions, and external devices are all used simultaneously; use of the methods may be temporary or permanent; methods vary widely in their use of technology; may be simple or complex devices including sophisticated computerized voice and speech synthesizers; useful for persons within varied diagnostic categories; all forms of communication described under this entry may be considered *augmentative* (not alternative) because individuals who use them have some vocal, gestural, or other typical means of communication no matter how limited.

Basic Terms of AAC

- *AAC system:* A group of components, symbols, aids, and strategies all integrated into a functional unit
- *AAC user:* The individual who has limited oral communication skills and thus needs to use a form of AAC
- *Access:* Means by which a communicator composes a message and manipulates (controls) the device
- *Aid or device:* Physical objects or instruments that transmit or receive messages; includes a note pad, message book, message boards, charts, mechanical equipment, or such electronic equipment as a microcomputer
- *Aided* and *unaided:* AAC strategies that either use some external device or equipment (aided; e.g., use of a communication board, symbol systems, computer-generated communication) or those that do not use such devices or equipment (unaided; e.g., gestures, sign languages)
- *Alternative:* Technically, a method of communication that replaces the typical oral communication; because this is not always true, all communication methods described under AAC may technically be *augmentative* (not alternative)
- *Augmentative:* Methods or devices that enhance or supplement the available means of typical communication (often oral communication); for example, a communication board that enhances or supplements oral communication
- *Communication Partner (CP):* Person or persons who interact with the AAC user
- *Direct selection:* Selecting a message by pointing, depressing an electronic key, touching a key pad, or touching an item or object within a selection set (contrasted with scanning)
- *Display (output):* Means by which a selection set (symbols, codes, signs, words, messages) is made available to the AAC user who then selects particular messages to be conveyed; includes such low-technology *fixed display* devices as communication boards or a high-technology *dynamic display* device as computer monitors
- *High-technology device:* An AAC method that uses electronic instruments including computers
- *Iconic* and *non-iconic symbol:* A picture or symbol that looks like the object it represents (iconic); a picture or symbol that does not look like the object it represents (noniconic); arbitrary symbols whose meaning has to be systematically taught are noniconic; the meaning of iconic symbols, though they too are arbitrary, will have been acquired in everyday interactions

- *Low-technology device:* An AAC method that does not use electronic instruments; such means as a message board or a note pad
- *Scanning:* Sequential offering of available messages by the communication partner or a mechanical device until the AAC user indicates the right message he or she wishes to convey (contrasted with direct selection); appropriate for those who cannot directly select a message from a selection set, typically because of impaired motor control
- *Selection set:* The entire collection of symbols, codes, signs, words, messages, and so forth that are displayed for the individual to select and communicate; a display of all the pictures that an individual uses to communicate is an example of a selection set; other selection sets include the computer keyboards on which symbols or messages are displayed or a communication board that includes the choices the individual can make.
- *Symbols:* Means of representation; includes drawings, photographs, objects, all kinds of gestures, manual signs, printed words, geometric shapes, Braille, and spoken words

Classification of AAC

Unaided Symbols. Form of AAC in which no instruments are used and communication is achieved through manual signs, gestures, and other patterned movement; may be accompanied by some speech, but the manual modes of communication play a major role in message transmission; gestures and manual signs may convey a letter, a phoneme, or a concept; the following are among the many varieties of gestural-unaided communication:

- American Sign Language (ASL or AMESLAN): Consists of manual signs for the 26 letters of the alphabet; can sign words or phrases; recognized as a language by itself; often used with oral speech (total communication)
- Sign languages that are specific to particular countries: The deaf community in different countries have their own unique sign language systems that may be appropriate as unaided communication modes for nondeaf individuals who have limited oral language skills
- Pidgin Sign English: Various forms of ASL that have evolved during interactions between deaf and hearing individuals; may include ASL sign, some invented or newer forms of signs, finger spelling, and oral speech or mouthing of words
- Signed English: A system of simple signs developed originally for preschoolers with hearing impairment; consists of 3,100 signs and some sign markers for grammatical morphemes (e.g., the present progressive, past tense inflections, plural inflections)
- Signing Exact English: A modified and supplemented ASL system of communication; includes roughly 4,000 signs and 70 morphological markers; requires greater motoric agility to produces the signs; system allows expansion by adding new signs
- Key-word signing: A method that combines speech with signing limited to major (key) words in a sentence; main nouns and verbs may be signed whereas smaller grammatical features (prepositions, articles, conjunctions)

may not be signed; the entire sentence or phrase is spoken while signing the key words
- Cued speech: A system of manual signs that supplement spoken language; includes eight hand shapes that represent categories of consonant sounds and four hand positions for vowels and diphthongs displayed around the face of the speaker
- American Indian Hand Talk (AMER-IND): A sign language system developed by North American Indians; includes gestures and movements to suggest ideas and concepts; not phonetic; complex ideas are expressed by a series of gestures.
- Left-hand manual alphabet: Similar to American Manual Alphabet, but more suitable for persons with right-sided paralysis; consists of concrete gestures that approximate printed letters of the alphabet
- Limited manual sign systems: Several systems with limited number of signs and gestures; useful for clients in medical settings; used to communicate basic needs, self-care needs, and to simply say *yes* or *no;* a variety of systems available
- Pantomime: Mostly the use of gestures and dynamic movements often involving the entire body; consists of facial expressions, transparent messages, and dramatizations of meanings expressed
- Eye blink encoding: Learning to transmit basic messages by specific number of blinks (e.g., one blink means *yes,* two blinks mean *no*)

Aided Symbols. Form of AAC in which gestures or movements are combined with a message display device or instrument; gestures may directly point to an object or message; gestures may select a message displayed or indirectly generate messages by providing input to an electronic unit resulting in a message display; displays include a board, screen, or computer monitor; aided because of the use of such external devices as objects or a display instrument; the following are among the many varieties of gestural-assisted (aided) communication:
- Symbol sets: Various symbols that stand for messages or symbols that may be associated with messages; include ordinary objects, miniature objects, pictures, and drawings; special set of symbols such as Blissymbols and rebuses; Premack-type plastic tokens; Yerkish language (LANA Lexigrams); printed letters and words; synthesized speech (messages stored in a device that the AAC user activates by touching a symbol or a sequence of symbols); natural-sounding digitized speech (natural speech recorded and stored, and activated by the AAC user); Morse code; and Braille alphabet
- Nonelectronic gestural-assisted AAC: Three major types: (1) Communication boards that display messages; the AAC user may confirm a message that CP scans; may directly point to a message; may gaze at a message; may select with a head pointer; may point to or otherwise select numbers or symbols that stand for specific messages; (2) symbols that the AAC user arranges or manipulates on a magnetic board to convey messages; and (3) symbols that the AAC user draws or writes to

communicate; blackboard, magic slate, paper, or other device may be used to write or draw on; AAC user may print words of a natural language and draw objects and symbols

- Electronic gestural-assisted AAC: Use of electronic devices to communicate with the help of a switching mechanism the AAC user manipulates; a central unit that processes the signals and the output device that displays the message; (1) switching mechanisms vary widely and include pushing or touching switches (e.g., keyboards, graphic tablets), sliding handles, wobblesticks, joysticks, squeeze bulbs, tip or tilt position switches, pneumatic switches that are blown into, and sound- and light-controlled switches; (2) display devices that show the message also vary and include noise and light generators; various kinds of matrix displays in which rows and columns contain messages; cathode-ray tube displays; LED and LCD displays; printer displays; typewriters; computer printers; and various speech generators; (3) the central or control units connect the switch to the display; store messages; and help display the selected messages by switch activation.

Neuro-Assisted (Aided). Form of AAC in which bioelectrical signals (e.g., muscle action potentials) help generate messages on a display device; aided because of the use of instrumentation; useful for severely impaired AAC user whose hand mobility is extremely limited and cannot operate a switching mechanism; bioelectrical potentials activate switches and thus the messages; electrodes attached to the user and connected to the instrument help activate switching mechanisms; equipment is expensive and sophisticated; less developed than the other systems; the method is the same as that of *gestural-assisted* except for the switching mechanisms which include the following:

- Muscle action potentials: Electrical activity of the muscles associated with their contraction is used to activate switching mechanisms; electrodes attached to the skin pick up electrical discharges which are amplified so that they can activate special kinds of switches called myoswitches or specific displays; the user gets feedback (e.g., onset of light or sound or changes in their intensity) when a switch or display is activated and thus learns to use muscle action potentials for activating messages (biofeedback learning)
- Brain waves: Alpha brain waves may be used to generate messages on a computer screen through Morse code patterns; still in the research phase

Beukelman, D. R., & Mirenda, P. (2005). *Augmentative and Alternative Communication: Supporting children and adults with complex communication needs*. Baltimore, MD: Paul H. Brookes Publishing.

Light, J. C., Beukelman, D. R., & Reichle, J. (2003). *Communicative competence for individuals who use AAC*. Baltimore, MD: Paul H. Brookes.

Schlosser, R. W. (2003). *The efficacy of augmentative and alternative communication*. San Diego, CA: Academic Press.

Silverman, F. H. (1995). *Communication for the speechless* (3rd ed.). Boston: Allyn and Bacon.

Aural Atresia. Closure or absence of the external auditory canal; a congenital anomaly, found in various genetic syndromes; tends to be associated with other ear structure abnormalities; hearing impairment is a consequence.

Autism Spectrum Disorders. A group of behavioral and developmental disorders that begin in childhood and persist into adulthood; most notably include autism and Asperger syndrome or disorder, but may also include the Rett syndrome or disorder, and the childhood disintegrative disorder; all four are included in the Pervasive Developmental Disorders, an alternative classification promoted by the American Psychiatric Association.

Asperger's Disorder (Syndrome). Often called a syndrome, but the *Diagnostic and Statistical Manual* of the American Psychiatric Association calls it a form of pervasive developmental disorder; an autism spectrum disorder; some considered it a separate disorder in the past, but the current opinion is that it is a milder form of autism; a crucial difference between the classical form of autism and Asperger's disorder is that the former is characterized by significant language impairment and IQs of 70 or lower, whereas the latter is characterized by better language skills and IQs that exceed 70; individuals with Asperger's disorder lack social tact and a sense of social appropriateness

Etiology
- Unclear etiology; it may be the same as that for autism
- Possibly biologically based, although no specific gene has been identified
- Multiple genetic and nongenetic factors are thought to be involved (as in autism)

Physical and Behavioral Symptoms
- No particular physical features characterize Asperger's disorder
- Severe impairment in social interaction is its dominant feature
- Developmental milestones may be normal or nearly normal
- No significant intellectual disabilities, although some subtle cognitive deficits may be present
- Some may possess superior intellectual skills; nonetheless, may exhibit reasoning deficits
- Repetitive and stereotyped behaviors similar to those found in autism
- Unusual social behaviors and inability to appreciate the thoughts and feelings of other people
- Intense interest in specific topics (e.g., snakes or planets), some of them nonfunctional (e.g., train schedules)
- Interested in social contacts or making friends, but may get rebuffed because of awkward social behavior
- Attainment of independent living skills (unlike persons with autism)

Speech, Language, and Hearing
- Usually no significant delay in speech and language acquisition
- Generally good speech and language skills; some may even have superior language skills
- Verbal behavior, however, may be socially inappropriate or completely tactless (e.g., to a clinician's question, *What would you like to be doing*

when you are a grown-up man?, a child is reported to have replied, *I don't know, but you will be dead by then!*")

- The child may be eager to talk about his or her special interests, but it is unlikely to be a conversation; it will be more like a monologue
- The child fails to understand the listener's verbal and nonverbal cues; may not understand that the listener is bored or wants to say something
- Possibly, language may appear somewhat more impaired as the child attains adulthood because abstract and more complex language learning may be more impaired than the early language learning

Autism (Autistic Disorder). A pervasive developmental disorder or an autism spectrum disorder that in a majority of children persists into adulthood; the *Diagnostic and Statistical Manual* of the American Psychiatric Association calls it *autistic disorder*; within the spectrum disorder, autism is much more severe than Asperger's disorder; abnormal verbal as well nonverbal behaviors characterize autism; some children are only autistic-like in their behavior; often associated with intellectual disabilities because most children with autism have an IQ below 70; communication disorders are a significant characteristic; lack of interest in people and communication is a dominant characteristic.

Epidemiology and Ethnocultural Variables of Autism

- Prevalence figures vary, depending on whether only autism is being considered or the whole spectrum, especially if Asperger's disorder is also included
- Prevalence of pure cases of autism has been historically reported as 4 to 5 children per 10,000; this has been an underestimation; the American Psychiatric Association (1994) suggests 2 to 20 cases per 10,000, a wide and unreliable range; even as early as 1979, the prevalence of classic autism was reported to be 20 per 10,000 children; therefore, it is likely that the prevalence of autism has always been 20 or more per 10,000 children
- From the school year 1991–1992 to 1998–1999, there has been a 500% increase in the number of children with autism receiving special education services in the U.S. schools
- The most recent data available for 2002 are reported by the Center for Disease Control (CDC) in February 2007; monitoring autistic disorder, Asperger disorder, and pervasive development disorder not otherwise specified in 8-year-old children living in 14 states, CDC concluded that the prevalence of autism spectrum disorder varies between 33 per 10,000 (3.3/1,000) in Alabama to 106 per 10,000 (10.6/1,000) in New Jersey— still a wide range to be reconciled through further research; roughly 1 in 150 children has an autism spectrum disorder
- Data document an increased demand for services, not increased incidence of autism spectrum disorders; historically, prevalence of Asperger and other disorders in the spectrum was included in the estimates; increased awareness of the spectrum disorders, especially Asperger's disorder, broader diagnostic criteria that include all disorders in the spectrum, and

increased funding for services may all have contributed to increased demand for services; prevalence of Asperger's disorder alone is 36 per 10,000 children, higher than that of classic autism

- More males than females are affected; however, autism in females tends to be more severe than in males
- Variability of prevalence across different ethnocultural populations has not been well established; there is no evidence to suggest that certain groups are especially vulnerable or immune to autism

Characteristics of Autism

- Onset typically takes place during infancy and early childhood; when severe, early signs may be evident during infancy
- A significant lack of affectionate or emotional response to people noted during infancy and early childhood
- Lack of concern about feelings of other people; no interest in understanding what others think and feel
- Disinterest in mother's or primary caretaker's voice
- Tendency to seek extraordinary level of comfort when ill
- Failure to engage in age-appropriate play activities; lack of imaginative play; bizarre, stereotypical, or idiosyncratic play
- Lack of interest in friends and human contacts; an important diagnostic feature
- Stereotypical body movements (e.g., endless rocking, examining their own bizarre hand gestures)
- Preoccupation with objects or body parts; rejection of social contacts
- Insistence on the same living arrangements all the time; liking for constant structure and arrangement of living environment; changes may provoke temper tantrums
- Perseveration with one or a few activities; prolonged preoccupation with idiosyncratic activities
- Preference for being left alone; tendency to isolate themselves in the midst of people
- Fascination with mechanical noises (such as those made by toys) while being disinterested in surrounding human voice and speech
- Reluctance to be hugged, held, or touched; rejection of loving, affectionate contacts
- Self-injurious behaviors (e.g., constant poking into their eyes, biting their fingers, and hitting their head against hard surfaces)
- Exceptional talent in a restricted area; unusual mathematical or musical talent; good writing skills in the context of poor speaking skills; precocious reading skills (*hyperlexia*)

Associated Problems

- Abnormal brain electrical activity and seizure disorders in approximately 25% of children with autism
- Fragile X Syndrome (see under Syndromes Associated With Communication Disorders) in 2% to 5% of children with autism

- Higher prevalence of hearing loss than that in the general population
- Occurrence of tuberose sclerosis, a genetic disorder with benign brain tumors, epilepsy, intellectual disabilities, and skin lesions, in 1% to 4% of children with autism
- Hypo- or hypersensitivity to sensory stimuli; while some soft sounds may alarm them, other loud sounds may fail to evoke a response from them
- Motor deficits; some children may lack normal gait or have difficulty with fine coordination
- High prevalence of intellectual disabilities; many children with autism have IQs below 70

Etiology of Autism

- The earliest theory of autism, proposed by Kanner, was that it is due to impaired maternal bonding; this theory is now discredited
- Current research increasingly points to the influence of genetic factors; several genes (including those on chromosomes 7, 15, and 17) are considered candidates, although none have been fully confirmed
- Different genes in different families and multiple genes in most cases may be involved
- Neurological basis is suggested by some evidence of left cerebral injury documented in a few cases; abnormalities in the brainstem, frontal lobes, limbic system, and cerebellum have been reported although their significance is unclear
- Atypical head growth, especially a smaller-than-the normal head circumference (Macrocephaly), has been noted in children with autism
- Pseudoscientific theories abound; in recent years, autism was attributed to measles, mumps, and rubella (MMR) vaccination without strong evidence; the disorder also was attributed to the presence of heavy metals in the bloodstream; these theories, too, are now discredited; but new popular theories keep emerging
- No theory of causation has been fully accepted

Communication Disorders Associated With Autism

- A general lack of interest in people and social interactions is associated with a similar lack of interest in communication
- Limited response or no response to speech is an early characteristic of autism
- Delayed acquisition of speech sounds and articulation disorders
- Responses may be better to pure tones than to speech stimuli
- Lack of interest in asking questions or pointing to things they want
- Constant production of stereotypical and meaningless speech that may or may not have a communicative effects on others
- Relatively easier acquisition of object names than words that express human emotions or expressions
- Generally, faster learning of concrete words than abstract words; paradoxically, some children acquire abstract words (e.g., *triangle* or *square*) faster than concrete words (e.g., names of family members)

- Words may be used only in certain restricted contexts, suggesting lack of generalization
- Marked difficulty in understanding relational meanings (e.g., inability to relate the words *needle* and *thread*)
- A tendency to reverse the personal pronouns (e.g., referring to self as *you* and to others as I)
- Simpler, shorter, and more concrete sentences (unless a special verbal talent is evident)
- Pronounced difficulty with grammar; word order may be wrong and syntactic structures may lack variety
- Omission of grammatical morphemes (e.g., the present progressive, plural and past tense inflections, auxiliaries, copulas, prepositions, conjunctions)
- Socially inappropriate or irrelevant language
- A variety of pragmatic language problems including lack of eye contact, failure to maintain topic of conversation, and interrupting the speaker or not speaking when it is appropriate (lack of turn taking during conversation)
- Limited understanding of what others tell them
- Repetition of previously heard speech, apparently without much meaning (e.g., repetition of television commercials heard before)
- Voice disorders including a high-pitched voice, lack of intonations (monotonous speech), and inappropriate vocal intensity (whispering or shouting)
- Prosodic problems including abnormal patterns of inflection and a sing-song rhythm
- Echolalia; parrot-like repetition of what others say

Childhood Disintegrative Disorder (CDD). One of the autism spectrum disorders (or pervasive developmental disorders); also called *Heller's syndrome, dementia infantilis,* or *disintegrative psychosis*; occurs much less frequently than autism; more males than females are affected; a disorder of early childhood, but at least 2 years of normal development precedes its onset; significant regression in behavior of a child who was developing normally is the hallmark of this disorder; regression should be evident after age 2 and before age 10 to diagnose this disorder; the disorder is characterized by:

- Relatively abrupt or insidious loss of skills
- Loss of voluntary hand skills, often occurring between the age of 5 and 30 months
- Stereotyped hand movements (e.g., hand-wringing and hand washing)
- Loss of interest in social interactions
- Poor motor coordination, including impaired gait or trunk movements
- Severe speech and language impairment; severely affected production and comprehension
- Loss of bowel or bladder control
- Loss of play activities
- Stereotypical and restricted activities, interests, and movements
- Associated conditions include severe intellectual disabilities, seizure disorders, and rarely such other medical diseases as Schilder's disease

- Some improvement in skills may be noted as the child grows older, but nothing remarkable; progressive loss of skill if a neurological disorder is also present
- Once the total symptom complex is established, children with CDD are indistinguishable from those with autism; therefore, some question the validity of a separate diagnostic category

Rett Syndrome (Disorder). A progressive neurodevelopmental disorder considered a part of autism spectrum disorder or pervasive developmental disorder; also known as the *Rett disorder*; almost exclusively affects females; incidence of Rett syndrome is 1 in 10,000 births; it is a common cause of profound intellectual disabilities in girls; development is typically normal until the age of 6 to 18 months; affected children begin to show speech impairment and inability to purposefully use their hands; other symptoms soon follow.

Etiology

- A gene abnormality on the long arm of chromosome X (Xq28); found in most but not all with the syndrome
- Although rare, boys may have Rett syndrome

Physical and Behavioral Symptoms

- Autistic-like behaviors in the early stage of the disorder, which tend to diminish over time; physical symptoms become more prominent
- Decelerated head growth, resulting in microcephaly
- Neuromotor disturbances including reduced muscle tone, gait disturbances, ataxia, spasticity, seizure disorders, tremors, and dystonia
- Wringing hand movements, clapping, and mouthing are characteristic stereotypic behaviors
- Arrested progress in language learning
- Impaired comprehension of spoken language
- Autistic-like behavior
- Breathing abnormalities such as hyperventilation and apnea

Speech, Language, and Hearing

- Lack of interest in social interactions (similar to autism)
- Regression of the limited language skills, acquired until the onset of the disorder
- Cognitive impairments and intellectual disabilities

American Psychiatric Association (1994). *Diagnostic and statistical manual of mental disorders* (*DSM-IV*, 4th ed. revised). Washington, DC: Author.

Center for Disease Control (February 9, 2007). Prevalence of autism spectrum disorders—autism and developmental disabilities monitoring network, 15 sites, United States 2002. *Morbidity and Mortality Weekly Report, 56*(SS01), 12–28; http://www.cdc.gov/mmwr_wk.htm

Hegde, M. N., & Maul, C. A. (2006). *Language disorders in children: An evidence-based approach to assessment and treatment.* Boston, MA: Allyn and Bacon.

Muhle, R., Trentacoste, S. V., & Rapin, I. (2004). The genetics of autism. *Pediatrics, 113*, 472–486.

Soko, D. K., & Edwards-Brown, M. (2004). Neuroimaging in autistic spectrum disorders (ASD). *Journal of Neuroimaging, 14*, 8–15.

Wing, L., & Potter, D. (2004). Notes on the prevalence of autism spectrum disorders. National Autistic Society. Retrieved on July 27, 2006 from http://www.nas.org.uk.

Automated Speech.   Overly learned verbal behavior, including the recitation of the days of the week, months, and seasons of the year; counting, recitation of the alphabet, and so forth; generally better preserved than more spontaneous speech in most adult disorders of communication (e.g., aphasia).

Autosomal Dominant.   Any chromosome apart from the sex chromosome is *autosomal*; autosomal chromosomes (1 through 22) are not sex-linked; autosomes are alike in males and females; the term *dominant* implies that the defective gene dominates its normal partner in its phenotypic expression; the probability (not certainty) that the defective gene may express is 50% for each pregnancy, regardless of the sex of the offspring.

Autosomal Recessive.   A genetic trait or defect not capable of expression unless coupled with a similar trait or defect by both members of a pair of homologous chromosomes; individuals carrying an autosomal recessive defect may not be affected by it; the defect may be transmitted with a 25% probability only if both the parents carry the mutant (defective) gene; there is a 50% chance that the children will be carriers of the defective gene.

B

Bardet-Biedl Syndrome. The same as Laurence-Moon Syndrome (see Syndromes Associated With Communication Disorders).

Basal Ganglia. Subcortical structures that include the caudate nucleus, putamen, and globus pallidus; part of the extrapyramidal system that controls tone and posture related to movement; injury is associated with Dysarthria (motor speech disorders).

Bifid Uvula. A split uvula that suggests an underlying submucous cleft covered by tissue.

Bilateral. Both sides of a paired structure; as in *bilateral hearing loss* (loss in both ears) or *bilateral brain injury* (injury to both the hemispheres of the brain).

Binswanger Disease. A neurodegenerative disorder associated with atrophy of the subcortical white matter that produces a variety of Vascular Dementia; see also Dementia.

Bolus. A portion of food placed in the mouth as well as a mass of masticated food; result of the activities of the oral preparatory phase of swallow; bolus preparation of solid and semisolid food is essential for normal swallowing; bolus formation may be impaired in swallowing disorders; see Dysphagia.

Botulinum Toxin. A biologic toxin that paralyzes muscles; used as a medical treatment in some cases (as in spasmodic dysphonia to paralyze a vocal fold that is hyperadducting or hyperabducting) and as a cosmetic procedure (e.g., to reduce facial wrinkles).

Bound Morphemes. Grammatical morphemes that cannot convey meaning by themselves; typically inflected (added) with other morphemes (usually free morphemes) to change meaning; such inflections as the present progressive *ing*, regular plural, and regular past are examples of bound morphemes; see Grammatical Morphemes of Language.

Brachman-de Lange Syndrome. The same as Cornelia de Lange Syndrome (see under Syndromes Associated With Communication Disorders).

Brachycephaly. Shortness of the head with a cephalic index of 81.0 to 85.4; characteristic of certain genetic syndromes.

Brachydactyly. Shortness of the fingers and toes; characteristic of certain genetic syndromes.

Bradykinesia. A movement disorder associated with neuromuscular impairments and characterized by slowness of movements; difficulty in stopping movement once initiated (perseveration); freezing of movement.

Brain Tumors. Also known as intracranial neoplasms, brain tumors are pathological growths within the cranial structures; space-occupying lesions that cause swelling in the surrounding tissue and lead to increased intracranial pressure; brain tumors are one of the causes of aphasia, although they produce an array of neurobehavioral symptoms that may overshadow aphasic symptoms; depending on how aggressively they grow, brain tumors are classified as Grade I, II, III, or IV; there are several kinds of brain tumors:

- Primary intracranial tumors: Originate in the brain; more common in the age group of 25–50 years than in other age groups; loss of a tumor suppressing gene, expression of a cancerous gene, or a combination of the two are the suspected causes; include gliomas, which affect the glia cells in the brain; astrocytomas, that affect the astrocytes, and oligodendrogliomas that arise from oligodendrocytes; glioblastoma multiforme, a form of glioma, is an especially malignant form of brain tumors associated with a high death rate
- Meningiomas: Another variety of intracranial tumors that grow within the meninges that cover the brain; these slow-growing tumors cause focal symptoms, and are often effectively surgically removed; also known as extra-cerebral tumors because they grow outside the brain (within the meninges)
- Secondary (metastatic) intracranial tumors: Have their origin elsewhere but have migrated into the brain and begin to grow there; *metastasis* is the migration or spreading of cancerous cells; cancer of the breast, lungs, pharynx, or larynx tend to metastasize into the cranial space; associated with a high mortality rate

Broca's Aphasia.   A type of nonfluent aphasia, characterized by telegraphic, agrammatic, dysfluent, effortful speech; a result of brain injury caused most often by strokes that damage Broca's area; see Aphasia.

Broca's Area.   The left, posterior, and lower portion of the frontal lobe on the inferior frontal gyrus at the juncture of the lateral and central fissures; a site of lesion that is controversially associated with Broca's aphasia; see Aphasia and Aphasia: Specific Types.

Broken Word.   A type of dysfluency characterized by a silent pause within a word; also called intralexical pause; see Stuttering under Fluency Disorders.

Buccofacial Apraxia.   Difficulty in performing buccofacial movements when requested; movements may be executed spontaneously; thought to be a motor planning and programming disorder; may be associated with Apraxia of Speech; see also Apraxia.

Bulbar Palsy.   A neurological disease of the lower motor neurons, cranial nerves, and neuromuscular junctions that create such problems as dysphagia, dysphonia, and dysarthria; multiple cranial nerve involvement that affects the jaw, face, lips, tongue, palate, pharynx, and larynx.

C

C

Canthi. Plural of *canthus*, *canthi* are the angles at which the lower and upper eyelids meet; may be nasal (inner) canthus or temporal (outer) canthus; wider canthi are a part of several genetic syndromes; (e.g., see Waardenburg Syndrome under Syndromes Associated With Communication Disorders).

Case History. A description of the origin, development, and progression of a disorder or disease, including the family, health, social, educational, occupational factors that affect it; includes a description of prior assessment and treatment and the effects of prior treatment; helps understand the disorder or disease; an initial step in assessment; see the companion volume, *Hegde's PocketGuide to Assessment in Speech-Language Pathology* (3rd ed.), for details.

Catatonic Motor Behavior. A symptom of schizophrenia, characterized by reduced reactivity to environmental stimuli, catatonic stupor (the person is totally unaware of the surroundings), rigid or bizarre posture, and resistance to movement; may also be found in other disorders including medication-induced movement disorder.

Central Aphasia. The same as Wernicke's Aphasia (see Aphasia: Specific Types).

Central Nervous System. The brain and the spinal cord; both are encased in bone.

Cerebellar Mutism. A form of transient speechlessness due to neurological involvement; affects mostly children who have had posterior fossa tumors surgically removed; when regained, speech is dysarthric, perhaps of the ataxic variety because of extensive cerebellar damage secondary to surgery; see also Mutism and Psychiatric Problems Associated With Communicative Disorders.

Cerebellum. Hindbrain; regulates motor movements; damage to cerebellum can cause such neurological impairments as ataxia and is associated with ataxic Dysarthria.

Cerebral Hemorrhage. Bleeding within the brain because of ruptured blood vessels; an immediate cause of aphasia (of the hemorrhagic type); due to various factors including weakened arterial walls (aneurysm), high and fluctuating blood pressure, and trauma to blood vessels; see Aphasia.

Cerebral Palsy (CP). A nonprogressive neuromotor disorder resulting from brain damage before, during, or shortly after birth; often described as a congenital disorder (noticed at birth), although the damage may occur sometime after birth; generally, damage to still-developing brain (up to age 16 years) resulting in neuromotor control problems that tend to improve with growth; multiple factors are associated with cerebral palsy; speech disorders, classified as Dysarthria or Developmental Dysarthria, are found in many, but not all children with CP; the symptom complex is highly varied; neuromuscular disorders are the hallmark of CP, but in addition, the disorder is associated with speech and language problems; impairments in respiration, laryngeal function, and general neuromotor control; intellectual disabilities in about 50% of children; a higher prevalence of hearing impairment than in the non-CP population; often associated with feeding problems; a common handicapping condition of early childhood.

C

Epidemiology and Ethnocultural Variables
- Incidence figures for CP vary across studies; early studies suggested an incidence of 6 in 1,000 live births
- More recent estimates suggest an incidence of 2 or 3 in 1,000 children
- Incidence of CP may have declined in recent years because of better prenatal and natal care
- No specific information is available on ethnocultural variables as they relate to the incidence and prevalence of CP
- Most children with CP grow into adulthood because the disease is static

Classification of Cerebral Palsy
- Some classifications are based on affected limbs (orthopedic-topographic classification); other classifications are based on affected neurological systems.
- Orthopedic-topographic classification is based on the limbs that are affected by the disorder; includes:
  - Diplegia: Bilateral paralysis or weakness (paresis) of like parts; both hands and both legs may be involved; generally the legs are more severely affected than the hands; spasticity is the most common neurological symptom; children have difficulty sitting, walking, and running; skilled hand movements may be normal
  - Monoplegia: Paralysis of one extremity, somewhat rare
  - Hemiplegia: Paralysis of one side of the body (arms and legs on either the left or right side); but arms are affected to a greater extent than the legs; damage to the extrapyramidal system causes hemiplegia
  - Paraplegia: Paralysis of the two lower extremities (legs); upper extremities are almost always normal, although the lower trunk may be involved to some extent; pyramidal tracts are affected; spasticity is common
  - Triplegia: Paralysis of three extremities, although one or more may be more severely affected; both legs and one arm may be affected
  - Quadriplegia: Paralysis of four extremities, although may be more severe in the upper extremities; may be paresis in four extremities; spasticity and weakness are the neurological symptoms; due to bilateral damage to the pyramidal and extrapyramidal tracts (bilateral cortical damage to the motor systems); the two sides of the body may not be equally affected; one side may function better than the other
- Classification based on the affected neurological system
  - Spastic cerebral palsy: Most common type of CP with increased tone and rigidity of muscles; may affect 50% to 70% of children with CP; pyramidal lesions with spasticity is the typical cause; spastic paraplegia, diplegia, or quadriplegia
  - Athetoid cerebral palsy: Damage to the extrapyramidal motor control system (particularly the basal ganglia) causes athetosis (slow, involuntary, worm-like movements), tremor, or both; disorders of posture and involuntary movements are the main neurological symptoms
  - Ataxic and dystonic cerebral palsy: Cerebellar lesions cause ataxia; pure ataxic type found in only about 5% of children with CP; ataxic-dystonic type may be found in about 10% of children with CP

C

o Mixed type of cerebral palsy: Lesions in both the pyramidal and extrapyramidal regions cause the mixed variety of CP; lesion in one of the structures may be dominant, however; this type occurs in almost 30% of cases; either the spastic symptoms or the athetotic symptoms may be dominant; the brain injury is usually extensive and the children tend to have additional serious problems (e.g., significant intellectual disabilities)

Etiologic Factors of Cerebral Palsy

- It is difficult to pinpoint the precise cause of CP in many children, although the neurological systems affected can be clearly delineated
- Direct and indirect motor system lesions are the primary and immediate causes of CP and the resulting associated problems, including communication disorders
- Preventable causes of brain injury that result in CP fall into three main categories: prenatal, perinatal, and postnatal.
- Some early signs of CP may be observed at, or some time after, birth; factors that may negatively affect the growth of the fetus include:
  o Maternal radiation exposure, especially repetitive and high dose
  o Intrauterine infections that damage the fetus (e.g., maternal HIV infection)
  o Fetal exposure to toxic drugs due to maternal drug abuse, including alcoholism
  o Maternal exposure to metal toxicity (e.g., mercury fumes)
  o Fetal anoxia (oxygen deprivation and resulting fetal brain damage); various factors, including maternal anemia, may cause fetal anoxia
  o Damage caused by blood infiltration of the nervous system
  o Genetic factors including chromosomal abnormalities
  o Abruptio placenta (premature detachment of the fetus)
  o Brain growth deficiency due to various reasons
- Perinatal factors (factors associated with birth) include:
  o Birth complications, including trauma to brain during birth (only in a small percentage of cases)
  o Cerebral hemorrhage due to trauma to the head during birth
- Postnatal factors (factors associated with an infant's physical development) include:
  o Prematurity and low birth weight are known risk factors; these, however, may reflect the influence of prenatal factors that cause brain injury in most cases
  o Asphyxia, which is lack of sufficient oxygen in respired air, causing brain damage
  o Sepsis (blood toxicity and microorganisms in the blood) in the newborn can seriously damage the brain and limit its growth
  o Cerebral hemorrhage, often due to vascular diseases, is a serious cause of brain injury in children as well as adults
  o Ischemia, also due to vascular diseases, causing reduced blood flow through the blood vessels in the brain; frequently associated with prematurity
  o Encephalitis and meningitis that cause swelling and brain damage
  o Traumatic brain injury, secondary to accidental falls, physical abuse, violence, vehicular accidents, shaken baby syndrome

Symptoms and Effects of Cerebral Palsy

- CP is a term for a multitude of symptoms; it is not the name of a disease; the symptoms may be grouped in various ways, including the one used here.
- Neuromotor symptoms
  - Persistence of primitive reflexes; these reflexes include *asymmetric tonic neck reflex* (also known as fenser's response), in which a head turn is accompanied by an extension of the arm and leg, parallel to the chin; *tonic labyrinthine reflex*, in which the shoulders retract and the legs extend when the head tilts back; *positive support reflex*, in which the legs straighten to support the weight of the body when someone bounces the baby; the sucking reflex (elicited by stroking an infant's cheek) and the Moro reflex (startle reflex) also may persist
  - Spasticity (increased tone) and rigidity of muscles; these are among the more persistent, common, and disabling neuromuscular symptoms of CP; the muscles are tight or excessively contracted with an exaggerated stretch reflex; caused by injury to the pyramidal motor pathways and the higher cortical motor control centers
  - Athetosis, characterized by slow, involuntary, writhing movements associated with injury to the extrapyramidal motor pathways, especially to the basal ganglia; currently, the term *dyskinesia*, rather than athetosis, is the preferred term
  - Ataxia, which is disturbed balance and uncoordinated movement; injury to the cerebellum, which modulates movement, is the main cause; may be an infrequently used diagnostic category
  - Tremors, which are similar to trembling and shaking, are involuntary, repetitive, rapid, and rhythmic movements; classified as *intentional* when they appear at the onset of volitional acts or *nonintentional* when they occur at rest and stop at the onset of volitional acts; only occasionally found in children and adults with cerebral palsy
  - Dysphagia (swallowing problems), early feeding difficulties, and drooling may be associated with cerebral palsy
- Motor development
  - Retarded neuromuscular development is the main and early characteristic
  - Motor skills improve as the child gets older, but the following kinds of motor development problems may be evident:
    - Ten to 24 months of delay in motor development
    - Permanent motor control problems associated with severe neurological damage
    - Delayed attainment of all motor milestones, including head control, sitting, crawling, standing, walking, and achieving hand movement control for skill acquisition
    - Slowness in initiating movement (a pervasive characteristic)
    - Motor development most seriously affected in quadriplegia and least seriously affected in hemiplegia
- Intellectual development
  - Because of brain injury, CP may be associated with intellectual disabilities in some, but not all, children

- o Combination of neuromuscular problems and limited intellectual skills may create more serious speech problems (dysarthria), and may increase the chances of language problems; generally:
  - Intelligence is below normal in 30% to 70% of children with CP
  - Intelligence may be normal or even above normal in the remaining cases
- Sensory impairments
  - o Frequent auditory and visual problems
  - o A combination of hearing impairment and neuromuscular problems cause serious speech and language difficulties; kinds of hearing loss associated with specific types of CP include:
    - Generally, hearing impairment is more common in children with CP than in children without it
    - Conductive hearing loss is frequently associated with CP; mostly due to the recurring middle ear infections
    - Spasticity may be more often associated with conductive hearing loss than with other types of loss
    - Athetosis may be associated with a greater degree of hearing loss and bilateral loss
    - Visual impairments are frequently associated with CP
- Perceptual and attentional problems
  - o Along with neuromotor impairments and intellectual disabilities, perceptual and attentional problems contribute to the child's academic learning disorders; the latter kinds of problems include:
    - Distractibility and short attention span
    - A preference for a rigid schedule (perceptual rigidity)
    - Disassociation—difficulty in integrating different aspects of the same event or experience
    - Disinhibition or random activity
- Emotional disturbances
  - o Emotional disturbances, which include:
    - Emotional lability (emotional instability or overreactivity) is found in a majority of adolescents and adults
    - Frequent episodes of emotional upsets may add to the emotional disorders in many cases
  - o Difficulty finding and sustaining employment, possibly due to emotional problems combined with below normal intellectual skills
- Educational problems
  - o Learning disorders, including:
    - Reading, writing, and arithmetic problems
    - Literacy problems complicated by neuromotor, intellectual, behavioral, and sensory deficits
  - o Behavioral problems, intellectual deficits, speech and language problems, and sensory limitations (e.g., hearing and visual impairments) may further limit the child's learning potential
- Communication problems: General considerations
  - o Communication disorders associated with CP are called <u>Dysarthria</u> (versus articulation and phonological disorders found in children without significant

neuromuscular impairments); dysarthria involves not only articulation of speech sounds, but also voice, resonance, and prosody
- o Dysarthria in CP may vary from nonexistent to severe; a few children and adults may have normal or even superior communication skills
- o Significant and persistent communication problems, especially speech production problems
- o The degree of neuromotor impairment, sensory limitations, intellectual deficits, and environmental factors (e.g., efficacy of rehabilitation and parental involvement) will affect the degree of communication impairment
- o Measures of speech intelligibility may be one of the indicators of communication deficits associated with CP
- Speech disorders (dysarthria)
  - o Spastic, athetoid, and ataxic types of cerebral palsy may show some unique features, but many types of speech disorders are common to the different types; speech disorders are common in children with spastic diplegia and quadriplegia
  - o Generally, the following kinds of speech disorders are associated with cerebral palsy:
    - Delayed but normal (typical) pattern of speech development
    - Greater difficulty on more complex sounds or complex phonetic sequences
    - Jerky, effortful, labored, and irregular speech production causing reduced intelligibility
    - No unique pattern of speech errors associated with different types of CP
    - More accurate production of labial sounds than dental and glottal sounds; nasals the least difficult and fricatives and glides the most difficult; voiceless sounds more difficult than voiced cognates
    - Muscle weakness, articulatory instability, and errors in attaining articulatory targets are common in the spastic variety of CP
    - Slightly more severe articulation disorders associated with athetosis than the spastic variety of CP; athetosis is associated with a large range of jaw movements during articulation, inappropriate tongue placement due to reduced range of movement, and prolonged transition time between articulatory movements
    - Irregular articulatory breakdowns, prolonged sound productions, and silent intervals during speech production are often associated with athetosis
    - More severe speech problems associated with hemiplegia and quadriplegia than with paraplegia
    - Difficulty phonating or prolonging speech sounds
    - Significant difficulty with tongue-tip sounds
    - Predominance of speech sound omissions over substitutions or distortions
    - Greater difficulty with sounds in word final positions than in other positions
    - Such Phonological Processes as consonant cluster deletion, stopping, depalatalization, fronting, and gliding
    - Slower diadachokinetic rates

- Language disorders
  - Whether a child with CP will have language disorders or not depends on the coexisting clinical conditions:
    - Children with CP may develop language normally unless they have other complicating clinical conditions
    - Language disorders in CP are associated with such coexisting conditions as hearing impairment and intellectual deficits
- Fluency problems
  - Limited fluency, mainly due to brain injury and intellectual disabilities
  - Fluency problems include:
    - A high prevalence of stuttering
    - Jerky and arrhythmic flow of speech because of extrapyramidal motor track lesions and spasticity
- Voice problems
  - Dysarthria is associated with phonatory and voice disorders
  - Common laryngeal muscle involvement may cause:
    - Weak voice, lacking in normal levels of loudness
    - Poor control of vocal loudness, resulting in irregular bursts in loudness
    - Loss of voice toward the end of sentences and phrases, resulting in whispers
    - Limited loudness and pitch variations, causing monotonous speech (voice)
    - High-pitched voice and frequent pitch breaks
    - Strained voice quality due to hyperadduction of vocal folds
    - Breathy voice due to hypoadduction of vocal folds
    - Delayed voice onset and harsh voice
    - Persistent aphonia in a few children
- Prosodic problems
  - Dysarthria in adults and children is associated with significant prosodic problems (dysprosody)
  - Dysprosody, a combination of the children's respiratory, articulatory, fluency, and voice problems is characterized by:
    - Generally arrhythmic speech with a monotone, lacking in forward flow, and devoid of variations in intonation
    - Speech rate variations, also contributing to dysprosody
    - Short phrases (possibly because of respiratory abnormalities), frequent silent pauses, and voice stoppages that also affect normal prosody
    - Abnormal linguistic stress patterns (often equal stress on all syllables)
- Respiratory problems
  - Dysarthria associated with CP includes respiratory problems that affect speech production
  - Slightly better respiratory control associated with spasticity than with athetosis; however, the two groups have:
    - Persistence of a rapid breathing rate beyond the first year of infancy (versus the normal slowdown of the rate during the second year)
    - Reduced respiratory reserve and vital capacity, although these problems by themselves may not cause impaired speech production; combination of respiratory, laryngeal, velopharyngeal, and articulatory abnormalities

- Excessive diaphragmatic activity and reduced activity of the chest and neck muscles during breathing (*belly-breathing*); also found in normal infants, may persist in CP
- Flattening or flaring of the rib cage and indented (sucked-in) sternum (*paradoxical breathing* or *reverse breathing*)
- Air wastage during speech production, causing short phrases or weak productions of final segments of sentences
- Resonance problems
  - Similar to dysarthria in adults, CP tends to be associated with several resonance problems:
    - Velopharyngeal function abnormalities that cause resonance disorders
    - Hypernasality due to inadequate velopharyngeal closure during the production of nonnasal speech sounds
    - Nasal emission
- Swallowing problems
  - Similar to dysarthria in adults, CP is associated with swallowing difficulties:
    - Early feeding problems in as many as 60% of children with CP, necessitating nonoral feeding
    - Problems related to sucking and swallowing during the child's first year
    - Increased risk of nutritional deficiencies and failure to gain weight
    - Swallowing disorders in all stages of swallow; premature leaking of food or liquid into the pharynx in the oral phase of swallow; delayed bolus preparation and organization; delayed pharyngeal phase of swallow; gastroesophageal reflux in the esophageal stage of swallow
    - Silent aspiration (airway aspiration of food or liquid without cough)
    - Difficulty coordinating breathing and swallowing while eating or drinking
    - Drooling during eating or breathing, caused by poor oral motor control, incomplete lip closure during swallow, low suction pressure, and delay in initiating the next stage of swallow

Hardy, J. C. (1983). *Cerebral palsy.* Englewood Cliffs, NJ: Prentice Hall.

Love, R. J. (2000). *Childhood motor speech disability* (2nd ed.). Boston, MA: Allyn and Bacon.

Mecham, M. J. (1996). *Cerebral palsy* (2nd ed.). Austin, TX: Pro-Ed.

Yorkston, K. M., Beukelman, D. R., & Bell, K. R. (1999). *Management of motor speech disorders in children and adults* (2nd ed.). Austin, TX: Pro-Ed.

Cerebrovascular Accidents (Strokes). The most common cause of aphasia; popularly known as "brain attacks"; the third leading cause of death in the United States; may be ischemic or hemorrhagic; ischemic strokes caused by interruption of blood supply to a part of the brain because of arterial thrombosis or embolism; hemorrhagic strokes are due to bleeding in the brain; see also Cerebral Hemorrhage, Stokes, and Aphasia.

Childhood Apraxia of Speech (CAS). A speech disorder in children characterized by problems in positioning and sequentially moving muscles for the volitional production of speech; also known as *developmental apraxia of* *speech* and *developmental verbal dyspraxia*; CAS is associated with articulation and prosodic problems; it is not caused by muscle weakness or neuromuscular slowness; CAS is described as a disorder of motor planning and programming for speech, although competing explanations abound; whether children with CAS have a unique pattern of speech disorders and whether their speech disorders systematically differ from other children who have phonological disorders have not been firmly established; CAS continues to be a controversial diagnostic category, because unlike Apraxia of Speech (AOS) in Adults, there is no demonstrated neuropathology in CAS; experts continue to present data to justify the existence of the disorder; some believe that language disorders, especially problems in syntax, are a part of the syndrome and should be called *developmental verbal apraxia*; others believe that it is strictly a disorder of motor speech control, although independent language and other problems may coexist with it; historically known as *developmental motor aphasia, executive aphasia, articulatory apraxia,* and *phonologic programming deficit syndrome*; some correctly believe that CAS does not necessarily suggest a specific neuropathology, but only describes specific speech motor control problems in children.

Epidemiology and Ethnocultural Variables

* The incidence, prevalence, and ethnocultural variables associated with CAS have not been fully studied
* Estimates of the prevalence of CAS vary and range between less than 1% to 1.3% of the population; compared to straightforward phonological disorders in 5% of school-age children, the incidence of CAS is lower
* Noticed in the early speech developmental period, although a specific age of onset is unclear
* Some children might improve without professional help
* More boys than girls are diagnosed with CAS, suggesting a possible genetic basis; suspected to be X-linked or X-influenced; although fewer girls may have CAS, their problems may be severe
* Familial aggregation of CAS; 80% or more children may have another affected member in the family; 55% to 60% of children may have an affected parent, more often the mother
* Lack of agreement on the symptom complex of CAS makes it difficult to find its genetic markers

Issues Related to CAS as a Diagnostic Category

* It is not clear whether CAS can be reliably distinguished from other phonological disorders or speech delays
* Except for inappropriate linguistic stress, CAS may be similar to other speech disorders
* CAS associated with inappropriate stress patterns may be a subtype, although there is no general agreement on this; one might as well argue that linguistic stress abnormalities are found in some children with phonological disorders (with no implication of CAS); in this interpretation, children with linguistic stress abnormalities form a subtype of phonological disorders, not CAS

- Almost all studies on CAS are open to criticism because it is not clear who were and who should be selected as participants for studying its characteristics; participant selection biases may be a problem with most studies
- CAS is a heterogeneous disorder; the older hypothesis that CAS is found only in children who are otherwise normal may be due to participant selection biases; CAS may be found in children with several associated disabilities including sensorineural hearing loss, intellectual disabilities, ataxic cerebral palsy and generalized hypotonia, developmental delay, and attention deficit disorders
- CAS is not necessarily the most severe form of articulation disorder; the severity may range from mild to severe, like any other disorder
- Although CAS is often classified as a motor programming disorder similar to apraxia of speech in adults, neuropathological factors found in adults with apraxia of speech are absent in CAS
- To make a valid diagnosis of CAS, the clinician may need to document not only a speech disorder, but also a nonverbal oral apraxia
- Many clinicians who typically diagnose CAS do not use a consistent set of diagnostic criteria; what follows is a summary of symptoms described in multiple sources, often with contradictory claims

Speech Disorders Associated with CAS

- Moderate to severe speech intelligibility problems
- Most frequent errors on consonant clusters followed by fricatives, affricates, stops, and nasals; persistence of errors on fricatives and affricates
- Articulatory groping and silent articulatory postures
- Inconsistent and variable articulatory errors; different patterns of errors on the repeated productions of the same word
- Atypical errors of articulation not found in children with functional articulation disorders; include unusual phonemic sequencing errors of the following kinds:
  - Metathetic errors (transposition or reversal of phoneme sequences; e.g., *maks* for *masks* or *soun* for *snow*)
  - Addition of phonemes (e.g., *applesaks* for *applesauce* or *clat* for *cat*)
  - Prolongation of speech sounds
  - Repetition of sounds and syllables, even the final sounds or syllables in words
  - Nonphonemic productions that cannot be transcribed
- Typical errors of articulation found in other children with phonological disorders; include the following kinds of common error types:
  - More frequent occurrence of omissions and substitutions
  - More prevalent distortions in some older children
  - Varied simplification of consonant blends (e.g., omission of one sound, substitution for another sound, correct production of one element, substitution of one sound for the entire cluster)
  - Voicing and devoicing errors
  - Vowel and diphthong errors (distorted vowels and diphthong reduction)

C

- Delayed speech development; speech production skills may lag behind
  - Language comprehension skills
  - Cognitive skills
- Resonance problems, including:
  - Hypernasality, hyponasality, or nasal emission
  - Variability in the presence of resonance
  - Possibly, poor velopharyngeal control which may explain the resonance problems
- Prosodic problems, including:
  - Abnormal prosody
  - Aprosodic speech (flat prosody)
  - Dysprosodic speech (presence of variation in frequency and duration, but inappropriate expression of them)
  - Inappropriate stress patterns
- Fluency problems also may be associated with CAS and include:
  - Increased frequency of dysfluencies, although information on specific types and their frequencies are unavailable

Associated Problems
- CAS may be associated with certain additional problems, including:
  - Delayed language development, in conjunction with delayed speech development
  - Hearing impairment
  - Intellectual disabilities
  - Neuromuscular disorders (e.g., cerebral palsy)
  - Gross and fine visual and motor skill deficits (e.g., problems of coordination in handwriting and typing)
  - Learning disabilities (academic difficulties)

Etiologic Factors and Neuropathology
- Etiologic factors are mostly presumed because of the absence of demonstrated neuropathology; by definition, CAS is a motor planning and programming disorder, but this disorder is not documented, but inferred from speech errors
- Although no gene abnormality or mechanism of inheritance has been demonstrated, the following observations suggest potential genetic influences:
  - A higher familial incidence of CAS
  - A greater prevalence among boys than girls
  - Association of CAS with certain syndromes, including Down syndrome and Fragile X syndrome (see Syndromes Associated With Communication Disorders) that have a genetic basis
  - Association of CAS with inborn errors of metabolism, also with a genetic basis
- No significant and consistent evidence of brain lesions in children diagnosed with CAS
- General clumsiness and lack of coordination is interpreted to support a neurological basis for CAS
- Oral apraxia, suggestive of a more general, nonverbal, oral motor control problem may or may not be associated with CAS

Theories of Childhood Apraxia of Speech

- The standard theory of apraxia of speech, regardless of whether it occurs in children or adults, is that it is a central motor planning and programming disorder; see Apraxia of Speech in Adults for the standard explanation; it is not clear whether the standard theory advanced to explain apraxia of speech in adults also applies to children; the implication is that it does, although there are competing theories of AOS in children; that the standard theory is speculative makes it equally suspect when applied to children with AOS

- An explanation that opposes a motor planning and programming theory of AOS is that it is a phonological disorder; a poor phonological representation may be the essence of the disorder; some evidence suggests that CAS is a part of a larger complex of symptoms which includes impaired language skills (e.g., lexical and syntactic impairments), impaired nonverbal or verbal oral movements, and lower verbal intelligence

- No theory or explanation of CAS is currently complete, generally accepted, or supported by convincing evidence; almost all evidence cited for theories are the disorders themselves; therefore, most theories are circular because the theories point out the disorder to support the explanation of the disorder

Forrest, K. (2003). Diagnostic criteria of developmental apraxia of speech used by clinical speech-language pathologists. *American Journal of Speech-Language Pathology, 12,* 376–380.

Hall, P. K., Jordan, L. S., & Robin, D. A. (1993). *Developmental apraxia of speech: Theory and clinical practice.* Austin, TX: Pro-Ed.

Hayden, D. A. (1994). Differential diagnosis of motor speech dysfunction in children. *Clinics in Communication Disorders, 4*(2), 119–141.

Hodge, M. M. (1994). Assessment of children with developmental apraxia of speech: A rationale. *Clinics in Communication Disorders, 4*(2), 91–101.

Hodge, M. M., & Hancock, H. R. (1994). Assessment of children with developmental apraxia of speech: A procedure. *Clinics in Communication Disorders, 4*(2), 102–118.

Lewis, B. A., Freebairn, L. A., Hansen, A. J., Iyengar, S. K., & Taylor, H. G. (2004). School-age follow-up of children with childhood apraxia of speech. *Language, Speech, and Hearing Services in Schools, 35,* 122–140.

Lewis, B. A., Freebairn, L. A., Hansen, A. J., Taylor, H. G., Iyengar, S. K., & Shriberg, L. D. (2004). Family pedigrees of children with suspected childhood apraxia of speech. *Journal of Communication Disorders, 37*(2), 157–175.

Love, R. J. (2000). *Childhood motor speech disability* (2nd ed.). Boston, MA: Allyn and Bacon.

Panagos, J. M., & Bobkoff, K. (1984). Beliefs about developmental apraxia of speech. *Australian Journal of Human Communication Disorders, 12*(2), 39–52.

Peña-Brooks, A., & Hegde, M. N. (2007). *Assessment and treatment of articulation and phonological disorders in children* (2nd ed.). Austin, TX: Pro-Ed.

C

Shriberg, L. D., Aram, D. M., & Kwiatkowski, J. (1997). Developmental apraxia of speech: I. Descriptive and theoretical perspectives. *Journal of Speech and Hearing Research, 40,* 273–286.

Waldron, C. M. (1998). Comments regarding the investigation of developmental apraxia of speech: Response to Shriberg, Aram, and Kwiatkowski. *Journal of Speech and Hearing Research, 41,* 958–960.

Childhood Disintegrative Disorders. A pervasive developmental disorder or one of the autism spectrum disorders; see under Autism Spectrum Disorders.

Cholinergic Neurons. Neurons that produce acetylcholine (Ach); a neurotransmitter that is negatively affected in neurodegenerative diseases; associated with various forms of Dementia.

Chorea. A movement disorder characterized by random and involuntary movements of the limbs, trunk, head, and neck; the movements are unpredictable and meaningless, and sometimes jerky; may involve gross movements of the body parts; individuals with mild cases may disguise these involuntary movements as purposeful; movements progress into serious and constant features, affecting walking, swallowing, speaking, and other finely coordinated movements and skills; caused by damage to the caudate and the putamen; may be due to neurodegenerative diseases (e.g., Huntington's Disease or infections and Sydenham's Chorea).

Choreiform Movements. A neurological movement disorder; jerky, irregular, involuntary, and rapid movements characterize chorea; observed during rest; associated with such degenerative neurological diseases as Huntington's Disease and infectious diseases as Sydenham's Chorea; also may be due to drug interactions, brain tumors, and vascular diseases; affects speech production (e.g., Hyperkinetic Dysarthria).

Cleft Lip. An opening in the lip, usually the upper lip and very rarely the lower lip; a congenital malformation associated with several syndromes; may be unilateral or bilateral; often associated with cleft of the palate; cleft lip may be associated with minor deviations in the alveolar ridge; etiologically, cleft lip and cleft palate are different entities because the embryonic disruptions that cause them occur at different stages of development; familial incidence may be predominantly of cleft palate, cleft lip, or a combination; the prevalence of cleft lip with or without cleft palate is anywhere between 1 in 250 births and 1 in 1,000 births; variations are due to different prevalence rates in varied ethnocultural groups.

Cleft Palate. Opening in the hard palate, the soft palate, or both due to various congenital malformations; clefts of the lip may be present in 50% of the cases; clefts are due to disruptions of the embryonic growth processes; due to such disruptions, palatal and lip structures fail to grow and fuse; clefts may be unilateral or bilateral; clefts are often a part of a genetic syndrome with other anomalies; other anomalies are more commonly associated with clefts of the palate than clefts of the lip; palatal clefts may be associated with various communication disorders; less severe clefts that are medically and surgically managed early in life may not produce significant communication disorders; the more severe the malformations and more delayed the surgical and medical intervention, the greater the severity of communication disorders; hearing impairment may create additional difficulties.

C

Epidemiology and Ethnocultural Variables

- Incidence figures vary, mostly because of different methods of counting children with clefts; inclusion or exclusion of minor clefts of the lip will change the numbers significantly; birth certificates are often used to count the number of children with clefts, but more than one-third of the certificates may fail to record clefts; when reported, their accuracy may be less than 50%; when other anomalies are present (as in genetic syndromes), the presence of cleft or other anomalies may be missed; submucous clefts may be entirely missed not only at birth, but until a few years after birth
- Various studies suggest a range of incidence of 1 in 500 to 1 in 750 live births; many factors, including the gender, the combination of the clefts of the palate and the lip, and some ethnocultural variables affect this general estimation for the population as a whole
- Nearly one-half show cleft of the palate and lip; thus, this combination has the highest incidence of all other varieties of cleft; one-fourth of children have cleft of the lip only; and another one-fourth have cleft of the palate only
- Cleft lip (with or without palatal clefts) is more likely to be unilateral than bilateral
- Gender has an influence on the differential incidence of different forms of clefts; frequency and severity of cleft lip (with or without cleft palate) is higher in males; frequency of palatal clefts (without the cleft lip) is higher in females; ethnocultural variables have an effect on these trends, as described later; compared to the males, the palatal shelves in the female embryo take more time to fuse during the embryonic growth, thus making the shelves more vulnerable to negative influences
- Generally, in both males and females, left unilateral clefts are more frequent than right unilateral clefts
- Among the different ethnic groups studied, the highest incidence of cleft lip with or without cleft palate is found among North American Indians and Asians; the lowest incidence is found among African Americans; generally, the incidence of clefts among Asians is double the incidence among Caucasians; the incidence among Caucasians is double that among African Americans; the incidence rate for Caucasians is in between; specifically, the ranges of incidence figures of *cleft lip with or without cleft palate* reported for each group are as follows:
  o 1 in 1,200 to 1 in 267 North American Indian children
  o 1 in 1,219 to 1 in 297 Japanese children
  o 1 in 689 to 1 in 247 Chinese children
  o 1 in 1,000 to 1 in 372 Caucasian children
  o 1 in 5,555 to 1 in 598 African American children
- The incidence of clefts of the palate only does not vary much across these ethnocultural groups; all groups are vulnerable to clefts of the secondary palate to roughly the same extent

- Familial prevalence of cleft lip, palate, or both poses greater risk for clefts in subsequently born children; for example, for a Caucasian family with no family history of clefts, the incidence of having a child with clefts is less than 1 in 1,000; with one parent and one already-affected child, a subsequent child being born with a cleft is 1 in 137 births
- The incidence of cleft uvula is affected by ethnocultural variables; the highest incidence is found among American Indians and the lowest among African Americans
- Minor abnormalities of the uvula with no clinical consequences is a relatively common finding in the general population; bifid uvula may be found in up to 3% of children
- Incidence of the *types of clefts* vary among different racial or ethnocultural groups and among males and females within each group; among African Americans, a slightly greater number of males than females have clefts of the palate (with or without the lip involvement); among the Chinese, the trend is reversed (slightly more females than males with clefts of the palate with or without the lip involvement)
- Maternal and paternal ethnocultural backgrounds of children may influence the incidence of different types of cleft; generally, the ethnocultural background of the mother seems to exert a greater influence than the same background of the father; for example, more Caucasian mothers than African American mothers may have children with cleft lip with or without cleft palate; the ethnocultural background of the father may not have an effect; in general, the ethnocultural background of both parents may influence the incidence of cleft lip with or without cleft palate, but have no influence on the incidence of cleft palate alone
- Genetic or neuroanatomic anomalies are more likely to be associated with clefts of the palate only
- Incidence of clefts may be on the rise mainly due to better prenatal, natal, and postnatal care, as well as improved chances of well-rehabilitated men and women (born with clefts) who are able to marry and have children; but their children may have a greater likelihood of having clefts, thus accounting for any real increase in the incidence of clefts
- The wide range of incidence reported for different ethnocultural groups and for variations across sexes and families with or without a history of clefts should be viewed with caution and any generalizations should always be qualified while counseling families

Classification of Clefts
- There are several classifications of clefts; none are accepted universally because each has its limitations; clefts of the lip and palate are complexly varied congenital conditions that are hard to classify except in some gross or general manner; clefts vary in extent (often measured in thirds (1/3, 2/3, and 3/3) and widths, lengths, severity, and the number of structures that are involved, making it difficult to classify; nonetheless, attempts to classify clefts abound

- Some experts simply describe clefts of the lip and clefts of the palate, and a combination of the two; others elaborate on this basic classification; the classification system (cleft lip through facial clefts) summarized here is similar to the one suggested by the American Cleft Palate Association:
- Cleft lip: Cleft of the lip may be complete or incomplete; it may be unilateral or bilateral
- Cleft of the alveolar process: This, too, may be unilateral, bilateral, median, and submucous
- Cleft of the prepalate: A combination of the previous types with or without prepalate protrusion or rotation
- Clefts of the palate: Clefts of the soft palate, clefts of the hard palate, and submucous clefts
- Clefts of the prepalate and palate: Any combination of clefts of the prepalate and palate
- Facial clefts that do not involve the prepalate and palate: Include such rare forms as horizontal clefts, lower mandibular clefts, lateral oro-ocular clefts, and naso-ocular clefts
- Microforms: Minimal expressions of clefts including hairline indentation of the lip or just a notch on the lip; palatal defects that are revealed only through laminographic examination; submucous clefts may be included

Communication Disorders Associated With Clefts

- The most significant communication disorders include articulation disorders, impaired resonance, and oral language skills; velopharyngeal inadequacy associated with the clefts of the soft palate contribute greatly to the communication problems
- Not all children who had clefts of the lip, palate, or both exhibit communication disorders; children with competent and early surgical treatment of the clefts may acquire speech and language skills as well as those without clefts
- Some children with surgically closed clefts may have speech disorders mainly due to serious dental or malocclusion problems; others may have such disorders because of delayed surgical procedures, inadequate surgical rehabilitation, inadequate speech-language services, and poor family support for speech-language and other services
- The same type of cleft with the same severity may produce differential effects on speech
- Cleft lip alone rarely results in serious misarticulations; bilateral complete clefts of the hard and soft palates create the most severe speech and resonance problems
- Articulation disorders
    - Articulation and phonological disorders or processes may be independent of clefts; see Articulation and Phonological Disorders for details; speech sound production errors that are due to the clefts (or other pure structural problems) are typically not characterized as *phonological;* the description offered here pertains to articulation disorders that are a function of the clefts and related anatomical, physiological, and auditory deficiencies

C

- o Cleft palate only is associated with relatively fewer errors than cleft lip and palate, complicated by maxillary and dental problems; fewest errors of articulation or even normal speech production may be associated with only the cleft of the lip with no significant involvement of the alveolar process
- o Articulatory skills vary from normal to significantly abnormal; estimates of percentages of children with surgically treated clefts who have articulation disorders varies between 50% and 90% of 5-year-olds or younger to about 15% to 25% of adolescents; usually, reported higher percentages are related to an absence of high-quality cleft palate team services
- o Articulation disorders associated with clefts include:
  - Predominantly substitutions and omissions, along with some sound distortions; distortions may be more common in older children and adults
  - Greater difficulty with unvoiced sounds than with voiced sounds; voiceless stops and affricates may be especially difficult for younger children, but this may not be true for fricatives; adolescents and adults may exhibit frequent misarticulations of voiceless stops and fricatives
  - Greater difficulty with sounds that require a build-up of intraoral pressure; this difficulty, due largely to velopharyngeal insufficiency, results in weak production of pressure consonants (e.g., stops, fricatives, and affricates)
  - Although somewhat unexpected, children with cleft plate may misarticulate /r/ and /l/, as well as liquids that do not require a buildup of intraoral air pressure; similarly, glides, too, may be misarticulated
  - Apparent substitutions of nasal sounds for nonnasal sounds; these may not be true substitutions because the added nasal resonance may be due to velopharyngeal incompetence or insufficiency
  - Increased difficulty producing consonant clusters than singletons, a trend similar to that found in misarticulating children without clefts; clusters that involve multiple sounds may be more difficult than those that involve only two sounds
  - Some distortion of vowels, more evident in isolated production than in continuous speech; vowel intelligibility is negatively affected in cleft palate speakers partly because of tongue position, restricted mouth opening, and hypernasality
  - A slower rate of speech; this may be a compensatory strategy to increase speech intelligibility
- o Compensatory errors, although they may be found in children without clefts; the frequency of errors or the number of children who make errors depend on the timing and the quality of the medical, surgical, and speech-language treatment offered to them; such errors, once common among children with clefts, are less frequently observed in U.S. children who receive competent and timely service from a team of specialists, including speech-language pathologists; still, some 25% of children with surgically closed clefts in the United States may have deviant articulation
- o Compensatory errors of articulation are those that are produced at unusual articulatory loci; sounds typically produced in the anterior oral region may be produced in the posterior region; errors are due to a shifting of the place of articulation because of organic problems, including

velopharyngeal insufficiency or incompetence, severe dental abnormalities, or extreme degrees of malocclusions; errors are often substitutions that help compensate for the inadequate anatomic and physiologic mechanisms; compensatory substitutions include:

- Substitution of stops, fricatives, and affricates with unusual (often posterior) movements and posture of the tongue to stop the air or to produce friction noise
- Generally, the place of articulation of oral sounds may be shifted to the pharyngeal, laryngeal, and velar loci of articulation
- Substitution of glottal stops for stop consonants
- Substitution of laryngeal stops for stop consonants and laryngeal fricatives for fricatives; such productions involve posterior postures of the tongue so as to move the epiglottis toward the pharynx to block the air or to create friction noise
- Substitution of pharyngeal stop for stop consonants and pharyngeal affricates for affricates; such productions involve the posterior movement of the tongue to make contact with the pharynx to build up pressure that is suddenly released or to constrict the air to create friction
- Substitution of posterior nasal fricative for fricative; the child uses the posterior dorsum of the tongue and the soft palate to create the friction sound
- Substitution of mid-dorsum palatal stop for /t/, /d/, /k/, and /g/; in such productions, the child attempts to build air pressure by raising the mid-dorsum of the tongue to the hard palate
- Substitution of mid-dorsum palatal fricatives and mid-dorsum palatal affricates for fricatives and affricates; in such productions, the mid-dorsum moves toward the hard palate to create friction or to increase air pressure
- Some children may have even more unusual patterns of compensatory articulation; for instance, substitution of a click-like sound for stop consonants; sibilant productions with an ingressive airflow; lateral movement of the mandible during the production of /s/; a nasal grimace, an attempt to narrow the nasal cavity to reduce the air escape through the nose
- Most gross substitutions are due to velopharyngeal inadequacy, palatal fistulae, or malocclusion; errors (mostly substitutions) are a means of coping with these problems

o Nasal emission is a special kind of problem frequently seen in children with clefts; although whether it is a resonance or an articulation disorder has been debated in the past, it most likely is a result of certain articulatory attempts and efforts in the context of inadequate velopharyngeal function; see Velopharyngeal Dysfunction; characteristics of nasal emission include:

- Audible or inaudible nasal air emission while producing many speech sounds
- Inaudible nasal emission is visible air escape through the nostrils with no sound; a cold mirror held below the nostrils will fog, thus making it visible even if inaudible; this is due to inefficient velopharyngeal function

C

- Audible nasal emission is due to the sound generated by the air that is escaping through the nose while producing speech; it adds an undesirable and distracting quality to speech; an inefficient velopharyngeal valve is the cause of this problem
  - A lateralized /s/ production may sound like nasal emission
- o Reduced speech intelligibility, which depends on all associated communication deficits, including the number and severity of misarticulations and the degree of velopharyngeal dysfunction
- o There generally is an improving trend in articulation skills as the child grows older
- Language disorders
  - o Generally, children with clefts may have delayed language development initially but may improve significantly as they grow older; many may attain normal or near-normal language by age 4 or so
  - o Babies with clefts vocalize less frequently than those without clefts; delayed onset of babbling; in excess of 3 months delay in producing the first few words and the first 50 words
  - o During the early language learning period, children may produce more words that begin with nasals, vowels, velars, labials, and glottals than those that begin with stops, fricatives, and affricates
  - o Shorter mean length of utterances, simpler or shorter words and sentences, restricted vocabulary, and limited syntactic variety associated especially with palatal clefts
  - o Slightly higher than the normal grammatical errors
  - o Slower mastery of social communication skills; passivity during conversation, suggesting a conversational turn-taking deficiency
  - o Significant language disorders if the clefts are associated with genetic syndromes; intellectual disabilities and hearing loss may be additional contributing factors
  - o Otitis media, which occurs more frequently in children with palatal clefts, may affect language learning during the early childhood years, but the evidence to date is weak
- Laryngeal pathologies and phonatory disorders
  - o Frequent development of bilateral vocal fold nodules, resulting in hoarseness of voice; hoarseness without vocal fold pathology in some children; the nodules and hoarseness are the result of velopharyngeal insufficiency and the resulting vocal hyperfunction
  - o Hypertrophy and edema of the vocal folds
  - o Soft voice because of velopharyngeal inadequacy; may partly be due to conductive hearing loss; vocal intensity decreases because of loss of pressure at the velopharyngeal port; the speech may be too soft to be understood in most social situations; may be a compensatory strategy to reduce the effects of hypernasality because of the association of hypernasality and nasal emission with increased vocal loudness
  - o Monotonous voice (limited pitch variation) in some children
  - o Generally, strangled voice quality (due to excessive effort and tension in producing voice to avoid hypernasality)

- Resonance disorders
  o Hypernasality on vowels and voiced oral consonants due to inadequate velopharyngeal closure and restricted mouth opening
  o Hyponasality (reduced nasal resonance) and denasality (near-complete lack of nasal resonance)
  o Both hyponasality and denasality are due to nasal obstructions caused by upper respiratory infections, abnormal growths in the nasal cavity, or a deviated nasal septum
  o See Velopharyngeal Dysfunction for details

Related Problems
- Various physical anomalies when associated with genetic syndromes; see Syndromes Associated With Communication Disorders.
- Hearing loss in nearly half of all children with cleft palates; more commonly, conductive hearing loss; infrequently, high-frequency loss

Etiologic Factors Related to Clefts
- Clefts of the lips may have different causes than clefts of the palate with or without the cleft lip; disruptions during the embryonic growth stages when the palatal shelves fuse are the main causes of clefts
- Genetic anomalies are the most frequent causes; although clefts may be found in children who do not have other genetic anomalies, many genetic syndromes (some 400 plus) are associated with clefts; see Syndromes Associated With Communication Disorders for more information
  o Clefts are associated with autosomal dominant syndromes in which a single gene is defective; even if only one parent has a defective gene, the probability is 50% that a child will inherit the condition; such syndromes include Apert Syndrome, Stickler Syndrome, Treacher Collins Syndrome, van der Wude Syndrome, Velocardiofacial Syndrome, and Waardenburg Syndrome, all described under Syndromes Associated With Communication Disorders
  o Clefts also are associated with recessive genetic syndromes (e.g., Oro-Facial-Digital Syndrome; for a recessive genetic syndrome to be expressed, the defective gene must be inherited from both parents
  o Clefts may be associated with X-linked (sex-linked) syndromes (e.g., Oto-Palatal-Digital Syndrome)
  o Other chromosomal abnormalities (e.g., trisomy 13)
- Environmental factors linked to clefts and associated anomalies include:
  o Alcohol consumed during pregnancy; clefts of both lips and palates are frequently found in children with Fetal Alcohol Syndrome (see Syndromes Associated With Communication Disorders)
  o Use of illegal drugs, including marijuana, cocaine, crack cocaine, and heroin, although the effects of particular drugs have not been isolated
  o Prescription drugs including anticonvulsant drugs and thalidomide (a sedative) that pregnant women take
  o Excessive maternal smoking, a suspected factor in inducing clefts and other birth defects

C

- Mechanical factors that interfere with the fetal growth and cause clefts include:
  - Intrauterine crowding (twins, triplets, etc.)
  - Uterine tumors and amniotic ruptures

Bzoch, K. R. (2004). *Communicative disorders related to cleft palate* (5th ed.). Austin, TX: Pro-Ed.

Kummer, A. W. (2001). *Cleft palate and craniofacial anomalies.* Clifton Park, NY: Thomson Delmar Learning.

Moller, K. T., & Starr, C. D. (1993). *Cleft palate: Interdisciplinary issues and treatment.* Austin, TX: Pro-Ed.

McWilliams, B. J., Morris, H. L., & Shelton, R. L. (1990). *Cleft palate speech* (2nd ed.). Philadelphia, PA: B. C. Decker.

Peterson-Falzone, S. J., Hardin-Jones, M. A., & Karnell, M. P. (2001). *Cleft palate speech* (3rd ed.). St. Louis, MO: Mosby.

Shprintzen, R. J., & Bardach, J. (1995). *Cleft palate speech management: A multidisciplinary approach.* St. Louis, MO: Mosby.

Closed-Head Injury.   A head injury in which the meninges remain intact; the skull may or may not be fractured; the same as Nonpenetrating Head Injury; see Traumatic Brain Injury for symptoms and causes.

Cluster Reduction.   A phonological process or articulation disorder characterized by omission of one or more sounds in a cluster (blend) of sounds; also called cluster simplification; see Articulation and Phonological Disorders.

Clusters.   Two or more consonant sounds produced adjacent to each other; also called *blends*; difficult for children with Articulation and Phonological Disorders.

Cluttering.   A disorder of fluency characterized by excessively fast speech rate, reduced speech intelligibility, increased dysfluencies, and possibly language and thought disorders; see Cluttering under Fluency Disorders.

Coloboma.   A defect in which portions of a structure, especially the eye, are missing; characteristic of Treacher-Collins syndrome (see Syndromes Associated With Communication Disorders).

Compensatory Behaviors (Strategies).   An action or skill that minimizes the negative effects of a disease or disorder; a learned behavior that improves actions that would otherwise be more deficient; compensatory behaviors may be naturally (without training) acquired as a coping strategy when more effective strategies are out of reach; such strategies may be clinically taught when certain residual effects of disorders cannot be eliminated.

Concordance Rate.   The frequency with which a clinical condition found in one member of an identical or fraternal twin also is found in the other twin member; higher concordance rates of clinical conditions have been used to support genetic etiology.

Conduction Aphasia.   Form of fluent aphasia characterized by paraphasic fluency, good comprehension of spoken speech, and impaired repetition; see under Aphasia: Specific Types.

Conductive Hearing Loss. Hearing loss due to a failure to conduct sound to the cochlea; see Hearing Impairment.

Confrontation Naming. Naming stimulus items when asked; naming in response to a typical question, "What is this?"; a difficult task for clients who have a naming problem; a characteristic of Aphasia.

Congenital. Any condition noticed at birth or soon thereafter; may be genetic or acquired.

Congenital Abducens-Facial Paralysis. The same as Moebius syndrome (see Syndromes Associated With Communication Disorders).

Congenital Apoculofacial Paralysis. The same as Moebius syndrome (see Syndromes Associated With Communication Disorders).

Congenital Facial Diplegia. The same as Moebius syndrome (see Syndromes Associated With Communication Disorders).

Congenital Palatopharyngeal Incompetence. A velopharyngeal mechanism that is functionally incompetent; it cannot close the velopharyngeal port for the production of nonnasal speech sounds; not due to clefts; hard palate, soft palate, or both may be too short or the nasopharynx may be too deep; speech is hypernasal; see Velopharyngeal Dysfunction for details and related conditions.

Consistency Effect. Stuttering that occurs on the same loci in repeated oral reading of a passage; some loci are consistent in evoking the same kind of dysfluency when the person who stutters repeatedly reads aloud a printed passage, usually up to five times; suggests that stuttering is stronger, more habitual, or more stimulus-bound than stuttering that shows the contrasted Adaptation Effect.

Consonant Deletion. A phonological process or an articulation error in which a consonant is deleted from a word production; the same as omission of consonants, although viewed from the standpoint of phonological processes; see Articulation and Phonological Disorders.

Consonantal Harmony. A phonological assimilation process that affects the manner or place of production; includes labial assimilation, velar assimilation, nasal assimilation, and alveolar assimilation; see Articulation and Phonological Disorders.

Constructional Apraxia. Difficulty in reconstructing such geometric designs as a block design; often associated with brain injury; see Constructional Impairment.

Constructional Impairment. Difficulty in visuospatial tasks; includes problems in constructing block designs, copying or drawing geometric figures, reproducing stick figures, and drawing human faces; often associated with Right Hemisphere Syndrome and Traumatic Brain Injury; also called Constructional Apraxia.

Conversational Repair Strategies. Several kinds of verbal behaviors that help reestablish broken communication links; part of pragmatic language skills; children and adults with language disorders often have difficulty with conversational repair strategies; see Language Disorders in Children; the normal repair strategies include:

- Request for clarification; typically, listeners who do not understand a speaker request clarification from the speaker; request for clarification may include such statements as "What do you mean?," "I am not sure what you mean," "Can you say it differently?," "I don't understand," "I didn't hear you," or "Can you say it louder?"
- Appropriate response to a listener's request for clarification; helpful responses to request for clarification include such speech modifications as saying the same thing in different words, in more elaborate terms, with examples, with simpler terms, and more loudly

Cough. An abrupt and forceful expulsion of air from the lungs; may be associated with aspiration and Dysphagia.

Craniocerebral Trauma. Trauma or injury to the head and the brain; see Traumatic Brain Injury for causes, consequences, and associated communication disorders.

Creutzfeldt-Jakob Disease (CJD). A rare degenerative disease that affects 1 in a million persons; thought to be caused by a virus called prion (proteinaceous infectious particle), although not microscopically identified; a form of fatal encephalopathy, associated with widespread spongiform state in the brain; characteristics of the disease include:

- Onset during the 60s and 70s; positive family history in about 10% of cases
- Partial degeneration of pyramidal and extrapyramidal systems
- Initial symptoms of sleeplessness, fatigue, apprehension, and impaired concentration
- Memory loss and other cognitive impairments along with psychiatric symptoms (anxiety, hallucinations, delusions) as the disease progresses
- Cerebellar ataxia, tremor, rigidity, chorea, athetosis, and visual problems
- Stupor, mutism, and vegetative state in the final stages
- Rapid course with certain fatality (mean duration of illness is 7 months)
- Associated with Apraxia, Dementia, and almost all types of Dysarthria.

Cystic Fibrosis. An inherited genetic disorder, commonly affecting Caucasian children; excessive secretion of the exocrine glands causes obstruction of passageways in the pancreas and the lungs.

D

Deaf. A person whose hearing impairment is severe enough to prevent normal oral language acquisition, production, and comprehension; a person with profound hearing loss that exceeds 90 dB HL.

Degenerative Neurological Disease. Progressive neurological diseases that do not have effective treatment; the diseases end in deterioration in health and behavior; terminal neurological diseases; associated with various kinds of communication and swallowing disorders; see Dementia, Dysarthria, and Dysphagia.

Deglutition. The same as swallowing. See Dysphagia.

de Lange Syndrome. The same as Cornelia de Lange Syndrome (see Syndromes Associated With Communication Disorders).

Deletion Processes. A phonological process similar to omission of sounds or syllables, although viewed from the standpoint of phonological theory; see Phonological Processes.

Dementia, Progressive. A neurodegenerative syndrome associated with deterioration in intellect, communication, and general behavior; a generic term that includes varied neuropathologies and their persistent and progressive consequences on intellectual skills and behavior; American Psychiatric Association's DSM-IV and its 2000 text revision requires memory impairments and at least one of the following impairments for diagnosis: Aphasia, Apraxia, Agnosia, or impaired Executive Functions; other definitions of dementia require impairments in three of the following: language, memory, visuospatial skills, emotion or personality, and cognition; except for reversible varieties of dementia, the deterioration should be sustained over a period of months or years and should be progressive; controversially classified as *cortical* and *subcortical*; varied etiologic factors, but often associated with such neurologic diseases as Alzheimer's Disease (AD), Huntington's Disease (HD), and Parkinson's Disease (PD); the most frequently occurring forms are associated with Alzheimer's disease (50% of the cases) and AIDS; also frequently associated with vascular diseases (15% to 20% of the cases); progressive and irreversible in most cases; static in a few cases and reversible in 10% to 20% of the cases; may be classified as primary degenerative, multi-infarct, and all other; also may be classified as cortical (degeneration primarily in neocortical association areas) with better preserved motor speech skills, subcortical (degeneration in the basal ganglia, thalamus, and brainstem) with better preserved language skills, and mixed; much of the information presented here about the neuropathology and communication disorders is associated with dementia in general; for specific information on dementia associated with Alzheimer's Disease (AD), Creutzfeldt-Jakob Disease, Parkinson's Disease (PD), Huntington's Disease (HD), Pick's Disease, Progressive Supranuclear Palsy (PS), and Wilson's Disease, see their respective alphabetical main entries; see also Vascular Dementia.

Epidemiology and Ethnocultural Variables
- Affects about 10% of the population over 65 years of age, although as high a prevalence rate of 25% has been suggested
- Approximately 6% to 20% of nursing home residents may have dementia

- After the age of 65, prevalence doubles every 5 years; while the prevalence rate during the early 60s is less than 1%, it is 30% during the mid to late 80s
- The rate of dementia may decline in the ninth decade of life (limited evidence)
- Dementia may be more common in urban regions than rural parts of the world
- Contrary to previous claims, women are not more prone than men to dementia
- Younger age of onset of reversible dementia and dementia due to acquired immune deficiency syndrome (AIDS)
- Increased prevalence of dementia as the population gets older
- Increased worldwide incidence of dementia as health care improves in many countries and longevity increases
- Dementia has varied causes, resulting in several types of dementia; incidence of different types of dementia vary somewhat across ethnocultural groups:
  o Dementia due to Alzheimer's disease may be more common among whites than in African Americans or Asian Americans
  o Dementia due to vascular diseases may be more common among African Americans and Asian Americans than white or Hispanic elderly
  o Asian Americans, African Americans, and Latinos may have a lower incidence of Lewy Body Dementia than whites
  o Incidence of dementia due to frontotemporal lobar degeneration may be similar in Asian Americans, Pacific Islanders, and whites, but be less common in African Americans and Latinos
  o Incidence of dementia due to progressive supranuclear palsy may be higher in Asian Americans and Pacific Islanders than in whites, but roughly the same in African Americans and Latinos
  o In Japan, vascular dementia is more common than other types; among the Caucasians living in Europe and the United States, vascular dementia is less common than that due to Alzheimer's disease
  o Late onset dementia may be more common among African Americans
  o Dementia may be uncommon in certain African countries; Nigerians are reported to have the lowest incidence; people living in the Kashmir region of India also are reported to have a low incidence of dementia
- Dementia is a serious and expensive health care problem; most clients with dementia need specialized care and treatment for up to 10 years
- In the 1990s, the cost of dementia treatment and care in the United States was in excess of $30 billion a year

Onset and Early Symptoms of Progressive Dementia
- Onset is slow and gradual, with mild symptoms that may be either missed or blamed on old age
- Subtle memory problems are among the earliest symptoms; impairment may be mild for remote events and more pronounced for recent events and for learning and remembering new information
- Reasoning problems and poor judgment may be the next set of symptoms to appear; more often than memory problems, lapses in reasoning and judgment are the ones noticed by family members

- Subtle deterioration in daily skills (e.g., cooking, checkbook balancing, or bill paying); the client may compensate for such deteriorations by assigning responsibility to others or by avoiding the difficult tasks
- Brief, subtle, or transitory problems of disorientation; sometimes ignored or not noticed by family members
- Mild depression and other mood changes
- Subtle language problems that include the following:
  o Mild naming problems that becomes progressively worse
  o Beginning of progressive decrease in vocabulary, possibly due to naming problems (production of fewer nouns)
  o Verbal paraphasia, as a consequence of naming difficulties; beating around the bush or describing instead of naming objects (circumlocution)
  o Subtle language comprehension problems, especially understanding implied meanings and humor
  o Impaired picture description; one of the early diagnostic features
  o Incorrect use of pronouns
  o Pragmatic language problems; difficulty in topic maintenance, failure to ask for clarification from speakers, or failure to respond appropriately when listeners ask for clarification
  o Repetitious speech
  o Intact automatic speech
  o Intact articulation and phonological skills
  o Intact syntactic skills
- Impaired pantomime recognition and expression
- Visuospatial problems, including difficulty in drawing simple figures or in copying three-dimensional drawings; problems in constructing block designs, or lacing one's own shoes

Progression/Advanced Characteristics of Progressive Dementia

- Severely impaired memory skills; memory for both remote and recent events may be severely affected, and the client may be unable to learn or retain any new information
- Severe visuospatial problems; difficulties found in the initial stages intensify to affect even the routine and automatic tasks, affecting such daily activities as dressing, eating, walking, and bathing
- Pronounced and generalized intellectual impairment eventually resulting in profound intellectual deterioration; the client may be unable to perform skills normally performed, including cooking, shopping, and managing personal and family affairs
- Inability to make decisions and rational judgments in all aspects of life
- Loss of mathematical skills; the client may totally lose even rudimentary arithmetic skills
- Profound agnosia; the client is unable to not only name objects, but recognize them for what they are; consequently, the client may try to eat with a pencil, or to drink with a plate
- Behavior changes of the early stage dementia may evolve into seriously aberrant behaviors; profoundly disturbing psychiatric symptoms emerge
  o Delusions and hallucinations

o Violent outbursts as a reaction to trivial incidents or situations
o Paranoid reactions, causing the client to make baseless accusations, hiding things, and stealing objects
o Socially inappropriate behavior including uncharacteristically tasteless humor and incongruous laughter; socially uninhibited behavior, including public masturbation and urination

D

o Restlessness, agitation, and hyperactivity resulting in aimless pacing, ritualistic and meaningless handling of objects in the house, and picking-up things for no apparent reason
o Profound disorientation to time, place, and person; the client may get lost in his or her own neighborhood, home, and other familiar surroundings; the client may repeatedly wander off; eventually may lose self-orientation (not knowing who he or she is)

- Periodic incontinence (urinary control problems) worsening to complete urinary and fecal incontinence
- Motor problems, apparent mostly in the advanced stage dementia, may include muscle spasticity, unstable gait, frequent falls, and a bewildered facial expression
- Diurnal rhythm disturbance in some cases; the client may be restless, anxious, and may wander during nights and try to sleep in the day time
- Intensification of communication problems seen in the early stage dementia; emergence of additional problems, including speech production problems
  o Rapidly diminishing vocabulary, eventually leading to mutism in the final stages of the disease
  o Severe naming problems, resulting in literal paraphasias, circumlocution, empty speech (expression of fewer ideas even when the number of words produced do not decline much), and beating around the bush
  o Jargon and stereotypical expressions, often a result of naming problems and paraphasia
  o Incoherent and irrelevant speech
  o Rapid rate of speech, sometimes hyperfluent, even though paraphasic or meaningless
  o Echolalic speech (meaningless repetition of what is heard) and palilalia (compulsive repetition of one's own speech, often with accelerating rate and decelerating loudness)
  o Seriously impaired speech and language comprehension; especially difficult for the client are instructions for performing sequenced tasks; comprehension skills diminish for even simple conversation as the disease advances
  o Pragmatic communication problems including difficulty initiating conversation, maintaining a topic of conversation, and taking turns during conversation
  o Inattention to such social conventions as greeting people, bidding farewell, and thanking others
  o Emergence of dysarthria as a consequence of deteriorating neurological status
  o Completely meaningless and confused speech
  o Muteness in the final stage

Etiologic Factors of Progressive Dementia

- Because progressive dementia is a category of many diseases and their effects, the etiologic factors are highly varied; many medical conditions and diseases may cause dementia in a small number of clients; in some individuals, dementia is due to multiple causes (e.g., Alzheimer's disease and a previous history of brain injury, history of drug abuse, and Parkinson's disease); major dementia forms with specific diseases that cause progressive dementia in significant numbers of clients have separate alphabetical entries and include:
  - o Alzheimer's Disease: The most common form of dementia in several ethnic groups; genetic factors are dominant but the role of environmental factors is also suspected
  - o Frontotemporal Dementia (PiD): A syndrome that now includes Pick's disease; caused by such neuropathological factors as Pick Bodies and Pick Cells
  - o Huntington's Disease (HD): A genetic, inherited, neurodegenerative disease; autosomal dominant inheritance expresses in half the offspring of an affected person; mutation may be found in the short arm of chromosome 4
  - o Infectious Dementia: Forms of dementia due to various infections of the central nervous system; include the human immunodeficiency virus (HIV) and the hypothesized prion infection that presumably causes Creutzfeldt-Jakob Disease
  - o Lewy Body Type Dementia: A relatively new diagnostic category, Lewy body dementia is caused by small pathologic spots found in the substantia negra, and are called intraneuronal cytoplasmic inclusions; such spots also are associated with Parkinson's disease
  - o Multiple Sclerosis and other demyelinating diseases: Demyelination of white matter results in a variety of neurological symptoms and may cause dementia
  - o Parkinson's Disease (PD): Neurodegenerative disease whose etiological factors are not well understood; genetic factors are suspected; 30% to 55% of clients with PD may develop dementia
  - o Pick's Disease: A form of dementia, now considered a part of the Frontotemporal Dementia; caused by such neuropathologies as Pick Bodies and Pick Cells
  - o Progressive Supranuclear Palsy: A degenerative neurological disease that mainly affects the basal ganglia and the brainstem; symptoms resemble those of Parkinson's disease
  - o Pseudodementias: Symptoms resembling dementia but are associated with such psychiatric disturbances as depression, schizophrenia, and mania; see Psychiatric Problems Associated With Communicative Disorders for details
  - o Traumatic Brain Injury—Dementia: Repeated traumatic brain injury, including what the professional boxers sustain: risk for developing dementia later in life
  - o Vascular Dementia: Vascular diseases resulting in repeated large vessel strokes and small arterial ruptures (lacunar state); dementia due to vascular diseases are second only to dementia due to Alzheimer's disease

o Wilson's Disease (WD): Inherited autosomal progressive neurodegenerative disease causing dementia as well as a form of dysarthria
- Toxic conditions including alcohol-related syndromes and multiple drug abuse, and toxicity due to various prescription drugs including anticonvulsive and antihypertensive drugs

D

Neuropathology of Progressive Dementia

- Neuropathology of progressive dementia is highly variable because of its multiple etiologic factors; each disease or cerebral trauma that causes dementia has its own neuropathological condition
  o Alzheimer's Disease: Neuropathologic factors include neurofibrillary tangles, neuritic plaques, neuronal cell loss, and neurochemical changes that reduce neural transmission
  o Frontotemporal Dementia (PiD): A heterogeneous group of diseases with a predominant pathology of neural degeneration in the frontal, temporal, or both regions of the brain; in Pick's disease, which causes the major form of frontotemporal dementia, the dense intracellular formations in the neuronal cytoplasm (Pick bodies) and ballooned, inflated, or enlarged neurons (Pick cells) are the two main pathological conditions; the Pick bodies are found especially in nonpyramidal cells in the cerebral layers 2, 3, and 6, whereas the Pick cells are found in the lower and middle cortical layers; dilation of ventricles and atrophy of cells in the left hemisphere also may be evident
  o Huntington's Disease (HD): Associated neuropathological conditions include neuronal loss in the basal ganglia; loss may be evident to some extent in the pallidus and the parietal lobe, but severe in the caudate nucleus and the putamen; reduced inhibitory neurotransmitters GABA and Acetylcholine contribute to the symptoms of dementia
  o Infectious Dementia: Acquired immune deficiency syndrome (AIDS) and the resulting neuropathological factors are associated with AIDS dementia complex; encephalopathy (degeneration) of subcortical white matter, the basal ganglia, and cortical layers are involved in AIDS dementia complex; diffuse and varied loss of neurons is associated with Creutzfeldt-Jakob disease caused by a presumed prion infection
  o Lewy Body Type Dementia: Intraneuronal cytoplasmic inclusions, also known as Lewy bodies, are the main neuropathological condition, common in the substantia negra
  o Multiple Sclerosis: Demyelination of white matter is the main neuropathological condition
  o Parkinson's Disease (PD): Degeneration of brainstem nuclei, widening of sulci especially in the frontal region, neuronal loss in substantia negra, neurofibrillary tangles, neuritic plaques, presence of Lewy bodies, and reduced dopamine are the main neuropathological conditions
  o Progressive Supranuclear Palsy: Neuropathological conditions mostly limited to the basal ganglia and the brainstem; neuronal loss, neurofibrillary tangles, granulovacuolar degeneration, demyelination, gliosis, and depletion of dopamine and an impaired cholinergic system are common pathological conditions

D

- Pseudodementias: Secondary to such psychiatric disorders as schizophrenia and depression; no specific neuropathological conditions that are found in neurodegenerative diseases; see Psychiatric Problems Associated With Communicative Disorders for details
- Traumatic Brain Injury—Dementia: Neuropathological conditions are unlike those in neurodegenerative diseases; injury to brain structures due to external trauma is the main pathological condition; diffuse axonal and vascular injury, primary brainstem injury, focal lesions, and such secondary effects as intracranial hematoma, increased intracranial pressure, ischemic brain damage, and infection are among the neuropathological conditions
- Vascular Dementia: Multiple neuropathological conditions due mainly to various vascular diseases; widespread cortical and subcortical damage due to repeated occurrences of thrombosis or embolism are the main neuropathology causing *multi-infarct dementia; lacunar states* are another form of neuropathological condition characterized by hollow spaces in neural structures due mostly to ischemic infarctions; atrophy of the subcortical white matter, which is associated with Binswanger's Disease
- Wilson's Disease (WD): Etiology is genetic; pathological factors include degeneration of the lenticular nuclei of the basal ganglia
- General neuropathological conditions associated with various forms of progressive dementia include:
  - Neurofibrillary tangles; twisted and tangled structures of dendrites and axons (especially in DAT)
  - Neuritic (senile) plaques; small areas of cortical and subcortical degeneration (especially in DAT)
  - Granulovacuolar degeneration; degeneration of nerve cells because of the formation of small fluid-filled cavities containing granular debris (especially in DAT)
  - Reduced gray and white matter of the brain; loss of large neurons in the frontal and temporal regions of the brain; about 10% loss of brain weight
  - Decreased dendritic connections
  - Neurochemical deficiencies in the brain that affect neurotransmission, especially cholinergic and dopamine deficiency along with deficient neuropeptides
  - Decreased cerebral metabolism
  - Reduced cerebral blood flow
  - Enlarged ventricles and widened sulci
  - Bilateral brain damage due to repeated CVA
  - Damaged subcortical structures due to multiple infarcts (Binswanger's disease)

Theories of Progressive Dementia

- Theories are varied, depending on the type of dementia and the underlying neuropathology; more research needed before any of the theories are accepted
- Genetic factors; may play a less important role in infectious dementias and dementia due to traumatic brain injury than in dementias associated with

neurodegenerative diseases (e.g., Alzheimer's, Huntington's, and Parkinson's diseases)
- Environmental factors, especially in infectious dementias
- Lifestyle factors that either protect (e.g., healthy eating habits or regular exercise) or pose additional risks (e.g., poor eating habits leading to vascular diseases and strokes; weight gain, diabetes, and other factors that increase the risk of diseases that eventually affect brain function)
- Personal characteristics; higher education and lifelong intellectual pursuits are thought to reduce the risk or delay the onset; lack of higher education and lack of interest in intellectual activities are thought to increase the chances of dementia or lead to an earlier onset; the evidence is mostly suggestive
- Interaction of genetic, environmental, and personal characteristics

Bayles, K. A., & Kaszniak, A. W. (1987). *Communication and cognition in normal aging and dementia.* Austin, TX: Pro-Ed.

Brookshire, R. H. (2003). *An introduction to neurogenic communication disorders* (6th ed.). St. Louis, MO: Mosby Year Book.

Bourgeois, M. (2005). Dementia. In L. L. LaPointe (Ed.), *Aphasia and other neurogenic language disorders* (3rd ed., pp. 199–213). New York: Thieme.

Cummings, J. L., & Benson, D. F. (1983). *Dementia: A clinical approach.* Boston, MA: Butterworth

Hegde, M. N. (2006). *A coursebook on aphasia and other neurogenic language disorders* (3rd ed.). Clifton Park, NY: Thomson Delmar Learning.

Hou, C. E., Yaffe, K., Perez-Stable, E. J., & Miller B. L. (2006). Frequency of dementia etiologies in four ethnic groups. *Dementia and Geriatric Cognitive Disorders, 22*(1), 42–47.

Lubinski, R. (1991). *Dementia and communication.* Philadelphia, PA: B. C. Decker.

Ripich, D. N. (1991). *Geriatric communication disorders.* Austin, TX: Pro-Ed.

Wells, C. E. (1980). The differential diagnosis of psychiatric disorders in the elderly. In J. Cole & J. Barrett (Eds.), *Psychopathology in the aged* (pp. 19–29). New York: Raven Press.

Dementia, Reversible. Temporary dementia due to various factors whose effects may be neutralized or greatly reduced by prompt and effective treatment; mostly due to treatable diseases or disorders (e.g., certain nutritional deficiencies or metabolic disorders); the degree to which dementia may be reversed with treatment varies and often is controversial; some residual intellectual and behavioral effects following what is considered successful treatment is typical; therefore, *reversible* may mean substantial improvement, no progressive deterioration, but no complete recovery in most cases.

Epidemiology and Ethnocultural Variables
- Incidence estimates of reversible dementia vary greatly; some studies suggest that of all the cases diagnosed with dementia, 10% to 20% may be reversible

D

- Some studies suggest that the incidence of reversible dementia may be lower than traditionally thought; there is some suggestion that the incidence of reversible dementia may be declining
- Some recent investigations have reported as high as 30% of cases of nondegenerative nonvascular dementia in clients with a younger age of onset (before the age of 70); in most cases, dementia was not completely reversed with treatment
- New cases of reversible dementia with hitherto unsuspected causes also are routinely reported
- Nonvascular, nondegenerative (reversible) dementia is generally more often reported in persons with younger age of onset than in those with older age
- No specific ethnocultural data on reversible dementia are available

Etiology of Reversible Dementia

- Various prescription drugs may lead to dementia; drugs known to induce reversible dementia include:
  o Lithium carbonate, used to treat manic depressive psychosis
  o Tricyclic antidepressants
  o Anticonvulsants used to treat epilepsy
  o Some antibiotics (e.g., penicillin)
  o Medications involving steroids
- Drug abuse is a known cause of reversible dementia
- Alcoholism may eventually lead to symptoms of dementia
- Metal toxicity (e.g., toxicity due to lead and mercury) that receives timely and effective medical management
- Long-standing lung and heart diseases and general anemia that lead to *postanoxic dementia* that may be reversed by treating the underlying disease or clinical condition
- Depression leading to symptoms of reversible dementia; often successfully treated
- Some metabolic disorders (e.g., encephalopathies from kidney or liver diseases that are successfully treated)
- Vitamin deficiencies, especially vitamin B_1 and B_{12} deficiencies that are medically managed; one of the more frequently cited causes of reversible dementia in developing countries where nutritional deficiencies are a problem
- Some endocrine disorders (e.g., thyroid deficiencies) that are successfully treated
- Head trauma that produces transient symptoms of dementia
- Normal pressure hydrocephalus, a neurological condition in which the flow of the cerebrospinal fluid is blocked, thus increasing the pressure within the cranium; factors that increase the risk of hydrocephalus include closed head injury, brain surgery, and subarachnoid hemorrhage accounting for about 5% of reversible dementia
- Various brain infections, including various forms of meningitis, including cryptococcal meningitis
- Certain brain tumors that are surgically or medically treated with temporary symptoms of dementia

- Some infections (e.g., meningitis and encephalitis that are medically managed)
- Inflammation of the brain tissue due to various reasons
- Chronic renal failure that may cause a form of reversible dementia called *uremic encephalopathy*
- Prolonged dialysis may lead to reversible *dialysis dementia*
- Certain infections that go untreated or inadequately treated (e.g., syphilis)
- Chronic subdural hematomas; the resulting dementia may be reversed with surgical treatment of hematomas
- Such endocrine disorders as hypothyroidism, hyperthyroidism, and hyper-parathyroidism may cause reversible dementia
- Chronic mental illness (e.g., schizophrenia) that lead to progressive mental deterioration
- Neurocysticercosis, a common parasitic infection of the central nervous system due to the tissue-invading larval forms of the pork tapeworm *Taenia solium*; also known as the pork tape worm disease; found mostly in children; formerly limited to regions of Latin America, Asia, and Africa, but currently found in the United States
- Low sodium and calcium and high calcium may lead to reversible symptoms of dementia
- Persistence of subtle deficits and development of more serious and progressive dementia later in life

Onset and Early Symptoms
- Similar symptoms in reversible and progressive dementias
- Whether reversible or progressive, diagnosed with the same diagnostic criteria
- Associated symptoms based on the underlying pathology are important in the diagnosis (e.g., renal failure, hydrocephalus, pork tape worm infection, subdural hematomas, endocrine disorders, schizophrenia, metabolic disorders, or drug toxicity—each producing its own symptom complex besides dementia)

Progression and Advanced Characteristics
- By definition, reversible dementia should not lead to progression of symptoms
- The degree to which dementia will advance will depend on the timing and efficiency of treatment
- Only untreated underlying pathology may lead to more advanced symptoms of dementia; in which case, the reversible form will have been transformed into an irreversible form

Ala, T. A., Doss, R. C., & Sullivan, J. C. (2004). Reversible dementia: a case of cryptococcal meningitis masquerading as Alzheimer's disease. *Journal of Alzheimer's Disorder, 7*(2), 99–100.

Bourgeois, M. (2005). Dementia. In L. L. LaPointe (Ed.), *Aphasia and other neurogenic language disorders* (3rd ed., pp. 199–213). New York: Thieme.

Charfield, A. M. (2003). The decreasing prevalence of reversible dementia: an updated meta-analysis, *Archives of Internal Medicine, 163*(18), 2219–2229.

Cummings, J. L., & Benson, D. F. (1983). *Dementia: A clinical approach.* Boston, MA: Butterworth

Knopman, D. S., Petersen, R. C., Cha, R. H., Edland, S. D., & Rocca, W. A. (2006). Incidence and causes of nondegenerative nonvascular dementia: a population-based study. *Archives of Neurology, 63*(2), 218–221.

Saks, O., & Shulman, M. (2005). Steroid dementia: an overlooked diagnosis? *Neurology, 10;66*(1), 155.

Srikanth, S., & Nagaraja, A. V. (2005). A prospective study of reversible dementia: frequency, causes, clinical profile, and results of treatment. *Neurology India, 53*(3), 294–296.

Denasality (Hyponasality). Lack of nasal resonance on nasal sounds; a disorder of resonance; often due to some form of obstruction that prevents nasal resonance of speech; specific causes include upper respiratory infections that cause swelling of the nasal passage; obstructing pharyngeal flap, palatal obturator, palatal cleft, deviated nasal septum, or neurological impairments that cause improper timing of velopharyngeal closure; found in various neurogenic communication disorders; see Dysarthria and Voice Disorders.

Developmental Dysarthria. A motor speech disorder found in children whose speech and language acquisition is still in progress, although it may be acquired later in childhood; often due to congenital disorders that affect the neuromuscular growth; various neuromuscular diseases and disorders are associated with dysarthria in children; site of lesions may include the lower motor neuron, upper motor neuron, extrapyramidal system, and the cerebellar system; for details on developmental dysarthria, see Cerebral Palsy.

Diagnosis. A clinical activity designed to find the causes of diseases or disorders, especially in medicine and medical speech-language pathology; in communicative disorders for which there is no known physical or neurological cause, diagnosis often is aimed at describing and assessing the degree of severity of the disorders; requires a precise and reliable measurement of communicative behaviors; sometimes means the same as Assessment; see the companion volume, *Hegde's PocketGuide to Assessment in Speech-Language Pathology* (3rd ed.); diagnosis consists of the following activities:
- Taking a case history
- Interviewing the client, family members, or both
- Screening hearing
- Conducting an orofacial examination
- Administering standardized tests that are culturally and linguistically appropriate for the client
- Designing and using client-specific procedures
- Taking a comprehensive speech-language sample
- Analyzing the results and making a clinical judgment
- Writing a diagnostic report that includes recommendations

Diplegia. Paralysis of either the legs or the arms; see Cerebral Palsy.

Diplophonia. Double voice resulting from differential vibration of the two folds or vibration of both the true and false vocal folds; a form of Voice Disorder; causes of diplophonia include:

- Abnormal growth on one vocal fold (e.g., a large polyp) that makes it heavier so that it vibrates at a different frequency than the other
- Other structural anomalies of the laryngeal areas, including the laryngeal web
- Paralysis of one vocal fold
- Simultaneous true and false (ventricular) vocal fold vibrations

Distinctive Features. Multiple properties of phonemes that help distinguish one phoneme from the other; a method for classifying phonemes based on their special and common features; an approach to analyzing and grouping errors of articulation; see the companion volume, *Hegde's PocketGuide to Assessment in Speech-Language Pathology* (3rd ed.) for a description of the features and application in assessment of articulation disorders.

Diverticulum. A sac-like formation on the wall of an organ; a bulge in the layers of an organ wall; esophageal diverticulum is associated with Dysphagia.

Dopamine. A neurotransmitter; its depletion is associated with various neurodegenerative diseases that cause Dementia; offered as a form of pharmacological treatment for clients with certain kinds of dementia.

Dynamic Aphasia. The same as transcortical motor aphasia (see Aphasia: Specific Types).

Dysarthrias in Adults. A group of motor speech disorders resulting from impaired muscular control of the speech mechanism because of damage to the peripheral or central nervous system; oral communication problems, mostly speech production problems, due to weakness, incoordination, or paralysis of speech musculature; physiologic characteristics include abnormal or disturbed strength, speed, range, steadiness, tone, and accuracy of muscle movements; communication characteristics include disturbed pitch, loudness, voice quality, resonance, respiratory support for speech, prosody, and articulation; may be congenital or acquired, although much of the information presented here is most relevant to acquired disorders in adults; may be chronic, improving, or exacerbating-remitting; progressive when associated with neurodegenerative diseases; associated with the diagnosis of a neurological condition or disease; the most frequently occurring disorder among the neurogenic communication disorders; to be distinguished from apraxia of speech, a central (cortical) speech planning and programming disorder with no impairment in the peripheral nerves and muscles of speech production; to be distinguished from aphasia, a language disorder due to recent brain injury; also to be distinguished from dementia associated with significant intellectual and behavioral impairments that are not found in dysarthria; may be a coexisting condition in aphasia, especially Broca's aphasia and dementia; classified into *ataxic dysarthria, flaccid dysarthria, hyperkinetic dysarthria, hypokinetic dysarthria, mixed dysarthria, spastic dysarthria,* and *unilateral upper motor neuron dysarthria*; see also, Dysarthria: Specific Types to distinguish among them; also found in children; see Dysarthrias in Children.

Epidemiology and Ethnocultural Variables

- Epidemiology and ethnocultural variables associated with dysarthrias are poorly researched; available information on these factors is limited; reliable rates of the incidence of dysarthrias in the general population have not been established
- Medical speech-language pathologists work with a significant number of adults with dysarthrias and apraxias (motor speech disorders); dysarthrias are a notable consequence of many neurological diseases:
  - Roughly 25% of people who experience lacunar (minor) strokes have dysarthria
  - About 30% of people who sustain traumatic brain injury may have dysarthria
  - Up to 60% of individuals with Parkinson's disease may have dysarthria; may be higher in the advanced stage of the disease
  - Amyotrophic lateral sclerosis is associated with dysarthria in the early stages
  - Motor speech disorders (including dysarthrias and apraxia of speech) may constitute more than 40% of all acquired adult communication disorders
  - Dysarthrias may be more common than aphasia or apraxia of speech combined
  - No specific information is available on the distribution of dysarthrias across males and females and across various socioeconomic or ethnocultural groups
- Dysarthria may be acquired at any age, although it is more common in older people who are susceptible to various neurological diseases (including strokes)
  - In adults, the age of onset can be relatively easily established with a careful history and clinical and neurological examination
  - Such conditions as strokes and tumors help establish the age of onset
- The course of dysarthrias in adults varies, depending on the underlying neuropathological factors
  - Dysarthria in adults is *chronic* and stable when it is due to such congenital or early childhood conditions as cerebral palsy
  - Dysarthria may be a *temporary* (transient) problem in strokes and traumatic brain injury; in such instances, dysarthric symptoms, even if they do not completely resolve, improve significantly
  - Dysarthria may be *progressive* if associated with degenerative neurological diseases (e.g., AIDS dementia complex, Parkinson's disease, Pick's disease, Huntington's disease, or Alzheimer's disease)
  - Dysarthria may be *cyclic,* with periods of improvement and exacerbation of symptoms when associated with such disorders as multiple sclerosis

Neurophysiological Symptoms in Dysarthria

- Neurophysiological symptoms associated with dysarthria depend on the site and extent of lesion or lesions
  - Lesions in the lower motor neurons (also known as the *final common pathway*) negatively affect the normal activation of the muscles; lower motor neurons originate in the brainstem and spinal cord and are responsible for muscle tone, movement, and reflexes

- o Damage to a single alpha motor neuron may cause muscle weakness (Paresis)
- o Damage to all motor neurons that supply a muscle may cause Paralysis
- o Other effects of lower motor neuron lesions include impaired reflex actions and decreased muscle tone
- o Atrophy of paralyzed muscles
- o Damage to the lower motor neuron causes Flaccid Dysarthria (see Dysarthria: Specific Types)
- Lesions in the upper motor neuron system cause varied symptoms depending on the site of the lesion that may be either the *direct activation pathways* or the *indirect activation pathways* that constitute the system; upper motor neurons have their origins in the cerebral cortex (both hemispheres) and reach cranial and spinal nerve nuclei
- Direct activation pathways of the upper motor neuron system (also known as the *pyramidal* system or tract) are responsible for voluntary skilled movements and lesions in the pathways that cause varied effects
- o Lesions in the direct activation pathways affect consciously controlled skilled movements; movements may be absent or reduced, although reflexes remain unaffected
- o The effects of unilateral lesions are on the opposite side of the body; speech muscles are only minimally affected because of the bilateral supply to nerves involved in speech, including respiratory functions; unilateral lesions are associated with Unilateral Upper Motor Neuron Dysarthria (see Dysarthria: Specific Types)
- o Bilateral lesions in the upper motor neuron system are associated with Spastic Dysarthria (see Dysarthria: Specific Types)
- Indirect activation pathways of the upper motor neuron system (also known as the *extrapyramidal* system or tract) are responsible for posture and muscle tone and provide appropriate background for normal muscle movements; lesions in the direct action pathways cause several effects, although they also involve the direct activation pathways:
- o Lesions cause spasticity of the muscles and hyperadduction of the vocal folds
- o Bilateral lesions cause Spastic Dysarthria (see Dysarthria: Specific Types)
- Lesions in the motor control circuits produce their own specific effects; control circuits integrate and coordinate the functions of different motor systems; they are not in direct contact with the lower motor neurons; the control circuits are found in the basal ganglia and the cerebellum; effects of lesions depend on the specific circuits that are affected:
- o Lesions in the basal ganglia control circuit produce either Hypokinesia (reduced movement) or Hyperkinesia (involuntary and excessive movements)
- o Hypokinesia is associated with Hypokinetic Dysarthria (see Dysarthria: Specific Types) whereas hyperkinesia is associated with Hyperkinetic Dysarthria (see Dysarthria: Specific Types)
- Generally, lesions in the motor systems cause weakness, spasticity, incoordination, rigidity, reduced range of movement, and involuntary and uncontrolled

movements; movements may also be variable in speed and force and unsteady and inaccurate

Communication Disorders Associated with Dysarthria

- Dysarthria affects all aspects of speech production, including respiration, phonation, resonation, articulation, and prosody; pure dysarthria does not affect syntactic and morphologic aspects of speech; dysarthria may coexist with aphasia or dementia; specific constellation of symptoms depend on the type of dysarthria, although the different types share many common symptoms; features unique to the different types are described under Dysarthria: Specific Types; what follows is an overview of common symptoms.
- Respiratory problems: Damage to nerves that supply respiratory muscles can weaken or impair the sustained air supply needed for continuous speech; consequences on speech include:
  - Forced inspirations and expirations that interrupt speech, resulting in shorter phrases and sentences
  - Irregular breathing rate that may affect speech loudness, rhythm, and the length of phrases produced
  - Shallow, rapid, or effortful breathing that affects speech production
  - Running out of air before starting the next exhalation which may reduce phrase lengths and loudness of voice
  - Reduced lung capacity that limits the amount and duration of speech output
- Phonatory disorders: These disorders are due to damage to the nerves that innervate the vocal folds and related structures in the larynx; impaired respiratory control also will be a factor in causing certain phonatory abnormalities; the laryngeal abduction may be excessively forceful, weak and inadequate, or unstable, causing a variety of undesirable phonatory effects, including:
  - Pitch that is too high or too low
  - Abrupt variations in pitch, resulting in frequent pitch breaks
  - Lack of variations in pitch (monopitch)
  - Shaky or tremulous voice
  - Diplophonia (simultaneous production of both a lower and a higher pitch)
  - Too soft or too loud speech
  - Lack of variation in loudness, resulting in monoloudness
  - Sudden and excessive variation in loudness resulting in too loud or too soft speech
  - Loudness decay or progressive decrease in loudness resulting in inadequate loudness toward the end of utterances
  - Alternating changes in loudness
  - Harsh, rough, gravely voice
  - Hoarse, "wet" voice which is "liquid sounding" wet hoarseness
  - Continuous or intermittent breathiness
  - Strained-strangled, effortful phonation
  - Sudden and uncontrolled cessation of voice
- Articulation disorders: Due to impairments in the muscles of the jaw, lips, tongue, velum, vocal folds, caused by neuromotor control problems; include:
  - Generally slow and weak movement of the articulators
  - Imprecise consonant productions and weak pressure consonants

o Phoneme prolongations and repetitions
o Irregular breakdowns in articulation
o Distortion of vowels
o Inappropriate silent periods during speech
- Prosodic disorders: Disorders of speech rate, linguistic stress patterns, length of phrases or utterances, overall rhythm of speech, loci and duration of pauses in speech, and so forth; these impairments result in unnatural-sounding speech; speakers with dysarthria may exhibit:
  o Slower than the normal speech rate
  o Excessively rapid speech rate
  o An overall fast speech rate
  o Progressive increase in rate in certain segments of speech
  o Variable speech rate
  o Shorter phrase lengths
  o Reduced stress on stressed syllables
  o Equal stress on stressed and unstressed syllables
  o Excessive stress on unstressed syllables
  o Prolongation of intervals between words or syllables
  o Inappropriate pauses (silent intervals) in speech
  o Short rushes of speech
- Resonance disorders: These disorders are a function of impaired velopharyngeal function due to neuromotor control problems; velopharyngeal closure during speech production may be mildly or severely compromised, causing:
  o Hypernasality: Excessive nasal resonance on nonnasal speech sounds; due to inadequate closure of the velopharyngeal port during the production of oral sounds
  o Hyponasality: Reduced nasal resonance on nasal sounds due to complete or partial blockage of the nasal cavity
  o Nasal Emission: Air escaping through the nose associated with the production of oral speech sounds; often associated with velopharyngeal dysfunction; may be a feature of articulation
- Other characteristics: Dysarthria may include:
  o Slow diadochokinetic rate or alternating motion rate (AMRs)
  o Fast diadochokinetic rate or AMRs
  o Irregular diadochokinetic rate or AMRs
  o Palilalia (compulsive repetition of one's own utterances with increasing rate and decreasing loudness)
- Global characteristics of communication: The effects of most of the impaired speech parameters, especially the articulatory and prosodic deficiencies, result in:
  o Decreased intelligibility of speech
  o Clinically judged bizarreness of speech because of its unusualness or peculiarity

Etiologic Factors in Dysarthrias
- Dysarthrias in adults are due to varied etiologic factors, including vascular, traumatic, infectious, neoplastic, metabolic, toxic, inflammatory, and degenerative neuropathological factors that eventually affect motor speech

control; variation in the etiological factors and site of lesions result in different types of dysarthria

- The site of lesions that cause dysarthrias may be the central nervous system, the peripheral nervous system, or both; specifically, lesions may be found in:
  o Various cerebral cortical regions
  o Peripheral and cranial nerves
  o The brainstem
  o The cerebellum
  o The neuromuscular junction
  o The basal ganglia
  o The pyramidal pathways
  o The extrapyramidal pathways
- Varied clinical conditions create lesions in the different parts of the brain; most clinical conditions produce a constellation of symptoms that include motor speech disorders; common clinical conditions that lead to dysarthria include:
  o Degenerative neurological diseases including Parkinson's disease, Pick's disease, Alzheimer's disease, Wilson's disease, progressive supranuclear palsy, dystonia, Huntington's disease, amyotrophic lateral sclerosis (ALS), multiple sclerosis, myasthenia gravis, Friedreich's ataxia, and progressive dysarthria
  o Vascular diseases that lead to strokes; although vascular disorders themselves do not directly cause dysarthria, cell death that may follow strokes due to either ischemia or hemorrhage may be associated with dysarthria; clients with stroke may also have a concomitant aphasia; neurobehavioral and communicative symptoms are likely to improve; see Aphasia
  o Brainstem strokes; nearly 50% of clients who suffer a brainstem stroke that causes lesions in the pons, midbrain, cerebellum, or medullar may have dysarthria
  o Infections that include meningitis, encephalitis, HIV, and hypothesized prion infection thought to cause Creutzfeldt-Jakob Disease; also associated with Dementia
  o Chronic and severe kidney and liver diseases that affect brain functions and impair motor speech control; progressive if not checked in the early stages
  o Traumatic brain injury (TBI); unlike neurodegenerative diseases that have a slow onset, TBI has a sudden onset, as does dysarthria, which tends to improve; see Traumatic Brain Injury
  o Surgical trauma or accidents
  o Congenital conditions including cerebral palsy and Moebius syndrome
  o Toxic effects on the brain from alcohol and drugs; severe vitamin deficiencies; improvement with effective and early medical treatment
  o Brain tumors; in some cases, cancerous cells from elsewhere in the body metastasize and begin to grow in the brain; other tumors originate in the brain itself

o Paraneoplastic cerebellar degeneration; *paraneoplastic* refers to the indirect clinical effects of cancer; condition is associated with cancer of the breast, lung, and ovary

o Such endocrine disorders as hypothyroidism

D

Theories of Dysarthria

- The classic 1975 publication by Darley, Aronson, and Brown characterized dysarthria as a motor speech disorder; the constellation of symptoms found in the different types of dysarthria was explained on the basis of impaired muscular control of speech production; damage to the central and peripheral nervous system involved in motor control is the primary cause of dysarthria; weakness, incoordination, and paralysis of speech muscles are the proximal causes of the speech disorders; the neural damage and resulting muscle impairments are explained on the basis of varied disease, toxic, and other conditions that affect the nervous system; motor planning and programming deficits, the basis of apraxia of speech, did not figure in classical theories of dysarthria

- Recent explanations of dysarthria include the possibility of motor speech planning and programming impairments; because movement programming is a major function of the basal ganglia and cerebellar circuits that are often involved in dysarthria, impaired motor planning may be inherent to dysarthric speech; because brain lesions affect movement, clients with dysarthria may be unable to (1) sustain a motor plan throughout the execution of a motor activity (including speech), (2) switch from one activity (motor plan) to another, and (3) modify or inhibit a response that has been initiated; a programmed movement plan may decay before the action is initiated or completed causing difficulty initiating speech, general slowness of speech, frequent pauses in speech, problems in smooth movement through an utterance, and impaired rhythm of speech

Darley, F. L., Aronson, A. E., & Brown, J. R. (1975). *Motor speech disorders.* Philadelphia, PA: W. B. Saunders.

Duffy, J. R. (2005). *Motor speech disorders: Substrates, differential diagnosis, and management* (2nd ed.). St. Louis, MO: Elsevier Mosby.

Freed, D. (2000). *Motor speech disorders.* Clifton Park, NY: Thomson Delmar Learning.

Kent, R. D., Duffy, J. R., Slama, A., Kent, J. F., & Clift, A. (2001). Clinicoanatomic studies in dysarthria: Review, critique, and directions for research. *Journal of Speech, Language, and Hearing Research, 44,* 535–551.

Kent, R. D., Kent, J. F., Weismer, G., & Duffy, J. R. (2000). What dysarthria can tell us about the neural control of speech. *Journal of Phonetics, 28,* 273–302.

Kent, R. D., Vorperian, K. K., Kent, J. F., & Duffy, J. R. (2003). Voice dysfunction in dysarthria: Application of the Multi-Dimensional Voice Program. *Journal of Communication Disorders, 36,* 281–306.

Paslawski, T., Duffy, J. R., & Vermino, S. (2005). Speech and language findings associated with paraneoplastic cerebellar degeneration. *American Journal of Speech-Language Pathology, 14,* 200–207.

Soliveri, P., Piacentini, S., Carella, F., Testa, D., Ciano, C., & Girotti, F. (2003). Progressive dysarthria: Definition and clinical follow-up. *Neurological Science, 24,* 211–212.

Spencer, K. A., & Rogers, M. A. (2005). Speech motor programming in hypokinetic and ataxic dysarthria. *Brain and Language, 94,* 347–366.

Stolberger, C., Finsterer, J., Bran, E., & Taschabitscher, D. (2001). Dysarthria as the leading symptom of hypothyroidism. *American Journal of Otolaryngology, 22*(1), 70–72.

Teasell, R., Foley, N., Doherty, T., & Finstone, H. (2002). Clinical characteristics of clients with brainstem strokes admitted to a rehabilitation unit. *Archives of Physical Medicine and Rehabilitation, 83*(7), 1013–1016.

Vogel, D., & Cannito, M. P. (2001). *Treating disordered speech motor control* (2nd ed.). Austin, TX: Pro-Ed.

Yorkston, K. M., Beukelman, D. R., Strand, E. A., & Bell, K. R. (1999). Management of motor speech disorders in children and adults (2nd ed.). Austin, TX: Pro-Ed.

Dysarthria: Specific Types. Variations in etiologic factors and symptoms of dysarthria allow for a typological classification; beyond the general symptoms and etiologic factors described under Dysarthria, specific and unique characteristics are associated with the different types of this complex speech disorder; the major types of dysarthria are described alphabetically.

Ataxic Dysarthria. Type of motor speech disorder involving damage to the cerebellar system; Ataxia is a major neurological symptom, hence the name; characterized by slow, inaccurate movement and Hypotonia; distinguished from other types by its dominant articulatory and prosodic problems and disturbances, especially in the timing and coordination of speech movements that overshadow muscle weakness and limited range of movement; the cause is bilateral or generalized cerebellar lesions; found in 10% of all cases of dysarthria.

Neuropathology of Ataxic Dysarthria

- Degenerative and hereditary diseases that affect the cerebellum and related structures, causing ataxia and ataxic dysarthria, include:
  o Friedreich's ataxia, an inherited ataxia with mortality in about 20 years; includes corticospinal tract pathology, limb and gait ataxia, and dysarthria
  o Olivopontocerebellar atrophy, a hereditary or sporadic disease that affects both the cerebellum and the inferior olive and pontine nuclei
  o Spinocerebellar atrophy, another hereditary disease that affects the cerebellum and spinal cord tracts
- Multiple sclerosis (MS) that affects the cerebellum; a demyelinating disease of the nerves, MS is not limited to cerebellar structures and the presence of dysarthria is uncommon; in some cases, may be associated with ataxic dysarthria as well as spastic and mixed types

- Vascular lesions that affect the cerebellum and cause ataxia and ataxic dysarthria include:
  - Strokes involving the posterior inferior cerebellar artery in the medullary region, the anterior inferior cerebellar artery in the pons region, and the superior cerebellar artery in the midbrain region
  - Cerebellar hemorrhage and artereovenous malformations
- Tumors of the cerebellum cause ataxia and ataxic dysarthria; metastatic cancerous cells that attach themselves to cerebellar tissue and begin to grow; other tumors may have their origins in the cerebellum itself
- Traumatic brain injury (TBI) that affects the cerebellum
- Toxic conditions that affect the cerebellum include chronic alcoholism, drug abuse, prescription drug toxicity, and anticonvulsant drugs
- Endocrine deficiencies, especially hypothyroidism
- Normal pressure hydrocephalus
- Inflammatory conditions including meningitis and encephalitis that affect the cerebellum

Major Neurological Symptoms of Ataxic Dysarthria

- Abnormal stance and gait; difficulty standing and walking; instability of the trunk and head; frequent falls; rotated or tilted head posture
- Tremors and rocking or rotary motions involving the trunk or head
- Hypotonia; decreased muscle tone and decreased resistance to movement
- Ocular motor abnormalities including nystagmus (lateral or upward gaze and rapid and jerky back-and-forth eye movements)
- Movement disorders including over- or undershooting of targets; discoordinated movements; jerky, inaccurate, slow, imprecise, and halting movements
- Impaired alternating motion rates or diadochokinetic rate involving the jaw, lips, and tongue; irregular movements
- Incoordination of movement, rather than weaknesses in individual muscles

Major Speech Disorders of Ataxic Dysarthria

- Articulation disorders: Due to lack of coordination in the movements of the jaw, lips, and tongue; articulatory inaccuracy (slurred speech) with the following main characteristics:
  - Imprecise production of consonants
  - Irregular breakdowns in articulation and compression of syllable durations (*telescoping* of syllables)
  - Distortion of vowels
- Prosodic disorders: Prosodic excess, a result of slowness of movement; may not be found in all clients; characterized by:
  - Excessive and even stress on syllables, which results in syllable segregation
  - Prolonged phonemes
  - Excessive intervals between words or syllables
  - Reduced speech rate

- Phonatory-Prosodic disorders: Interrelated disorders of communication, caused by hypotonia of the muscles of phonation and respiration, resulting in:
  - Monopitch
  - Monoloudness
  - Explosive loudness in a few cases
  - Harshness
  - Drunken speech quality
  - Voice tremor (infrequent; atypical of ataxic dysarthria)
  - Uncommon resonance disorders, except for an occasional hyponasality
- Prominent articulatory problems in some, prosodic excess in others

Flaccid Dysarthria. A type of motor speech disorder due to damage to the motor units of the cranial or spinal nerves that supply speech muscles (involvement of the lower motor neuron or final common pathway); neurologists tend to describe this as bulbar palsy; flaccid (hypotonic) muscles are the main characteristic; causes include various degenerative, vascular, traumatic, infectious, neoplastic, metabolic, and toxic factors, and other factors cause the neuropathology; may account for about 9% of all types of dysarthrias combined; may affect only a single muscle group that controls either the articulatory or phonatory functions or may affect many muscle groups resulting in more generalized effects on speech; lesions in the brainstem and spinal cord affecting the muscles of speech are common to all subvarieties of flaccid dysarthria.

Neuropathology of Flaccid Dysarthria

- Neuropathologies affect the cranial nerves involved in speech production and the spinal nerves that directly control breathing and perhaps indirectly contribute to voice, speech, and resonance characteristics
- Cranial nerves that may be damaged include:
  - Trigeminal nerve (cranial V)
  - Facial nerve (cranial VII); unilateral and bilateral damage can cause articulation disorders involving bilabial and labiodental sounds; client may be unable to produce them; pressure consonants may be weak
  - Vagus nerve (cranial X)
  - Accessory nerve (cranial XI)
  - Hypoglossal nerve (cranial XII)
- Spinal nerves that may be damaged include:
  - Phrenic nerve
  - Thoracic and spinal nerves
- Physical trauma in nearly one-third of clients; surgical trauma during neurosurgery, laryngeal and facial surgery, head and neck surgery, plastic and dental surgery, and chest or cardiac surgery may damage the cranial nerves of speech; traumatic brain injury and neck injury due to automobile accidents, job-related accidents, personal violence, and falls
- Diseases of neuromuscular junction (loci of lower motor neuron and muscle tissue contact) associated with flaccid dysarthria include:
  - Myasthenia Gravis (MG); disease that causes fatigue with muscle contractions; recovery with rest

126

- o Botulism; disease involving botulinum toxins, affecting the neuromuscular transmission of messages
- Vascular diseases and brainstem strokes that directly affect the cranial nerves whose nuclei are located in the brainstem (lower motor neuron cell bodies); severe strokes may damage more than one cranial nerve involved in speech, causing a more severe form of flaccid dysarthria
- Infections, including:
  - o Polio that affects spinal nerves
  - o Secondary infections in AIDS clients
  - o Herpes zoster (a viral infection that tends to affect the V and VII cranial nerve ganglia)
- Demyelinating diseases including Guillain-Barre syndrome (degeneration of the myelin sheath around axons); infections may precede the onset; affected motor neurons cause facial muscle weakness, swallowing problems, and flaccid dysarthria
- Inherited muscle diseases, including:
  - o Myotonic Muscular Dystrophy, an autosomal dominant disease that affects muscle contractions
  - o Muscular Dystrophy, a genetic disorder of the skeletal muscles
- Degenerative diseases including motor neuron diseases, Progressive Bulbar Palsy, Amyotrophic Lateral Sclerosis (ALS), and Spinal Muscle Atrophies may cause flaccid dysarthria in about 13% of cases
- In about one-fourth of cases, the cranial nerve damage may be evident, but the cause may be unknown

Major Neurological Symptoms of Flaccid Dysarthria
- Because of the lesions in the final common pathway, reflexive, automatic, and voluntary movements are all affected
- Muscle weakness, hypotonia, muscle atrophy, and diminished reflexes
- Fasciculations (isolated twitches of resting muscles) and fibrillations (contractions of individual muscles)
- Possible muscle atrophy due to lesions in the spinal or cranial nerve nuclei
- Rapid and progressive weakness with use; recovery with rest (found in all neuromuscular junction diseases)

Major Speech Disorders of Flaccid Dysarthria
- Flaccid dysarthria is complex and varied because of the multiple cranial and spinal nerves that may be damaged with different combinations of symptoms
  - o Facial (VII) nerve damage: Unilateral and bilateral damage can cause articulation disorders involving bilabial and labiodental sounds; client may be unable to produce them; pressure consonants may be weak
  - o Glossopharyngeal (IX) nerve: Isolated damage is uncommon; damage is usually associated with a lesion in nerve X; effects on speech is not fully understood
  - o Vagus (X) nerve: Lesions cause breathiness, diplophonia, reduced pitch, pitch breaks, reduced loudness, short phrases, and mild to moderate hypernasality

D

- o Accessory (XI) nerve: Effects on speech are unclear or minimal; any effect it has is intertwined with that of nerve X
- o Hypoglossal (XII) nerve: Imprecise articulation
- o Multiple cranial nerve damage (bulbar palsy): A combination of effects depending on the specific nerves involved
- o Spinal nerve lesions: Possible indirect effects on respiration
- Respiratory disorders: May or may not be evident; damage to cervical and thoracic spinal nerves may cause:
  - o Respiratory weakness
  - o Decreased inhalation
  - o Disturbed exhalation during speech production
  - o Reduced subglottal air pressure
- Phonatory disorders: May be prominent signs, especially when combined with hypernasality
  - o Breathy voice, due to inadequate abduction of vocal folds during speech production
  - o Audible inspiration
  - o Strained vocal quality if respiration is affected
- Resonance disorders: Prominent symptoms include:
  - o Hypernasality, a prominent sign of flaccid dysarthria
  - o Nasal emission, due to velopharyngeal closure problems
- Phonatory-Prosodic disorders: Likely due to hypotonic laryngeal muscles
  - o Harsh voice
  - o Monopitch (lack of pitch variations)
  - o Monoloudness (lack of loudness variations)
  - o Reduced loudness if respiration is affected
  - o Short phrases if respiration is affected
- Articulation disorders
  - o Imprecise production of consonants, perhaps partly due to a prominent hypernasality
  - o Articulation disorders may be significant especially with lesions of cranial nerves V, VII, and X

Hyperkinetic Dysarthria. A type of motor speech disorder caused by damage to the basal ganglia (extrapyramidal system); the term *hyperkinetic* implies abnormal, excessive, and normally modulated or inhibited muscle activity; damage to the basal ganglia results in such abnormal involuntary movements as tics, chorea, myoclonus, tremor, and dystonia that interferes with speech production; hypotonic to hypertonic muscles; dominant speech symptoms include impaired loudness and rate of speech and frequently interrupted phonation; up to 22% of all cases of dysarthria may exhibit this type; varied causes including degenerative, vascular, traumatic, infectious, neoplastic, and metabolic factors; also caused by neuroleptic and antipsychotic drugs that cause dyskinesia and dystonia and such degenerative diseases as Huntington's Disease; causes are unknown in a majority of cases (about 67%); affected structures include the muscles of the face, jaw, tongue, palate, larynx, and respiration

Neuropathology of Hyperkinetic Dysarthria

- Damage to the basal ganglia and its controlled circuits; affects the typical function of refining and smoothing out the motor impulses generated in the cortex; results in uncontrolled involuntary movements
- Impaired balance between excitatory and inhibitory neurotransmitters within the basal ganglia control circuits; either an excess of dopamine or too little acetylcholine may cause excessive excitation; other brain chemicals may be involved in this disorder; see also Hypokinetic Dysarthria, in which the similar basal ganglia damage causes opposite motor effects
- Various diseases and disorders that cause damage to the basal ganglia include:
  - Toxic metabolic conditions; negative effects of neuroleptic and antipsychotic drugs that reduce or block dopamine production; high prevalence of tardive dyskinesia in individuals with schizophrenia who take antipsychotic drugs; antidepressants and cocaine also may cause dyskinesia
  - Oral contraceptives, alcohol withdrawal, hyperthyroidism, hypoglycemia, and hypoparathyroidism, among others, may cause chorea by affecting the functioning of the basal ganglia
  - Mercury, lead, and marijuana, among other toxic agents, may cause myoclonus associated with hyperkinetic dysarthria
- Various diseases that affect the nervous system, some progressive; prominent among them are:
  - Huntington's Disease, a progressive neurodegenerative autosomal inherited disease; affects both cortical structures and the basal ganglia; chorea is a major symptom
  - Sydenham's chorea, an infectious disease that causes chorea in children and young adults; not progressive and clears in most cases, but while it is active, chorea and dysarthria may both be present
  - Diphtheria, rubella, and Acquired Immune Deficiency Syndrome (AIDS)
- Strokes at the level of the basal ganglia and strokes that affect cerebellar control circuits
- Tumors in the basal ganglia and the thalamus

Major Neurological Symptoms of Hyperkinetic Dysarthria

- Predominance of movement disorders (*dyskinesia*); mostly because of damage to the basal ganglia control circuit
- Orofacial dyskinesia; abnormal and involuntary movements limited to facial and oral muscles
- Myoclonus; involuntary jerks of body parts, due to basal ganglia pathology; single or repetitive, rhythmic or nonrhythmic jerks
- Tics of the face and shoulders; voluntarily controllable, although typically occur without an effort to control them; some complex tics include jumping, making noises, lip smacking, and touching
- Tremors; involuntary and rhythmic movement of a body part; may be *resting tremors* that occur when the body is relaxed (repose), *postural tremors* that occur when the body is in a relatively stable position, and *essential tremor*, which occurs during sustained postures or actions

D

- Chorea; random, rapid, and apparently meaningless movements of the limbs, trunk, head, and neck
- Spasm; sudden and involuntary contraction of a muscle or group of muscles; may be tonic (prolonged or continuous) or clonic (repetitive, rapid, brief in duration)
- Dystonia; contractions of antagonistic muscles resulting in abnormal postures; *spasmodic torticollis* is intermittent dystonia and spasm of the neck muscles; *blepharospasm* is characterized by forceful and sustained closure of the eyes due to spasms of the orbicularis oculi muscle
- Athetosis; movement disorder which includes writhing, involuntary, slow, and purposeless movements, often of the hands

Major Speech Disorders of Hyperkinetic Dysarthria

- Dysarthric symptom complex depends on the dominant neurological symptoms or specific combinations of such symptoms; the nature of communication disorders depends on whether the dominant neurological condition is chorea, dystonia, athetosis, myoclonus, spasmodic torticollis, and so forth
- Dysarthria associated with **chorea** as a dominant neurological symptom has the following characteristics:
  - Unpredictable errors in speech because chorea that affects the speech and related muscles strikes unpredictably
  - Involvement of different speech muscles at different times
  - Minimal impairments in speech for brief durations
  - Prominent prosodic disorders with chorea; include prolonged intervals, variable speech rate, monopitch, inappropriate silence during speech, and monoloudness or excess variations in loudness
  - Imprecise articulation of consonants; distorted vowels; prolonged phonemes
  - Harsh vocal quality, excess loudness variation, and strained-strangled voice quality
  - Rapid and unpredictable inhalations and exhalations that affect speech rhythm
  - Hypernasality, although on occasion the speech may sound hyponasal
- Dysarthria associated with **myoclonus** (involuntary contractions of muscles) is typically not severe and may be characterized by:
  - Occasional cessation of voice due to adduction of the vocal folds
  - Slow rate of articulation
  - Imprecise articulation when the speech rate is increased
  - Reluctance to speak at a faster rate, possibly because of the client's awareness of imprecise articulation at increased rates
  - Intermittent hypernasality
  - Imprecise consonants
  - Brief phonatory interruptions
- Dysarthria associated with isolated **tic disorders**, or as a part of Tourette's Syndrome, may be accompanied by such psychiatric symptoms

as obsessive-compulsive behaviors, phobias, hyperactivity, and attention deficits; speech may be characterized by:
- o Echolalia (repetition of what is heard)
- o Palilalia (repetition of one's own utterances)
- o Coprolalia (compulsive production of obscene words)
- o Grunting, yelling, screaming, and moaning
- o Humming and whistling
- o Throat clearing and coughing
- Dysarthria associated with **voice tremors** or Essential (Organic) Tremors may be significant especially if vocal folds are affected by tremors; characteristics include:
  - o Quivering of voice
  - o Rhythmic waxing and waning of voice during speech production
  - o Abrupt voice arrests
  - o Tremor while prolonging vowels
  - o Tremor of the lips, tongue, or neck associated with vocal tremors
- Dysarthria associated with **dystonia** is characterized by:
  - o Imprecise production of consonants and distorted vowels; irregular articulatory breakdowns
  - o Harsh, strained-strangled voice quality
  - o Monopitch and monoloudness; inappropriate silence during speech production; excess loudness variations; short phrases; prolonged phonemes; reduced stress; and slower rate
- Generally, hyperkinetic dysarthria is characterized by:
  - o Voice tremor; intermittently strained voice; voice stoppage; vocal noise; harsh voice
  - o Intermittent hypernasality
  - o Slower rate; excess loudness variations; prolonged inter-word intervals; inappropriate silent intervals; equal stress
  - o Audible inspiration; forced and sudden inspiration/expiration
  - o Imprecise consonants; distortion of vowels; inconsistent articulatory errors

Hypokinetic Dysarthria. A type of motor speech disorder caused by damage to the basal ganglia (extrapyramidal system); respiratory, phonatory, articulatory, and prosodic features may all be affected; prominent speech characteristics include voice, articulation, and prosodic disorders, especially impaired rate of speech; called *hypokinetic* because markedly restricted range of movement; rigidity of muscles and slowed movement also are important features; found in roughly 8% of all individuals with dysarthrias; damage to basal ganglia and degenerative neurological diseases account for a majority of cases; *hypokinetic* muscles are not to be confused with *hypotonic* muscles; hypokinetic muscles are slow to move, not of reduced tone; hypokinesia is characterized by increased tone and rigidity of muscles whereas hypotonia is characterized by decreased tone and flabby muscles.

D

Neuropathology of Hypokinetic Dysarthria
- Varied factors that result in damage to the basal ganglia control circuits
- Perhaps in more than a third, hypokinetic dysarthria is associated with idiopathic and degenerative Parkinson's Disease; in up to 30% of cases, Parkinson's disease terminates in dementia; of unknown cause (idiopathic) but clients respond to levodopa treatment; dopamine-producing cells in the substantia negra are degenerated; basal ganglia damage can have opposite effects in different individuals; in Parkinson's disease, basal ganglia damage is associated with reduced dopamine levels, leading to hypokinesia and hypokinetic dysarthria; in Huntington's Disease, the similar basal ganglia damage results in hyperkinesia and hyperkinetic dysarthria presumably because of either too much dopamine or too little acetylcholine that have an excitatory effect
- In about a quarter of individuals who have hypokinetic dysarthria, the cause may be Parkinsonism, which shares some common symptoms with the idiopathic Parkinson's disease, but the two are etiologically different; parkinsonism refers only to a pattern of symptoms that may have varied and known etiology (unlike Parkinson's disease); parkinsonian symptoms may be associated with some strokes, Alzheimer's disease, and drug-induced clinical conditions; drugs used to treat psychotic conditions and Tourette's syndrome (and other dyskinesias) may induce parkinsonian symptoms; withdrawal of these drugs will reduce or eliminate the symptoms
- Strokes that produce diffuse frontal lobe damage
- Cerebral hypoxia and carbon monoxide poisoning
- Heavy metal toxicity (e.g., manganese) or chemical toxicity (e.g., carbon disulfide, cyanide, and methanol)
- Alcohol withdrawal that cause parkinsonian symptoms that eventually clear
- Traumatic brain injury and repeated brain injury (e.g., of the kind boxers experience)
- Among infections, Acquired Immune Deficiency Syndrome (AIDS)
- Normal pressure hydrocephalus and obstructive hydrocephalus

Major Neurological Symptoms of Hypokinetic Dysarthria
- Most of the neurological symptoms described are found in Parkinson's disease or parkinsonism
- Tremor at rest; clients may have tremors in relaxed facial, mouth, and limb structures that diminish when moved voluntarily
- *Pill-rolling* movement between the thumb and forefinger is a hallmark of parkinsonian symptom complex
- Rigidity (resistance to passive stretch)
- Bradykinesia (delayed or slow initiation of movement); reduce speed of movement; sudden freezing of movement
- Lack of facial expression (mask-like face); infrequent blinking; lack of smiling; reduced hand and facial movements during speech
- Micrographic writing (small print)

- Walking disorders (slow to begin, then short, rapid, shuffling steps known as *festinating gait*)
- Postural disturbances (involuntary flexion of the head, trunk, and arm; difficulty changing positions)
- Decreased swallowing resulting in accumulated saliva in the mouth, possibly drooling

D

Major Speech Disorders of Hypokinetic Dysarthria

- Most of the speech disorders of hypokinetic dysarthria have been observed in clients with Parkinson's disease or those with parkinsonian symptoms
- Phonatory disorders: Hoarse, rough, unsteady, and breathy voice; monopitch and monoloudness; periodic aphonia (complete loss of phonation); inadequate adduction of the vocal folds; may be prominent or even presenting symptoms
- Prosodic disorders: Phonatory disorders have an effect on prosodic features of speech; for example, monoloudness and monopitch negatively affect the intonational patterns that characterize normal speech prosody; reduced linguistic stress, inappropriate silent intervals in speech, short rushes of speech, variable and increased speech rate in segments, and short phrases
- Articulation disorders: Imprecise consonants; stops, fricatives, and affricates, and especially stops, may be most often misarticulated; repeated phonemes
- Resonance disorders: Only mild hypernasality may be present in up to 25% of cases
- Respiratory problems: Reduced vital capacity, irregular breathing, faster rate of respiration, and shallow breathing due to limited movements of respiratory muscles
- Fluency problems: Repetition of phonemes; repetition of own words and phrases (palilalia) with increasing rate and decreasing loudness; dysfluencies that may sound like prolongations

Mixed Dysarthria. A type of motor speech disorder that is a combination of two or more pure dysarthrias; varied and multiple neuropathology; any and all combinations of pure dysarthrias are possible; two types are mixed in about 84% of cases; three types may be mixed in about 12%; flaccid-spastic combination is the most common (42% of the mixed cases), followed by the ataxic-spastic (23%) combination; varied patterns of speech disorders depending on the types of pure dysarthrias that are mixed; more common than the pure types of dysarthria because about 30% of all dysarthria clients have the mixed type, possibly because cerebral damage often has widespread effects, involving both the upper and lower motor neurons and different divisions of the nervous system.

Neuropathology of Mixed Dysarthria

- Multiple etiologic factors in the same client; multiple strokes or coexistence of strokes and Parkinson's disease; diseases that affect all of the motor systems and different parts of the nervous system

D

- Multiple Sclerosis (MS), progressive demyelinating disease with an unpredictable course affecting the brainstem, cerebellum, cerebral hemispheres, and spinal cord; demyelination of fibers in only one or the other structure is possible and produces focal symptoms; gait, visual, and sensory problems
- Various motor neuron diseases, which damage or destroy upper motor neurons, lower motor neurons, or both; spinal muscle atrophies, progressive bulbar palsy, primary lateral sclerosis, and Amyotrophic Lateral Sclerosis (ALS) are among the specific motor neuron diseases; of these, ALS is the most common disease associated with flaccid-spastic mixed dysarthria, although it may be a single type in the beginning stage of the disease
- Multisystems atrophy, a varied group of degenerative neurological disorders; spastic-ataxic-hypokinetic, hypokinetic-ataxic, and ataxic-spastic dysarthrias may be found in Shy-Drager syndrome; mixed hypokinetic-spastic dysarthrias are common in progressive supranuclear palsy; features of ataxic, spastic, flaccid, or hypokinetic types may be combined in olivopontocerebellar atrophy
- Among the toxic-metabolic conditions, Wilson's Disease is notable; a rare form of hereditary disorder that impairs copper metabolism; associated with hypokinetic, spastic, and ataxic dysarthrias; speech disorder may be the early sign of the disease
- Friedreich's Ataxia, an inherited neurodegenerative disease that affects the cerebellum, brainstem, and spinal cord with the predominance of ataxia, may cause ataxic-spastic dysarthria
- Tumors and traumatic brain injury

Major Neurological Symptoms of Mixed Dysarthria

- Neurological symptoms associated with mixed dysarthria are highly varied, depending on the underlying neurological disease or disorder
- In some individuals, damage to certain specific components of the motor system may be more severe than damage to other components; functions associated with the more severely damaged part of the motor system will be prominent compared to the functions of the less severely damaged part
- Multiple sclerosis, characterized by such focal symptoms as ataxia in some persons, and such varied and generalized symptoms as visual problems (e.g., diplopia and impaired central vision), chronic fatigue, weakness and painful spasticity in the limbs, especially in the legs, and sensory impairments (numbness, itching, and tingling)
- Amyotrophic lateral sclerosis; with spinal nerve damage, weakness in arms and legs, hypotonia, and muscle atrophy; with cranial nerve damage, facial and oral weakness along with dysphagia; weakness and spasticity associated with upper motor neuron involvement
- Neurological symptoms of clients with Wilson's disease include rigidity, bradykinesia, tremor, limb apraxia, and dysphagia; personality change and cognitive impairments
- Neurological symptoms of clients with Friedreich's ataxia include weakness and muscle atrophy in the arms and legs; initial symptoms of unsteady and clumsy movements

- Olivopontocerebellar atrophy causes ataxia and uncoordinated movements of the arms and legs along with tremor and numbness in the extremities
- Progressive supranuclear palsy limits voluntary eye movements; such parkinsonian symptoms as difficulty walking and rigidity of muscles, and spasticity of the limbs, face, or neck are additional features
- Shy-Drager syndrome that causes bradykinesia, akinesia, and rigidity; tremors are not typical; limbs may be mildly spastic; ataxia may be present in some individuals

Major Speech Disorders of Mixed Dysarthria

- The constellation of speech disorders depend on the individual (pure) types of dysarthria that are mixed; major symptoms of each type may be evident; in some cases, the symptoms of the two (or more) mixed types may all be equally evident; in other cases, symptoms of one pure type may be more prominent than the symptoms of the other type
- Depending on the disease process underlying dysarthria, the symptom complex may change over time from pure to mixed to mixed with dominant symptoms of one type to equally dominant symptoms of the mixed types; for instance, in the degenerative motor neuron disease amyotrophic lateral sclerosis (ALS), the initial involvement is lower motor neurons, resulting in relatively pure flaccid dysarthria; the disease eventually affects upper motor neurons, causing flaccid-spastic mixed dysarthria, with dominant flaccid symptoms; further progression of the disease into the upper motor neurons will result in somewhat equally prominent flaccid and spastic symptoms
- Constellation of symptoms of mixed flaccid-spastic dysarthria associated with ALS include (in their order of importance or frequency) imprecise production of consonants, hypernasality, harsh voice, slow rate, monopitch, short phrases, distorted vowels, low pitch, monoloudness, excess and equal stress or reduced stress, prolonged intervals, prolonged phonemes, strained-strangled quality, breathiness, audible inspiration, inappropriate silences, and nasal emission
- Constellation of speech problems associated with MS is a combination of ataxic and spastic dysarthrias; a majority of clients with MS have normal speech or only minor impairments; significant speech problems, when present, include (in their order of importance or frequency), impaired loudness control, harsh voice quality, imprecise articulation, impaired emphasis, decreased vital capacity, hypernasality, inappropriate pitch level, breathiness, increased breathing rate, and sudden articulatory breakdowns
- Wilson's disease is associated with symptoms of ataxic, spastic, and hypokinetic dysarthrias; speech disorders include (in their order of importance and frequency) imprecise consonant production, hypernasality, harsh voice quality, slow rate, monopitch, short phrases, distorted vowels, low pitch, monoloudness, and excess and equal stress

Spastic Dysarthria. A type of motor speech disorder caused by bilateral damage to the upper motor neuron (direct and indirect motor pathways);

neurologists tend to describe this as *pseudobulbar palsy* because of the paralysis of the bulbar muscles and similarity of symptoms with bulbar palsy and flaccid dysarthria caused by lower motor neuron lesions; varied causes of neuropathology causing lesions in multiple cortical and subcortical areas; neuropathology affects respiratory, phonatory, resonatory, and articulatory aspects of speech production; muscle spasticity (increased tone) is the major neurological symptom, and hence the name; approximately 8% of all clients with dysarthria may have the spastic type.

Neuropathology of Spastic Dysarthria
- Damage to the pyramidal (direct activation) and extrapyramidal (indirect activation) pathways or tracts of the upper motor neuron
- Pyramidal system contains two main tracts; one leads to cranial nerve nuclei (corticobulbar tract) and the other leads to spinal nerve nuclei (corticospinal tract) in the brainstem and spinal cord; damage to the pyramidal system impairs fine motor skills, including speech; movements of the tongue, lips, and velum will be affected
- Extrapyramidal system, a complex system of interconnections in the basal ganglia, cerebellum, reticular formation, vestibular nuclei, and red nucleus, helps maintain posture and tone and provides appropriate background for efficiently executed skilled movements; damage to this system causes weakness, spasticity (too much muscle tone), and impaired reflexes; to cause spastic dysarthria, the damage must be bilateral (both the left and right tracts of the two systems) because most of the speech structures (except for the tongue and the lower face) receive bilateral innervation; unilateral damage causes a milder form of dysarthria (called unilateral upper motor neuron dysarthria)
- Strokes due to vascular disorders; more often associated with spastic dysarthria than with other types
  o A single stroke within the brainstem where both the right and left pyramidal and extrapyramidal system fibers are found
  o Two strokes, one in each hemisphere; but not a single stroke in either hemisphere
  o A single stroke in one hemisphere combined with an old damage in the other hemisphere (due to previous trauma, tumor, or stroke)
  o Multiple small strokes in such deeper structures as the basal ganglia and the thalamus (lacunar states)
- Degenerative diseases, primarily amyotrophic lateral sclerosis; in many individuals, unknown or unspecified degenerative diseases
- Extensive traumatic head injury that affects the pyramidal and extrapyramidal systems
- Multiple sclerosis, brainstem tumors, and viral and bacterial infections of the brain

Major Neurological Symptoms of Spastic Dysarthria
- Spasticity (increased muscle tone) is the dominant neurological symptom; may be especially evident in the laryngeal muscles and in the velum to some extent

- Muscle weakness, especially bilateral facial weakness; may be especially noticeable in the tongue and lips; the jaw strength may be normal and lower face weakness may be less pronounced
- Slowness of movement; especially noticeable in the tongue and lips; restricted range of movements; slow nonspeech alternating motion rates
- Hyperactive gag reflex; such pathological reflexes as sucking
- Loss of fine, skilled movement; increased muscle tone
- Generally, impaired movement patterns, not weakness of individual muscles
- Hyperadduction of vocal folds and inadequate closure of the velopharyngeal port
- Dysphagia (swallowing disorders) and drooling
- Pathological laughing or crying; mismatch between emotional experiences and expressions

Major Speech Disorders of Spastic Dysarthria

- All aspects of speech production may be impaired to varying degrees in spastic dysarthria
- Prosodic disorders: Excess and equal stress, slow rate of speech, monopitch and monoloudness, reduced stress, and short phrases
- Articulation disorders: Imprecise production of consonants and distorted vowels
- Phonatory disorders: Continuous breathy voice, harshness, low pitch, pitch breaks, strained-strangled voice quality, and short phrases
- Resonance disorders: <u>Hypernasality</u>

Unilateral Upper Motor Neuron (UUMN) Dysarthria. Type of motor speech disorder caused by damage to the upper motor neurons, impairing the function of cranial and spinal nerves involved in speech production; face and tongue weakness; frequent causes are vascular disorders; with the left hemisphere lesion, may coexist with <u>Aphasia</u> or <u>Apraxia</u>; with the right hemisphere lesion, may coexist with <u>Right Hemisphere Syndrome</u>; temporary speech disorder in some, lasting in others; articulation, phonation, and prosodic features; dominant muscle weakness and some spasticity and incoordination; less well understood than other types of dysarthria because it is the latest type of dysarthria to be recognized; it may be found in about 8% of all clients diagnosed with dysarthria; the incidence may be higher if UUMN dysarthria is counted in people with aphasia and apraxia.

Neuropathology of UUMN Dysarthria

- The bilateral upper motor neuron system originates in both hemispheres and has two sets of pathways: the direct (pyramidal) and the indirect (extrapyramidal); when both are damaged, the result in spastic dysarthria; when only one side of the upper motor neurons are damaged, the result is the UUMN type
- Unilateral damage to upper motor neurons produces less severe speech consequences because most of the cranial nerves supplying the speech muscles (except for those of the lower face and tongue) are supplied bilaterally, and thus will remain supplied from the undamaged side of the brain

D

- The muscles of the lower face and tongue that do not have bilateral supply will be the most affected in UUMN lesions; the side opposite the brain damage will be the most affected; left UUMN lesions produce marked weakness on the right side of the lower face and tongue and vice versa
- Vascular diseases that lead to strokes are the most frequent causes of UUMN dysarthria (in about 90% of cases diagnosed with this type of dysarthria)
- Tumors and traumatic brain injuries, including accidental surgical injuries, add up to another 8% of clients with UUMN dysarthria
- Degenerative, inflammatory, and toxic-metabolic diseases are not the common causes of UUNM dysarthria because such clinical conditions produce more diffuse effects, which are unlike the more focal effects of UUMN damage
- Most clients are likely to have lesions in their left hemispheres whereas some will have them in their right hemispheres; when the lesions are large, the left hemisphere is rarely spared

Major Neurological Symptoms of UUMN Dysarthria

- Neurological symptoms are evident on the body side that is contralateral to the side of brain damage
- Hemiplegia and hemiparesis are common neurological symptoms, found in nearly 80% of cases
- Unilateral lower face weakness is the most dominant neurological symptom, found in excess of 80% of clients
- Unilateral tongue weakness is found in more than 50% of clients
- Unilateral palatal weakness and sensory deficits may be found in a small number of individuals

Major Speech Disorders of UUMN Dysarthria

- Less than 20% of clients with UUMN lesions may have dysarthria, although its presence may be masked in clients who have such other disorders as aphasia and apraxia
- Articulation disorders: Imprecise consonants are the most common speech disorder found across a vast majority of clients with UUMN dysarthria; irregular articulatory breakdowns and vowel distortions
- Phonatory disorders: Harsh voice, reduced loudness, sometimes excess loudness variation, strained-harshness, wet hoarseness, monoloudness, monopitch, unsteady voice, and breathiness constitute the phonatory disorders although harshness is the most frequently observed phonatory feature
- Prosodic disorders: A slow rate of speech with increased rate in segments, excess and equal stress, sometimes reduced stress, short phrases
- Resonance disorders: Hypernasality, nasal resonance, or both

Darley, F. L., Aronson, A. E., & Brown, J. R. (1975). *Motor speech disorders*. Philadelphia, PA: W. B. Saunders.

Darley, F. L., Aronson, A. E., & Brown, J. R. (1969a). Differential diagnostic patterns of dysarthria. *Journal of Speech and Hearing Research, 12*, 246–269.

Darley, F. L., Aronson, A. E., & Brown, J. R. (1969b). Clusters of deviant speech dimensions in the dysarthrias. *Journal of Speech and Hearing Research, 12,* 462–496.

Duffy, J. R. (2005). *Motor speech disorders* (2nd ed.). St. Louis, MO: C. V. Mosby.

Freed, D. (2000). *Motor speech disorders.* Clifton Park, NY: Thomson Delmar Learning.

D

Dysfluencies. Speech characteristics that interrupt fluency; may be measured in diagnosing stuttering; include such specific types as repetitions, prolongations, interjections, revisions, and incomplete phrases; may constitute a fluency disorder if the frequency exceeds normal limits (often 5% of the words spoken); see Stuttering under Fluency Disorders for a description of different forms.

Dysgraphia. Writing problems due to neurological injury; it is not due to lack of education or inadequate instruction; the same as Agraphia.

Dyskinesia. Muscle movement disorder due to brain injury; aberrant and involuntary movements; caused by a variety of etiological factors; speech disorders associated with muscle movement impairments are described under Dysarthria; common varieties of dyskinesias include:

- Orofacial dyskinesia: Abnormal involuntary movements of oral and facial muscles; seriously affect speech production; often due to lesions in the basal ganglia
- Tardive dyskinesia: A form of orofacial dyskinesia due to long-term use of antipsychotic drugs, resulting in oro-buccal-lingual dyskinesia characterized by involuntary and repetitive lip smacking and puffing, tongue protrusion, and uncontrolled jaw movements
- Akathisia: Restless movements (pacing, constant weight shitting) associated with Parkinson's disease

Dysostosis. Abnormal ossification; anomalous ossification of fetal cartilages; characteristic of several Syndromes Associated With Communication Disorders.

Dysphagia. Disorders of swallowing; problems in the execution of the oral, pharyngeal, and/or esophageal stages of swallow; problems in chewing food, preparing it for swallow, initiating the swallow, propelling the bolus through the pharynx, and in passing the food through the esophagus; speech-language pathologists assess and treat oropharyngeal disorders of swallowing; esophageal swallowing disorders are handled medically, although speech-language pathologists play a role in their overall clinical management; causes include a variety of diseases, including neuropathologies, cancer and the consequent surgical treatment (laryngectomy), mechanical obstructions within the swallowing mechanism, and brain injury; a majority of clients with dysphagia are assessed and treated in medical settings because of the associated diseases and the need for medical management; may be life threatening if not managed properly; the disorders occur at any age although more common in the elderly; may be unrecognized in some clients who do not complain of swallowing difficulty, possibly because the clients compensate for the problems.

D

Epidemiology and Ethnocultural Variables

- Dysphagia is not a unitary disorder that exists by itself; coexists with a multitude of other neurophysiological and behavioral symptoms; dysphagia is a result of several diseases and brain injury that produce a complex set of varied symptoms; therefore, it is hard to establish its incidence and prevalence in the general and specific ethnocultural populations
- In a large, comprehensive rehabilitation facility, nearly one-third of all clients may have swallowing difficulties
- In excess of 60% of clients in neuropsychiatric hospitals who cannot feed themselves may have swallowing problems
- Clients who have had head and neck surgery tend to have a high prevalence of swallowing disorders (close to 60%), followed by those who have had strokes (just under 50%); most clients with dementia have dysphagia; closed head injury, spinal cord injury, and degenerative neurological diseases also are contributors
- The prevalence of dysphagia is the highest in older people (age 65 and older) because of increased incidence of neurological diseases with which dysphagia is associated; although normal aging affects the efficiency of the swallowing mechanism, it typically does not create clinically significant swallowing difficulties

Normal Swallow

- Feeding versus swallowing: As activities, self-feeding or feeding by others and swallowing are interrelated; feeding is the transportation of food from the plate to the mouth; it is essential for the swallowing processes, which is the transportation of food from the mouth to the stomach; although self-feeding may be impaired in otherwise normal or healthy individuals (as in the case of injured hands placed in casts), feeding and swallowing disorders may coexist in many cases; see Feeding Disorders
- Mastication versus swallowing: Chewing solid or semisolid foods is called mastication; mastication is a part of the oral preparatory phase of the swallow; it is an activity that precedes swallowing (deglutition)
- Normal swallow has been described as a series of activities within four phases: Oral preparatory, oral, pharyngeal, and esophageal, although some experts consider the oral preparatory and oral phases as the single oral phase; the act of swallow does not take place in a series of discrete stages; a phase may be divided into subphases (see the *oral preparatory phase*), but phases and subphases are interrelated; oral preparatory and oral phases are not discrete; there is an overlap between the activities of the oral and pharyngeal phases of swallow; the concept of phases is retained only as a descriptive tool
- Oral preparatory phase: Food is prepared for swallow; food placed in the mouth and prepared for swallow is called a *bolus*; solid or semisolid food placed in the mouth needs to be transformed into a chewed and soft mass that is mixed with saliva; if the food requires chewing, the oral preparatory phase is sometimes subdivided into a *transport phase* during which the tongue moves the food posteriorly, places it between the molars, and a *reduction phase* in which the food is masticated into a cohesive bolus;

obviously, these subphases are not discrete acts; in the case of food that requires mastication, the following activities are parts of the oral preparatory phase in which the food is manipulated in the mouth:

o After the placement of the food in the mouth, the lips close to create a lip seal

o The tongue moves laterally to transport the food to the grinding surface of the teeth (the molars) so the person can chew the food

o The tongue moves vertically, mixes the food with saliva to make it easier to swallow and form the bolus as preparation for swallowing (hence the name, *oral preparatory*)

o The bolus, prepared through mastication and salivary mixing, is again placed on the tongue, transported to the oropharynx to initiate swallowing through the pharynx and the esophagus; elevation of the velum, contractions of the lips and the buccal muscles, posterior tongue depression, and pressing of the tonge against the hard palate are among the movements necessary for oral transport of the bolus

o If the food to be swallowed is liquid, it may be briefly held between the tongue and the anterior hard palate before initiating its pharyngeal swallow; some individuals hold their liquid bolus on the tongue surface and others on the floor of the mouth

o Cranial nerves V, VII, IX, and X provide sensory information (taste and smell) about the food that is essential for swallow; cranial nerves V, VII, IX, X, and XII control the muscles involved in the oral preparatory (and oral) phases of swallow

• Oral phase: Tongue action is the critical feature of this phase; swallowing begins with the tongue action that moves the bolus posteriorly; an anterior to posterior rolling action of the tongue is involved in moving the food toward the back of the mouth; the phase ends as the pharyngeal swallow reflex is initiated; the following activities consist of the oral phase:

o A labial seal is maintained through the closed lips; the lateral and anterior margins of the tongue are pressed against the alveolar ridge to form a seal

o The midline of the tongue moves the bolus posteriorly through a squeezing action; the sides and the tip of the tongue are positioned against the alveolar ridge to induce a sucking action; the greater the thickness of the bolus, the higher the tongue pressure needed to move the bolus back

o The buccal muscles act to keep the food out of the lateral sulcus

o The soft palate is then elevated so that the bolus can pass through the anterior faucial pillars; the soft palate and the posterior pharyngeal wall come into contact to prevent food or liquid from entering the nasal cavity

o The oral phase of swallow for a bolus is completed in 1 to 1.5 seconds

o Cranial nerves specified in the oral preparatory phase also are involved in the oral phase because the same structures are involved in both phases

• Pharyngeal phase: Reflex actions of the swallow that are triggered by the contact the food makes with the anterior faucial pillars is the beginning of the pharyngeal phase of the swallow; includes such functions as the velophryngeal closure, laryngeal closure by an elevated larynx that seals the airway, and the consequent interruption in breathing; reflexive relaxation of the

D

cricopharyngeal muscle for the bolus to inter; reflexive contractions of the pharyngeal contractors to move the bolus down and eventually into the esophagus; the main actions (movements) of this phase are as follows:

o Sensory information about the bolus to be swallowed, received by the brainstem and the cortical regions, is thought to trigger the actions involved in the pharyngeal phase of the swallow

o The pharyngeal swallow reflex is triggered when the tip of the bolus passes the anterior faucial pillars in younger people and at a lower point in middle-aged adults (the point where the tongue base crosses the lower edge of the mandible)

o The velopharyngeal port is closed by an elevated velum that moves back to make contact with the pharyngeal wall to prevent the entry of food or liquid into the nasopharynx

o Elevation of the larynx and the hyoid bone and the closure of the larynx at the level of the true vocal folds, false vocal folds, and the epiglottis help prevent aspiration

o Relaxation and opening of the cricopharyngeal sphincter allows food and liquid to move from the pharynx to the esophagus

o The tongue assumes a ramp-like shape to transport the bolus toward the pharynx; when the tail end of the bolus reaches the tongue base, the tongue base retracts and the pharyngeal wall contracts; the tongue base and the pharyngeal wall make contact

o Pharyngeal wall contractions keep the bolus moving through the pharynx until it reaches the upper esophageal spincter, which then begins to move the bolus down (the beginning of the esophageal phase of swallow); the transit time for the pharyngeal phase of swallow is about 1 second

o It is thought that both voluntary and reflexive actions are involved in the pharyngeal phase (as well as oral phase) swallow

o Cranial nerves V, VII, IX, and X carry sensory information about the swallow to the brainstem's swallowing center; cranial nerves IX, X, and XI are mainly responsible for the motor aspect of pharyngeal swallow

• Esophageal phase: This is an involuntary swallowing phase; the esophagus is a muscular tube that helps transmit food from the pharynx to the stomach; at both ends, the tube has short segments that contract to move the food down; the esophagus is narrower at the top and wider as it reaches the stomach; this phase of swallow begins when the food arrives at the orifice of the esophagus (the cricopharyngeal juncture or sphincter); peristaltic action of the esophagus propels the food into the stomach; this movement is aided by gravity; bolus entry into the esophagus results in restored breathing and a depressed larynx and soft palate; in swallowing, the main actions (movements) of this phase are as follows:

o Two important actions of the esophagus are the peristaltic movements that propel the bolus down and relaxation of the segments of the muscular tube just below the bolus that facilitates smooth movement of the bolus

o Peristaltic movements are sequential and continue until the food reaches the lower esophageal sphincter which opens to receive the bolus; the bolus then reaches the stomach

- o The esophageal bolus transmit time is about 8 to 20 seconds
- o The actions of the esophagus, being involuntary (reflexive), are controlled mostly by the vagus nerve (cranial nerve X), which has sensory, motor, and autonomic fibers; the recurrent laryngeal branches of nerve X innervate the cervical and the thoracic sections of the esophagus; in addition, the thoracic section of the esophagus is innervated by the main fibers of cranial nerve X; the esophagus has both sympathetic and parasympathetic innervations

Swallowing Disorders

- Swallowing disorders of the oral preparatory phase: These include the disorders of mastication, sometimes described separately; a wide range of disorders may be observed during the oral preparatory phase of swallow; major disorders of this phase and their main causes are as follows:
  - o Problems in chewing food; causes include reduced range of lateral and vertical tongue movement, reduced range of lateral mandibular movement, reduced buccal tension, and poor alignment of mandible and maxilla
  - o Difficulty holding food in the anterior portion of the mouth; mostly likely cause is the weak lips that cannot close firmly or because the client is a mouth breather who needs to keep the mouth open during this stage of swallow
  - o Difficulty holding the bolus; the bolus, especially if it is liquid or of paste consistency, needs to be held in the mouth before it enters the pharynx; difficulty holding the bolus in the mouth can send the food prematurely to the pharynx, potentially causing aspiration; reduced tongue movement and coordination is the main reason for this difficulty
  - o Difficulty forming a bolus before swallow; mostly due to weakness of the tongue that prevents the gathering of masticated food into a bolus
  - o Abnormal holding of the bolus; the bolus is held for a short duration either between the tongue and the hard palate or in the floor of the mouth; poor tongue control may lead to holding the bolus in an abnormal position, leading to impaired swallowing
  - o Food falling into the anterior sulcus because of labial and facial muscle weakness, and food falling into the lateral sulcus because of weakness of the buccal muscles which typically close the sulcus; these problems may occur as soon as the food is placed in the mouth or during mastication
- Swallowing disorders of the oral phase: The main disorder of this phase of the swallow is a failure to move the bolus toward the posterior portion of the mouth to trigger the pharyngeal swallow; the tongue is the prime mover of the bolus; the specific disorders of this phase of swallow and their potential causes include:
  - o Delayed or searching tongue movements, sometimes described as apraxia of swallow, refer to lack of prompt tongue movements when food is placed in the mouth, disorganized tongue movements, or lack of movement; bolus formation is impeded; tongue weakness is the main cause, although the range of motion is not affected
  - o Tongue thrust; a forward movement of the tongue may push the food forward in the mouth, a movement direction opposite to normal; anterior

instead of posterior tongue movement; neurological involvement is the main cause

o Food residue in various places (anterior and lateral sulcus, floor of the mouth, tongue surface, hard palate) indicating incomplete swallow or failure to move the bolus completely into the pharyngeal area; mostly due to tongue and buccal muscle weakness or tongue scarring (due to surgery) that may hold food; reduced tongue elevation and contact with the hard palate, and random (versus systematic front to back and lateral) movement of the tongue contribute to most of these problems

o Premature loss of liquid or pudding into the pharynx without triggering the pharyngeal swallow; when the oral preparatory or oral phase of the swallow is not yet completed, part of all of the material may fall into the pharynx; mostly due to a failure of the soft palate and the back of the tongue not getting sealed to prevent the premature loss of the bolus into the pharynx; tongue weakness is an important factor; may cause aspiration or the material may get collected in the valleculae (space between the base of the tongue and epiglottis) or pyriform sinuses

o Piecemeal swallow; attempting to swallow small amounts in succession, even though the bolus is small enough to be swallowed in a single try; may be due to client's compensatory behavior to avoid aspiration

• Disorders of the pharyngeal phase: Begins when the bolus head passes through the base of the tongue; problems in triggering the pharyngeal swallow and propelling the bolus through the pharynx and into the P-E segment characterize the pharyngeal phase disorders; lack of a trigger for the pharyngeal phase can cause aspiration; generally, there is a delay in pharyngeal transmit time; various symptoms and their causes include:

o Delayed or absent swallowing reflex; the laryngeal swallow fails to trigger; most evident in swallowing liquids that quickly splash into the pharynx; the liquid is likely to enter the open airway; food also may fall into the valleculae or pyriform sinuses;

o a 2-second delay in triggering the pharyngeal swallow is significant; delayed trigger or absence of pharyngeal swallow reflex is due mainly to brainstem injury

o Nasal penetration of food; mostly caused by inadequate velopharyngeal closure, which occurs briefly as the bolus passes the nasopharynx

o Food coating on the pharyngeal walls, especially on the side that is especially weak; if pharyngeal contractions are impaired bilaterally, food may coat the walls of the pharynx; such coating is minimal or totally absent in healthy individuals

o Food residue in valleculae, largely because of lack of efficient tongue movement

o Food residue on top of airway, largely because the larynx is not elevated enough during swallow; food on top of the airway may be aspirated

o Food residue in pyriform sinuses, due largely to weak anterior movement of the larynx; cricoarytenoid dysfunction also may cause this condition

- o Aspiration during swallow; aspiration is the penetration of food and liquid into the airway that occurs below the true vocal folds; due to a failure of the true vocal folds to close during swallow
- o Laryngeal penetration of food; unlike aspiration, laryngeal penetration of food occurs at any level except for the level below the true folds; airway penetration may occur at the middle of the arytenoid cartilage, at the surface of the false folds, or at the level, but not below that of, the true folds
- o Other factors include cervical osteophytes (bony outgrowth of the cervical vertebrae) that interfere with normal swallow, and mucosal fold at the base of the tongue (found in clients who have had a total laryngectomy) which restricts the pharyngeal passage and makes it difficult for the food to pass through

- Disorders of the esophageal phase: Problems in passing the bolus through the cricopharyngeus muscle and past the seventh cervical vertebra; due to a reduction of involuntary peristaltic movements within the esophagus; the main symptom is backflow of food from the esophagus to the pharynx; the main symptoms and their potential causes include:
  - o *Gastroesophageal reflux disease;* lack of esophageal peristaltic movements and a failure and weakness of the lower esophageal sphincter cause this condition; result is a backflow of food and stomach acids to the pharynx
  - o Formation of *tracheoesophageal fistula*, often between the first and third thoracic vertebrae; it is an abnormal channel or a hole between the trachea and the esophagus; food and liquid may flow back from the esophagus to the trachea
  - o Diverticulum (a pouch or pocket that collects food), especially Zenker's Diverticulum, which forms in the region of the upper esophageal sphincter or the cricopharyngeal region; excessive pharyngeal force or pressure in pushing the food down may cause herniation and diverticulum; food that falls into the diverticulum may enter the airway; the result is aspiration after the swallow
  - o A variety of causes and clinical conditions can result in esophageal swallowing disorders; reduced esophageal contractions and its efficiency to transport food may be due to surgery, neurologic damage, radiation therapy for cancer, caustic damage to the esophagus (ingestion of such corrosive chemicals as household cleansers, sulfuric acid, batteries that contain mercury), such esophageal infections as candida esophagitis or HIV infection, esophageal cancer, formation of esophageal webs or rings, esophageal obstruction due to benign tumors or foreign bodies that are accidentally or intentionally ingested, and compressed esophagus because of cancerous growths in the structures adjacent to it (e.g., lungs and lymph nodes)

General Etiologic Factors and Neurophysiological Variables

- In addition to the specific clinical conditions associated with swallowing disorders of particular phases, there are many general etiologic factors

- Strokes, especially brainstem and anterior cortical strokes resulting in poor motor control of the structures involved in swallowing (including the tongue and cricopharyngeal structures)
- Several neurological disorders and neurodegenerative diseases, including vocal fold paralysis, meningitis, brain tumors, Alzheimer's disease, Parkinson's disease, Huntington's disease, Wilson's disease, amyotrophic lateral sclerosis, multiple sclerosis, progressive supranuclear palsy, myasthenia gravis, muscular dystrophy, and various forms of dystonia including torticollis
- Tumors in the oral cavity, larynx, pharynx, or esophagus
- Surgical treatment of oral, pharyngeal, laryngeal, and esophageal cancer, and cervical spinal surgery, resulting in reduced efficiency of the remaining structures
- Any form of head, neck, skull base, and gastrointestinal surgery poses a high risk for dysphagia
- Tongue, lip, mandibular, and palatal surgery
- Radiation therapy for oral, pharyngeal, and laryngeal cancer, similar to surgical treatment, may weaken the structures involved in swallowing
- Traumatic brain injury in which the brain, brainstem, or cranial nerves are damaged
- Cerebral palsy
- Drugs prescribed for spasticity and psychosis (e.g., schizophrenia)

Carrau, R. L., & Murry, T. (2006). *Comprehensive management of swallowing disorders*. San Diego, CA: Plural Publishing.

Corbin-Lewis, K., Liss, J. M., & Sciortino, K. L. (2005). *Clinical anatomy and physiology of the swallow mechanism*. Clifton Park, NY: Thomson Delmar Learning.

Groher, M. E. (Ed.) (1997). *Dysphagia: Diagnosis and management*. Boston, MA: Butterworth-Heinemann.

Logemann, J. A. (1998). *Evaluation and treatment of swallowing disorders* (2nd ed.). Austin, TX: Pro-Ed.

Logemann, J. A. (1993). *A manual of videofluoroscopic evaluation of swallowing* (2nd ed.). Austin, TX: Pro-Ed.

Miller, R. M. (1992). Clinical examination for dysphagia. In M. E. Groher, (Ed.), *Dysphagia: Diagnosis and management* (pp. 143–162). Boston, MA: Butterworth-Heinemann.

Murry, T., & Carrau, R. L. (2006). *Clinical Management of Swallowing Disorders* (2nd ed.). San Diego, CA: Plural Publishing Inc.

Perlman, A., & Schultze-Delrieu, K. (1997). *Deglutition and its disorders: Anatomy, physiology, clinical diagnosis and management*: San Diego, CA: Singular Publishing Group.

Provencio-Arambula, M., Provencio, D., & Hegde, M. N. (2007a). *Assessment of dysphagia: Resources and protocols in English and Spanish*. San Diego, CA: Plural Publishing.

Provencio-Arambula, M., Provencio, D., & Hegde, M. N. (2007b). *Treatment of dysphagia: Resources and protocols in English and Spanish*. San Diego, CA: Plural Publishing.

Dysphonia. A general term for disordered voice; any voice disorder with the exception of Aphonia; see Voice Disorders.

Dysplasia. Abnormal growth and development; unusual shape and size of body parts; there are various forms of dysplasias; for example, in *anteroposterior facial dysplasia*, there is an abnormal anteroposterior relationship between the maxilla and the mandible.

Dystonia. Involuntary movements that are repetitive, slow, twisting, writhing, and flexing; abnormal postures; may affect a single group or multiple groups of muscles; in orofacial dystonia, only the muscles and the face may be affected; uncontrolled adductor and abductor laryngeal spasms, leading to breathy, strained, and hoarse voice may be associated with it; lesions or cell loss in basal ganglia are the potential causes; associated with Hyperkinetic Dysarthria (see also under Dysarthria).

E

Echolalia. Parrot-like repetition of what is heard; children who are autistic exhibit echolalia to a great extent and sometimes may imply communication (as when a child says "What do you want candy" to the question, "What do you want?"); even in clients with neurological diseases, echolalia may suggest that the client does understand what is being repeated (as when the client responds "What do I want to eat?" to the question "What do you want to eat?"); some clients may repeat television commercials or other statements that are heard; to be distinguished from imitation, which is purposeful reproduction of what is modeled; associated with autism and schizophrenia, various neuropathological and genetic conditions (e.g., strokes, Pick's disease, dementias, and Tourette's syndrome), carbon monoxide poisoning, and period during which a person emerges from a coma.

Ectoderm. Embryo's outermost germ layer; gives rise to nails, hair, enamel of teeth, sweat glands, nervous system, and such sense organs as the ear and eye; ectodermal deformities are a part of some genetic syndromes including ectrodactyly-ectodermal dysplasia-clefting syndrome; see Syndromes Associated With Communication Disorders.

Ectodermal Dysplasia. Underdevelopment of organs or tissue that are derived from the Ectoderm; due to hereditary or genetic disorders; see Syndromes Associated With Communication Disorders.

Ectrodactyly. Congenital absence of fingers or toes; part of some genetic syndromes including ectrodactyly-ectodermal dysplasia-clefting syndrome; see Syndromes Associated With Communication Disorders.

Edema. Swelling of tissue due to an accumulation of fluid; cerebral edema is found in clients who have had strokes or traumatic brain injury; cerebral edema increases intracranial pressure; associated with communication disorders.

Efferent Nerves. Nerves that carry motor impulses from the central nervous system to the peripheral muscles.

Embolism. A sudden blocking of blood flow within an artery by a clot or a mass of foreign material that had its origin elsewhere and traveled through the bloodstream to the site of blockage; a common cause of stroke and the resulting aphasia.

Epicanthal Fold. A vertical layer of skin covering the inner canthus on either side of the nose; normal in individuals of certain races and a physical characteristic in certain syndromes, the prominent being the Down syndrome (see Syndromes Associated With Communication Disorders)

Epilepsy. Neurological disorders due to transient electrical disturbances in brain functions; a single episode of such disturbance is called a *seizure*; epileptic attacks may include a loss of consciousness, convulsions, and other motor impairments; may be preceded by certain sensory experiences (e.g., a flash of light), headache, and so forth; may be due to focal or more generalized lesions in the brain.

Esophageal Spasm. Painful contractions of the esophagus; may be associated with Dysphagia.

Esophagitis. Inflammation of the esophagus; a common cause is gastroesophageal reflux; may be associated with Dysphagia.

Essential (Organic) Tremors. A hyperkinetic movement disorder of no known cause (idiopathic); may be familial in about 50% of cases; affects 300 persons per 100,000 individuals; affects the hands, arms, and head; most prominent when performing actions (such as drinking from a glass or writing); reduced when the muscles are at rest; a variation is *essential voice tremor;* associated with Hyperkinetic Dysarthria.

E

Ethnocultural Variables Associated with Communication Disorders.

Ethnic, cultural, and linguistic background that affect communication; affect how disorders of communication are viewed; whether to diagnose a disorder of communication (especially speech and language disorders) and whether to offer clinical services or not will depend on the individual's ethnocultural background and the language status; variables that are especially important in understanding communication and its disorders in people who speak dialectal variations of English (e.g., Black English or Spanish-influenced English); ethnocultural variables relevant to communication disorder are described under the main entry for each disorder; assessment issues related to ethnocultural (multicultural) factors are described in the companion volume, *Hegde's PocketGuide to Assessment in Speech-Language Pathology* (3rd ed.); treatment issues related to the topic are described in the companion volume, *Hegde's PocketGuide to Treatment in Speech-Language Pathology* (3rd ed.); see the following cited resources.

Battle, D. E. (2002). *Communication disorders in multicultural populations* (3rd ed.). Boston, MA: Andover Medical Publishers.

Cheng, L. L. (1995). *Integrating language and learning for inclusion.* San Diego, CA: Singular Publishing Group.

Goldstein, B. A. (2004). *Bilingual development and disorders in Spanish-English speakers.* Baltimore, MD: Paul H. Brookes.

Kamhi, A. G., Pollock, K. E., & Harris, J. L. (1996). *Communication development and disorders in African American Children.* Baltimore, MD: Paul H. Brookes.

Kayser, H. (1998). *Assessment and intervention resources for Hispanic children.* San Diego, CA: Singular Publishing Group.

Payne, J. C. (1997). *Adult neurogenic language disorders: Assessment and treatment.* San Diego, CA: Singular Publishing Group

Roseberry-McKibbin, C. (2002). *Multicultural students with special language needs* (2nd ed.). Ocean Side, CA: Academic Communication Associates.

Expressive Aphasia. A type of aphasia with predominant problems in language expression versus comprehension; the same as Broca's aphasia; see Aphasia: Specific Types.

Extrapyramidal System. Upper motor neuron system originating in the cerebral cortex (of the right and left hemispheres); takes a more indirect route to its destination in the brainstem and spinal cord; also known as indirect pathway or indirect motor system; it courses through the basal ganglia, cerebellum, reticular formation, vestibular nuclei, and the red nucleus; the system regulates reflexes, posture, and muscle tone; lesions result in a failure to inhibit and modulate movement, causing increased muscle tone, spasticity, and overactive reflexes; disorders of this system are associated with various kinds of <u>Dysarthrias</u>, especially <u>Spastic Dysarthria</u>.

F

F

Facio-Auriculo-Vertebral Syndrome. A genetic syndrome also known as Goldenhar Syndrome; see Syndromes Associated With Communication Disorders.

Factitious Disorders. Physical or psychological symptoms consciously and intentionally developed for no apparent gain; if gain is involved, it would be called Malingering; individuals apparently seek to be medical patients and are reinforced for their role as patients, but no other gains are evident; some patients may ingest certain medications that cause them problems, only to seek treatment for the consequences of their planned actions; hints of a factitious disorder are found in dramatic symptoms and extensive consultation in multiple medical centers in different cities; the disorder they present may have a wide range of possibilities, including neurological, abdominal, and dermatological problems; of relevance to speech-language pathologist, the patients may present voice disorders, aphonia, stuttering, or stuttering-like fluency problems; see Psychiatric Problems Associated With Communication Disorders for additional information.

Familial Incidence. Frequency with which a disease or disorder is found among blood relatives; many disorders (e.g., stuttering) show a higher familial incidence; a higher familial incidence means that a person with a given disorder is likely to have one or more blood relatives with the same disorder; autosomal dominant, autosomal recessive, and other genetic mechanisms may be involved in familial incidence; in most cases of behavioral disorders (such as stuttering), influence of environmental variables cannot be ruled out by studying merely the familial incidence of a disorder.

Feeding Disorders. Problems in transporting food from the plate to the mouth; difficulty in placing food in one's own mouth; to be distinguished from Swallowing Disorders; whereas feeding disorders may impair the transport of food from the plate to the mouth, swallowing disorders impair the transport of food from the mouth to the stomach; feeding disorders have multiple causes, including neurodegenerative disorders, paralysis of the hands, traumatic brain injury, dementia, various sensory deficits; cognitive impairments, and postural problems; most clients who have feeding problems also may have swallowing disorders; feeding problems may be due to paralysis of the hands in otherwise healthy, competent, and alert individuals; typically part of a complex of neurobehavioral symptoms due to various factors

- Neurodegenerative diseases that cause motor impairments as well as cognitive deficits
- Strokes that may impair motor skills needed to self-feed
- Sensory deficits; hearing loss that may affect a client's comprehension of instructions during eating; recent vision loss that will make it difficult for the client to see and judge the bite size of food; visuo-spatial difficulties associated with brain injury that affect accurate spatial judgments about food and its transport to the mouth; impaired taste or smell that may make food taste bitter, sour, or too sweet
- Cognitive deficits; limited attention span leading to impulsive self-feeding; lack of awareness, causing inadequate nutritional intake; impaired judgment that may lead to self-feeding nonfood items

- Psychiatric problems (e.g., schizophrenia) that may be associated with refusal to eat, insistence on being fed by others, uncooperative or aggressive behavior during meal time, and throwing or spilling food
- Postural problems; not being able to sit straight during eating, causing feeding difficulties; wrong posture, making it difficult to see the food that is being transported to the mouth
- Communication problems; inability to express food or liquid preferences and dislikes; failure to ask for assistance when needed; missing various cues used during meal times

Fetal Alcohol Syndrome. Congenital syndrome in children born to mothers who consumed alcohol during pregnancy; see Syndromes Associated With Communication Disorders.

Final Consonant Deletion. Omission of final consonants in words; a phonological process; see Articulation and Phonological Disorders.

First and Second Bronchial Arch Syndrome. Genetic syndrome also known as the Goldenhar Syndrome; see Syndromes Associated With Communication Disorders.

Fistula. An abnormal opening, passage, or channel between two internal organs; the passage may be opened from an internal organ to the surface of the body; for example, a small opening left after palatal surgery or a pharyngeal fistula which is an abnormal communicating channel to the pharynx; may be surgically created for a specific purpose as in tracheoesophageal puncture or fistulization, which helps clients with laryngectomy produce tracheoesophageal speech with the help of a voice prosthesis.

Flaccid Dysarthria. Motor speech disorder due to damage to the motor units of spinal or cranial nerves (lower motor neuron involvement); symptoms vary depending on the nerve or nerves affected; see Dysarthria: Specific Types.

Flaccid Paralysis. Soft and flabby muscles; muscle weakness, hypotonia, muscle atrophy, and diminished reflexes; associated with a type of dysarthria; see Dysarthria: Specific Types.

Fluency Disorders. A group of speech disorders whose main characteristic is reduced or impaired fluency of speech; include cluttering, stuttering, and neurogenic stuttering; each variety has certain unique features, although an excessive amount or duration of dysfluencies is a common feature; cluttering and stuttering begin in early childhood with late onset being unusual; neurogenic stuttering is typically of late onset and associated with neuropathology of recent origin; some forms may have a psychiatric basis; see Psychiatric Problems Associated With Communication Disorders for malingered stuttering and psychogenic stuttering.

Cluttering. Primarily a disorder of fluency and rate of speech but additional features are significant; may involve language and thought processes, but this is controversial; a fluency disorder related to, but different from, Stuttering; may coexist with stuttering; characterized by rapid and irregular speech rate and indistinct articulation; generally hurried speech even under normal circumstances; also known as *tachyphemia*; possibly underdiagnosed in the United States; epidemiological information, including its prevalence rate and distribution across different segments of the general population, is not well established in the United States

Description of Cluttering

- Experts differ on the specific set of symptoms that are essential to cluttering; some assign to it few mandatory symptoms, whereas others offer a long list of symptoms that include problems in fluency, speech rate variations, reduced speech intelligibility, impaired cognitive skills, emotional behavior disorders, neurological deficits, reading and writing impairments, disorganized thinking and behavior, deviant conversational speech skills, and prosodic problems, just to sample a few; there is no agreement on the core symptoms and associated conditions
- Excessively fast and somewhat variable rate of speech and increased frequency of dysfluencies are probably among the most essential features of cluttering; reduced intelligibility of cluttered speech is a necessary consequence of these two features
- The rate of speech may be variable in speakers who clutter; at times, the speech rate may increase rapidly with further reductions in intelligibility; in some cases, there might be a progressively faster rate of speech (festinating rate)
- Cluttering is associated with errors of articulation; however, these are not true articulation problems and people who clutter are not diagnosed with an articulation disorder unless it exists as an independent disorder; at a slower rate of speech, people who clutter can produce the speech sounds correctly; therefore, articulatory breakdowns are a function of the abnormal rate of speech; these errors include:
  o Omission of sounds, syllables, and even words
  o Sound transpositions within words
  o Inversion of the order of sounds
  o Compression of syllable durations (*syllable telescoping*)
- A significant and essential feature of cluttering is an increased frequency of dysfluencies; dysfluencies may be relatively effortless and may contain many units; various kinds of dysfluencies observed in people with cluttering include:
  o Repetition of initial sounds and syllables
  o Repetition of words
  o Repetition of phrases
  o Revisions
  o Interjections
  o Sound prolongations
- Dysfluencies may worsen when the person who clutters is relaxed or when reading a well-known text
- Fluency of people who clutter may improve when speaking under stress, when attention is drawn to dysfluencies, and while giving short answers, talking in a foreign language, and speaking after an interruption

- Several other features may be found in some but not all individuals who clutter, and include:
  o Dysrhythmic respiration
  o Motor incoordination
  o Disorganized thought processes
  o Language difficulties including poor syntactic structures, run-on sentences, and incorrect use of prepositions and pronouns; such social communication problems as inappropriate turn taking and topic initiation, abrupt termination of conversation, poor topic maintenance, and poor conversational repair strategies; difficulty comprehending spoken language
  o Reading and writing problems including poor spelling in writing, disorganized, sprawling writing, writing full of deletions and repetitions, misuse or absence of punctuation, and transposition of words
  o Monotonous speech due to lack of appropriate intonational patterns
  o Academic problems and learning disabilities
- A unique symptom much discussed in the literature is the clients' lack of awareness of their speech problem; it is suggested that people who clutter are unaware of their communication problem, a suggestion not entirely credible because of negative feedback they are likely to receive from listeners; it is more likely that they are unconcerned about their speech problem and its effects on listeners; generally, they tend to do less about their problem than people who stutter
- Some clinicians believe that persons who clutter are impulsive, careless, inattentive, and have poor self-monitoring skills

Etiology of Cluttering

- Genetic factors may be important in cluttering, although no specific genetic basis has been identified; familial incidence is thought to be high
- Neurophysiological abnormalities as suggested by deviant electroencephalographic (EEG) findings; however, only about 50% of clutterers show EEG abnormalities that have not been related to known neuropathologies
- Basal ganglia dysfunction may be involved in cluttering

Neurogenic Stuttering. Somewhat varied problems of fluency that resemble stuttering of early childhood onset, but have a demonstrated neurological basis and differential characteristics; stuttering or, more aptly, stuttering-like behaviors may be an isolated symptom of neuropathology and exist without associated speech or language disturbances; also known as acquired stuttering, or cortical stuttering; not all acquired stuttering may be of neurological origin; neurogenic stuttering may be associated with aphasia or apraxia of speech; may be evident in stroke clients who do not have aphasia, although more commonly associated with aphasia; to be distinguished from stuttering of early childhood onset (developmental) with no history of recent neuropathological events; may be persistent or transient; the same symptom complex may be associated with varied neuropathology.

Etiologic Factors of Neurogenic Stuttering

- Common etiologic factors of neurogenic stuttering include:
  - Strokes (with or without aphasia)
  - Many clinical conditions that cause apraxia of speech
  - Variety of clinical conditions that cause dysarthria, especially hypokinetic dysarthria
  - Head trauma
  - Extrapyramidal diseases, especially Parkinson's disease
  - Progressive supranuclear palsy
  - Brain tumors
  - Brain surgery, including bilateral thalamotomy
  - Thalamic stimulation
  - Seizure disorders
  - Dementia, especially dialysis dementia
  - Drug toxicity, especially from drugs prescribed for asthma, depression, schizophrenia, and anxiety
  - Cerebral anoxia due to a variety of clinical conditions (including vascular diseases) may cause neurogenic stuttering in some individuals
- Transient and persistent neurogenic stuttering have different neuropathologies
  - Bilateral brain damage often results in persistent neurogenic stuttering
  - Multiple lesions of a single hemisphere often results in transient neurogenic stuttering
  - Neurogenic stuttering due to drug toxicity may be transitory; it may dissipate when the drugs are withdrawn
- Left hemisphere damage in any form may increase the dysfluency rates; almost all types of aphasia have, as their characteristic, increased frequency of dysfluencies due to anomia
- Stuttering of early onset that has been well under control may re-emerge in individuals who experience left hemisphere stokes and at the onset of Parkinson's disease, Alzheimer's disease, or olivopontocerebellar atrophy
- Strangely, stuttering of early childhood onset may be remediated with certain neurological insults; traumatic brain injury, multiple sclerosis with cerebellar lesions, bilateral thalamic strokes, seizures, and neurosurgery for tumors or vascular disorders have been reported to reduce or eliminate stuttering in some cases

Neuropathology of Neurogenic Stuttering

- Neuroanatomic sites of lesion or lesions may be highly varied across individuals with neurogenic stuttering
- Stimulation of most cortical areas, except for the occipital lobe, may elicit part-word and whole word repetitions
- Single lesions are less often associated with neurogenic stuttering than are multiple (especially bilateral) lesions
- In many individuals, lesion location may remain undetermined
- Common neuropathology includes:
  - Lesions in the frontal, temporal, and parietal lobes

o Left cerebral damage in a majority of individuals; right hemisphere injury in a few
o Subcortical lesions; strokes within the basal ganglia; damage to the basal ganglia and its control circuits, causing neurogenic stuttering associated with Parkinson's disease
o Lesions to the supplementary motor area, thalamus, and midbrain

Characteristics of Neurogenic Stuttering

- Neurological symptoms consistent with the underlying neurological diseases or trauma distinguish this form of fluency disorder from that of the early childhood onset; may be difficult to distinguish neurogenic stuttering from stuttering of early childhood onset on the basis of dysfluency types alone
- Onset of stuttering is typically in later years, often in older people with documented neuropathology or history suggestive of neuropathology; neurogenic stuttering due to traumatic brain injury, drug toxicity, and neurosurgery may be evident at any age
- Both positive and negative signs or symptoms are important characteristics of neurogenic stuttering
- Positive signs of neurogenic stuttering include:
  o Repetitions of medial and final syllables in words, somewhat unusual in stuttering of early onset
  o Dysfluent production of function words, unusual in adults with early onset stuttering
  o Dysfluencies in imitated speech, observed much less frequently in stuttering of early childhood onset
  o Frozen articulatory positions (possibly, silent prolongations); common to both neurogenic stuttering and stuttering of early onset
  o Rapid speech rate
- Negative signs of neurogenic stuttering are those that are present in stuttering of early childhood onset but absent or infrequent in neurogenic stuttering
  o Lack of the Adaptation Effect, which is a reliable characteristic of early onset stuttering; neurogenic stuttering not characterized by reduction in stuttering upon repeated oral reading of the same passage
  o Few associated motor behaviors (e.g., facial grimacing and foot stamping) in neurogenic stuttering
  o Minimal or no effects of delayed auditory feedback, masking noise, rhythmic speech, choral reading, shadowing, singing, and such other variables that tend to reduce stuttering of early onset
  o No significant sign of anxiety associated with speech or speaking situations, a feature that is common to stuttering of childhood onset
  o No significant attempts at avoiding speech or speaking situations
- General characteristics that may not distinguish neurogenic stuttering from early onset stuttering
  o Pauses, revisions, incomplete phrases, and prolongation of sounds
  o Other kinds of dysfluencies that may not distinguish neurogenic stuttering from early onset stuttering

- General symptoms suggestive of brain injury
  - Problems in copying and drawing
  - Problems in copying block designs
  - Problems in sequential hand positions
  - Problems in tapping out rhythms and executing rhythmic movements
  - Such other problems as dysphagia, seizures, and paresis or paralysis
  - Other symptoms that are typically associated with Aphasia, Apraxia of Speech, Traumatic Brain Injury, and Dementia

F

Stuttering. A disorder of fluency and rhythm; a disorder of early childhood onset; generally, clinicians have little or no difficulty diagnosing stuttering, especially in adults, but have difficulty measuring it reliably; most parents diagnose stuttering reliably in their children; nonetheless, definitions vary; some definitions are descriptions of observable behaviors, whereas others are descriptions of covert processes; still others are descriptions of presumed etiological factors with very little reference to symptoms or behaviors; dysfluencies play some role in most, if not all, definitions or their descriptive expansions; some definitions include only certain kinds of dysfluencies (e.g., part-word repetitions and speech sound prolongations); other definitions include all kinds of dysfluencies; still other definitions mention moments or events of stuttering with no description of observable behaviors; some definitions do not specify a quantitative criterion for dysfluencies to diagnose stuttering; other definitions specify a 5% or a 10% dysfluency rate; many clinicians diagnose stuttering based on excessive amounts of dysfluencies, excessive durations of dysfluencies, unusually fast tempo of dysfluencies, and unusual amount of muscular effort associated with dysfluent speech production; may be associated with avoidance of certain words and speaking situations, experience of negative emotions, and expression of negative verbalizations about himself or herself and about listeners; the final diagnosis is based on multiple factors including the types, amounts, and characteristics of dysfluencies, avoidance and negative emotions, and struggle and tension associated with dysfluent speech production; another fluency disorder, Cluttering, may coexist with stuttering.

Epidemiology and Ethnocultural Variables

- The earliest age of reported onset is about 18 months; most children who begin to stutter do so before age 4; the rate of onset begins to taper off after age 6 or so; onset is rare in the teenage and subsequent years; adult onset of stuttering is suspected to have a neurological basis; see Neurogenic Fluency Disorders
- More common in males than in females; a general male:female ratio of 3:1 is often reported, but the ratio varies across studies and age groups; generally, the younger the age group, the closer the male:female ratios and vice versa; preschool male:female ratio is reportedly 1.4:1 or even 1:1, whereas the same ratio for children in the 11th grade might be much higher (perhaps as high as 5.5: 1); different sex ratios at different age levels may be a function of more girls recovering from stuttering and stuttering emerging anew in more boys than girls

- Prevalence rate is about 1% in the general population; the lifetime incidence (persons who have ever stuttered during their life time) is higher, between 5% and 10%; prevalence rates are influenced by gender and familial distribution
- Familial prevalence of stuttering is higher than that in the general population; 40% to 50% of individuals who stutter are likely to have another member in the family (mostly fathers or siblings) who also stutters; familial prevalence may be as high as three times the prevalence in the general population; perhaps up to 65% of those who stutter may have distant relatives who stutter
- The Concordance Rate of stuttering in identical twins is higher than that in fraternal twins, which is higher than that in ordinary siblings; however, if one member of an identical twin pair stutters, it does not mean that the other member will invariably stutter, although the chances that both will are higher than they are for ordinary siblings; that there is a slightly higher concordance rate for identical twins suggests that environmental variables play a role in the prevalence of stuttering in all twin pairs—including identical twin pairs
- Some children spontaneously recover from stuttering; estimates of spontaneous recovery vary between 30% and 80%; spontaneous recovery rates are a debated issue on which strong and opposing views are common; a more realistic estimate may be less than 50%; higher estimates of spontaneous recovery may be evident if children are allowed to stutter up to 4 years or more; it is not clear what kind of formal or informal intervention may occur during this extended period of time; most importantly, it is difficult to predict who will and who will not recover spontaneously because the statistics apply to group data; new cases replace spontaneously recovered cases throughout early childhood
- There is no strong and convincing evidence that parents of children who stutter are systematically different from parents of children who do not stutter; some parents may be anxious and overprotective of their children; such parental reactions may be due to the child's stuttering and may not play any causative role
- Stuttering has not been found to be absent in any culture, although some anthropologists have claimed that it does not exist in certain societies (e.g., people of New Guinea or Polar Eskimos); reported prevalence rates differ somewhat, but it is difficult to claim that the prevalence is significantly related to ethnocultural variables; once-advocated theory that the Native Americans did not stutter has now been discredited; available evidence suggests that stuttering exists in American, Native American, European, Asian, and African societies; it exists in rural as well as urban societies
- Although stuttering exists in all societies, the incidence rates may vary; the reliability of incidence data across cultures and studies is difficult to assess
- Some studies suggest that stuttering may be more common among African Americans than among whites; the dysfluency types may be roughly the same in the two ethnocultural groups

161

- The relationship between socioeconomic levels and stuttering is unclear
- Children and adults who stutter may have any level of intelligence as measured through IQ tests; when people with diagnosed intellectual disabilities are excluded, people who stutter may score about 95, which is 5 points below the average; nonetheless, among people who stutter, the range of IQ may vary from below normal to well above average; stuttering has not prevented many persons from outstanding artistic, scientific, and professional achievements
- The prevalence of stuttering may be slightly higher in children and adults with diagnosed intellectual disabilities; in people with Down syndrome, the prevalence is reported to be as high as 53%; even the lowest prevalence level reported, 15%, is much higher than that for the general population (about 1% to 1.5%)
- Stuttering and phonological acquisition and disorders may be correlated; the number of children who have phonological disorders along with persistent stuttering varies from a low of 16% to a high of 70%; even at the lowest level reported, phonological disorders are more common among children who stutter than among children who do not stutter; however, phonological disorders may resolve themselves without professional help; children who stutter do not have a unique pattern of phonological acquisition
- Stuttering and language skills may be correlated, but the evidence is currently contradictory; earlier studies reported that children who stutter may have deficient language skills; more recent studies have contradicted this, in fact suggesting that children who stutter may score even higher than normally fluent children on language tests

Characteristics of Stuttering

- Impairment of fluency: Stuttering is a disorder of fluency; dysfluencies impair fluency; although all speakers exhibit dysfluencies at some frequency (often below 5% of the words spoken), children and adults who stutter have an increased frequency of all types of dysfluencies
- Types of dysfluencies: Although there is some disagreement about the clinical (diagnostic) significance of different dysfluency types, clinicians should be aware of all types so they can formulate their own diagnostic criteria
  o Repetitions
    - Sound/syllable repetitions or part-word repetitions ("t-t-t-time"; "sa-sa-saturday"; "abou-abou-about")
    - Word repetitions: monosyllabic or multisyllabic ("I-I-I will go with you"; "his cousin-cousin came today")
    - Phrase repetitions ("how is-how is-how is it done?")
  o Prolongations
    - Sound prolongations ("Sssssoup, please"; "Mmmmommy")
    - Silent prolongations or articulatory postures without voicing (a silent period with a tensed articulatory posture for the initial sound in saying a word such as "Bob")

- o Broken words of intralexical pauses
  - Silent intervals within words ("g-(silent pause)-oing")
  - Contrasted with silent intervals between words, called *pauses*
- o Interjections
  - Sound/syllable interjections ("he was um going to do it")
  - Word interjections ("I can well do it")
  - Phrase interjections ("It is you know-you know well done")
- o Pauses
  - Excessively long silent intervals at inappropriate loci in speech ("I was [long pause] going to tell you")
  - To be distinguished from within-word pauses (broken words or intralexical pauses)
- o Revisions
  - Productions that retain the same idea but with word changes ("I will take a cab—bus")
  - To be distinguished from incomplete phrases
- o Incomplete phrases
  - Productions that suggest that the speaker dropped the idea he or she was going to express ("I was going to—but let me just say this")
  - To be distinguished from revisions
- Stuttering vs. nonstuttering dysfluencies: Some experts believe that stuttering is characterized by certain kinds of dysfluencies, whereas other kinds of dysfluencies are a part of normally fluent speech; there is no complete agreement as to what kinds of dysfluencies are stuttering; historically, part-word repetitions and speech sound prolongations were considered stuttering types; more recently, single-syllable word repetitions have been added to this short list; it is not clear why broken words, a very abnormal type, should not be added
- All types of dysfluencies are clinically significant: Some other experts believe that stuttering implies an increase in all kinds of dysfluencies—not just certain kinds—if they exceed their normal range (e.g., 5% of speech or some other quantitative criterion); there is evidence that when all kinds of dysfluencies increase beyond 5%, listeners consider the speech as either dysfluent or stuttered; therefore, all kinds of dysfluencies are of clinical significance if they exceed the range of normal frequency
- Subjective judgments: Still other experts believe in making a subjective judgment that a speaker is a stutterer or not a stutterer; "moments" and "events" may be measured without specifying what is measured
- Muscle tension: Dysfluent speech of persons who stutter may be distinguished from increased muscular tension and effort that are absent in their own normally fluent productions or the low-frequency dysfluencies of normally fluent speakers; some experts believe that dysfluencies produced without muscular tension and effort are normal; sound prolongations and part-word repetitions may be produced especially with a noticeable degree of tension and rapidity; tension may be evident in facial, chest, neck, and shoulder muscles; sometimes the entire body posture may be tensed

F

- Breathing abnormalities: Stuttering may be associated with breathing abnormalities; no inherent respiratory problems cause stuttering but stuttered speech productions and breathing abnormalities may coexist; such abnormalities are nonexistent during fluent speech production; these abnormalities may be more appropriately called airflow management problems than breathing abnormalities, and include the following:
  - o Attempts at speaking on limited or shallow inhalation
  - o Attempts at speaking during exhalation
  - o Running out of air at the end of phrases and sentences
  - o Apparent efforts to squeeze the air out of lungs to continue talking
  - o Inhalations and exhalations that interrupt each other
  - o Impounding of inhaled air with a sudden closure of the glottis and apparent attempts to speak while the air is impounded
  - o Sudden cessation of breathing during speech production
  - o Dysrhythmic respiration
  - o Audible inhalation, exhalation, or both
  - o Difficulty in maintaining an even airflow throughout an utterance
- Variability in stuttering: Although stuttering is highly variable within and across individuals, there are factors that account for that variability; for example, a portion of stuttering tends to occur on the same words or same loci in oral reading (the consistency effect); increases in the audience size increases stuttering frequency; repeated reading of a passage reduces its frequency; delayed auditory feedback, masking noise, choral reading, and shadowing reduce its frequency
- Associated motor behaviors: These are extraneous motor (nonspeech) behaviors that accompany dysfluencies or stutterings; a variety of associated motor behaviors may be seen in children and adults who stutter, although their frequency and severity may be higher in adults than in children; the associated motor behaviors may be more attention-drawing than the dysfluencies themselves, and include:
  - o Rapid and tense eye blink
  - o Tensed and prolonged shutting of the eyelids
  - o Rapid upward, downward, or lateral movement of the eyes
  - o Knitting of the eyebrows
  - o Nose wrinkling and flaring
  - o Pursing or quivering of the lips
  - o Tongue clicking
  - o Teeth clenching, grinding, and clicking
  - o Tension in facial muscles
  - o Wrinkling of the forehead
  - o Clenched jaw or jerky, slow, or tensed movement of the jaws
  - o Jaw opening or closing unrelated to target speech production
  - o Tension in chest, shoulder, and neck muscles including twitching and extraneous movements
  - o Head movements including turns, shakes, jerks, and lateral, upward, and downward movements

o Tensed and jerky hand movements including fist clenching and hand wringing

o Tensed and jerky arm movements including tapping on the thighs or pressing against the sides of the abdomen

o Tensed and jerky leg movements including kicking motions

o Tensed and jerky feet movements including grinding, pressing, rubbing, or circular movements on the floor

o Generally tense body postures

- Negative emotions: The stuttering symptom complex includes a variety of negative emotions and avoidance reactions; the more severe the stuttering, the longer its duration of persistence, and more socially handicapping it is, the greater the frequency and severity of emotional reactions and attending avoidance behaviors; not all speakers who stutter will exhibit all or even most of the following, but they need to be understood

o Anxiety or fear about speaking situations, although most people who stutter would not be diagnosed as clinically anxious or phobic, needing psychiatric or behavioral treatment

o Self-reported feelings of frustration in not being able to speak freely, spontaneously, and fluently

o Self-reported negative statements about himself or herself, especially as a competent speaker

o A sense of helplessness when unable to move forward with fluent expressions

o Feelings of unpleasantness associated with speech and speaking situations

o Belief or impression that listeners are impatient, critical, or unsympathetic

o Feelings of embarrassment in social situations

o "Stutterer" as the dominant self-concept; many adults who stutter describe themselves as "stutterers" and some describe that they stutter in their dreams which reinforces their self-concept of a stuttering person

o Belief that their stuttering may be due to some external, uncontrollable, and inexplicable force

o Self-reported lack of self-confidence in speaking situations

o Anxious or dreaded expectation of stuttering on certain words and in certain speaking situations (expectancy)

- Avoidance reactions: Largely because of the negative experiences and unpleasant emotional reactions associated with stuttering, people who stutter develop a variety of avoidance behaviors; the number and frequency of avoidance behaviors vary, but they tend to be stronger and more persistent in people who have a consistent tendency to stutter on certain words and in certain speaking situations:

o Avoidance of certain speaking situations; people who stutter are especially prone to avoid speaking on the telephone, ordering in restaurants, buying something at a counter, speaking to a group, introducing self, verbally giving personal phone numbers or addresses, saying one's own name, responding to roll calls, and asking for directions when lost

o Avoidance of certain conversation partners, including strangers, authority figures, supervisors or bosses, and persons of the opposite sex

o Avoidance of certain words; common among children and adults who stutter; most adults can list sounds or words that give them particular difficulty; they become adept at word substitutions and circumlocutions that help them avoid difficult sounds or words

o Avoidance of talking about their stuttering and their emotional experiences associated with it; it may be that such talk is unpleasant or that they would stutter more if they do

o Avoidance of eye contact; may be a sign of social embarrassment due to stuttering

o Avoidance of talking as much as possible; some may reduce verbal output

o Dependence on others to talk for them; persons who stutter may have a spouse or friend order at restaurants, gesture others to pick up the telephone, or take a friend along on shopping trips to avoid talking to the store clerks

Onset and Progression of Stuttering

- As noted, stuttering has its onset in early childhood; preschool years evidence the greatest incidence of new cases

- Stuttering may begin as an increase in the frequency of dysfluencies; although some dysfluencies (e.g., sound prolongations and part-word repetitions) may be more notable than others, any and all forms of dysfluencies may increase; a preschool child may repeat phrases (e.g., *I-do, I-do, I-do*), often half a dozen or more times at the onset of stuttering; in some children, excessive word or phrase repetitions may be the dominant symptoms that prompt the parents to seek help

- Increased frequency of dysfluencies at the time of onset and soon thereafter may or may not be associated with a significant level of muscle tension; whereas some preschoolers who stutter repeat much without a marked degree of oral and facial tension, others may show some degree of tension even during the early onset period; tensed dysfluencies are often accompanied by associated motor behaviors

- Severity of stuttering (measured by either the frequency or duration of individual instances of stuttering) tends to vary at or soon after the onset, suggesting that stuttering is not always a linearly progressing disorder; soon after the onset, a child's stuttering may be much more severe than that of an adult with a long history of stuttering; a severe initial stuttering may change into a mild or moderate but persistent stuttering; an initially mild stuttering may escalate in frequency and other features (e.g., associated motor behaviors), while still fluctuating across time and situations

- Close to the onset, periods of normal or near-normal fluency that reassures the parents may be alternated with periods of excessive and persistent dysfluency rates that alarm the parents and dash their hope that the problem has gone away

- Although most children do not show significant associated motor behaviors at or soon after the onset of stuttering, other children may
- There is no evidence to suggest that children at any age are unaware of their speech difficulties; preschoolers at age 2 or 2.5, with a recent onset of stuttering, may already show signs of avoidance behaviors, implying not only awareness of stuttering, but also the development of compensatory strategies to deal with it; some preschool children, following a severe instance of stuttering may say, "I don't want to talk"; others might simply stay quiet or say only a few words when urged; some children may begin to talk very softly; others may even resort to whispering; some may begin to talk with exaggerated articulation or cartoon character role playing to enhance fluency—all indications of awareness
- Emotional reactions, though strongly and unequivocally articulated by older students and adults, are present in preschool children as well; younger children's emotional reactions tend to be specific to situations, whereas another child usually gives negative feedback to the child about his or her stuttering problem
- Negative reactions evident sometime after the onset of stuttering may increase as the child grows, provided that stuttering persists and perhaps increases in severity; these reactions, too, are not always linear in their development; some adults who continue to stutter may have fewer negative emotional reactions than a teenager; some adults may have empathy for the listener instead of resentment toward them, and accept their problem without fighting an emotional battle even as they seek treatment for it
- Avoidance behaviors, as noted in the context of awareness of the problem, may be noticed at any age, although they be absent soon after the onset in some children; some avoidance strategies may be noticed in even as young a child as 2 years of age; avoidance behaviors increase as the child who stutters grows older, encounters more unpleasant speaking situations, and develops a variety of avoidance reactions
- Avoidance behaviors are not linearly progressive in all cases; teenagers and young adults who have an extensive collection of avoidance reactions may be forced to face situations previously avoided as soon as employment is secured; repeatedly facing the difficult situations out of necessity, some of the avoidance reactions may be extinguished even if the stuttering did not
- Whether children who stutter have serious social or academic problems has not been clearly established; some social limitations and academic difficulties may be expected especially when the teachers are not fully supportive of the child
- Adults who stutter experience occupational difficulties; they may avoid jobs that require much talking or formal oral presentations; may remain somewhat unhappy in such jobs; some adults may face employment discrimination even though such discrimination is illegal

- In essence, severity of stuttering and the number of complicating factors (e.g., associated motor behaviors, negative emotional experiences, and avoidance tactics) are not necessarily related to the onset and progression, nor to the age, of the client; if some older children and adults show a wider array of emotional and avoidance reactions than preschoolers, it is because of their larger communication playing field

Theories of Stuttering

- The causes of stuttering are not clearly understood; theories are based mostly on the differential prevalence of stuttering in subgroups of populations and comparative analysis of stuttering versus nonstuttering groups; in general, etiologic theories remain somewhat speculative; theories range from genetic to environmental to interactionist positions with very little agreement among theorists
- Genetic factors are thought to play an important role in stuttering etiology; but extensive as it is, the genetic research has used the population genetics techniques (epidemiological), not the molecular genetic techniques that seek to find the genetic abnormalities; therefore, genetic research has mostly identified susceptibility to stuttering, not genes; no inheritance pattern has been clearly established; available observations thought to support a genetic theory of stuttering include:
  - A higher familial incidence of stuttering, suggesting the influence of genetic susceptibility to stuttering; however, familial incidence does not rule out the influence of environmental factors
  - Greater concordance rate in monozygotic (identical) twins than in ordinary siblings, suggesting the influence of genes in the etiology of stuttering; concordance rates among identical twins reared in the same environment does not rule out the influence of environmental variables; that fraternal concordance is slightly higher than the rate for ordinary siblings suggests the importance of environmental variables
  - Interaction between gender and familial incidence; highest familial incidence with a female who stutters in the family, also suggests the influence of genetic factors; however, such incidences are no direct evidence of genetic factors
- Neurophysiological factors also figure prominently in several theoretical explanations; the basic hypothesis is that persons who stutter have a different neurophysiological makeup than those who do not stutter; neurophysiological explanations are mostly based on the evidence that individuals who stutter and those who are normally fluent differ on certain variables (e.g., voice initiation and onset reaction times, speech muscle movement parameters); however, such group differences do not constitute experimental evidence supportive of theoretical explanations; therefore, neurophysiological explanations specify differences, but do not explain why there are differences; as evidence, neurophysiological theorists point out
  - Subtle abnormality in the electrical activity of the brain in some individuals who stutter; although such abnormalities have been documented,

evidence for them are not strong and uniform enough to sustain a theory of stuttering

o Atypical cerebral language processing; either a lack of left hemisphere dominance for language processing or possible dual hemisphere language processing; evidence is weak and equivocal

o Subtle and variable problems in neuromotor speech control; these problems have led to the motor control theory of stuttering; subtle abnormalities in the speed, velocity, force, and latency of speech movements (including the movements of the lips, jaw, and laryngeal mechanism) have been demonstrated in some but not all individuals who stutter; most of these abnormalities tend to disappear with repeated trials or practice; however, such speech-movement problems themselves do not show that there is a motor control problem; they may be a part of subtle and unobserved stuttering or the effects of years of stuttering; independent evidence for motor control that is not the problems to be explained has not been marshaled

o Auditory feedback problems based on the effects of delayed auditory feedback and masking noise effects; reduction of stuttering under these two variables has been the basis to suggest that people who stutter may have a speech-related auditory feedback deficiency; however, this hypothesis has been largely discounted because delayed auditory feedback (DAF) and masking noise may reduce stuttering by slowing the speech, not by correcting any presumed auditory feedback deficit

o Subtle central auditory processing problems; such central auditory processing problems as poorer performance on dichotic listening tests or distorted speech recognition tasks have been suggested as evidence that there a deficient central auditory mechanism that is responsible for stuttering; the evidence is weak and variable across individuals who stutter; the theory is not well supported

o Elevated autonomic nervous system activity; this observation is used to suggest that anxiety may be causally involved in the development of stuttering; however, anxiety and other emotional reactivity of persons who stutter may be a part of their symptom complex or a consequence of their stuttering; at the time of onset, many preschoolers repeat and prolong speech sounds without any sign of anxiety

• Linguistic factors are important in certain theories of stuttering; a version of such theories is the covert repair hypothesis; this theory suggests errors occur when speech production is planned or programmed; these programming errors must be corrected; in the process of such corrections, dysfluencies are produced; as the speaker corrects those programming errors internally, the forward flow of speech is interrupted, resulting in dysfluencies; people who stutter, unlike those who do not, need to make multiple repairs to their programming errors, resulting in multiple repetitions, unusual prolongations, long silent pauses, and other severe forms of dysfluencies; in this theory, the errors in speech programming and the resulting covert repairs of those errors are both unobserved and presumed; difficult to verify this speculative theory

F

- Environmental contingencies or factors figure prominently in other theories of stuttering; advocates of this approach claim that stuttering may be a learned behavior or an "acquired" disorder
  - An early environmental explanation of stuttering was Johnson's diagnosogenic theory which stated that the child is normally fluent (or normally dysfluent), but overly critical parents diagnose stuttering when none existed; consequent to this diagnosis, the child begins to experience anticipation and apprehension about potential parental criticism of normal speech; the child then becomes tense in speaking situations and develops avoidance reactions, which are indeed stutterings (not the dysfluencies, which are normal); there is no evidence that parents misdiagnose stuttering in normally fluent child; stuttering is diagnosed when a child's dysfluency rate clearly exceeds the normal limits; increased dysfluencies may have other characteristics, including tension, avoidance reactions, emotional responses, and so forth
  - A variation of Johnson's theory is Bloodstein's anticipatory struggle hypothesis, which says that for various reasons, the child who stutters may come to believe that speech is a difficult task; anticipates difficulties and begins to struggle; such struggles in speech production are stutterings; this hypothesis assigns importance to environmental variables in the genesis of stuttering and includes such potential factors as language difficulties, articulation problems, cluttering, and many other conditions that may lead to the belief that speech is a difficult task; such a belief then causes the child to put unusual amounts of efforts into the speaking task
  - Higher concordance rate in dizygotic (fraternal) twins than in ordinary siblings; this suggests that the fraternal twins may be more similarly reacted to than the ordinary siblings, thus causing greater concordance rates in them; twins (both mono- and dizygotic) receive more similar reactions from others than ordinary siblings; however, the possibility that twins are reacted to similarly is not strong evidence of environmental variables; it is still not clear what kinds of reactions from others may be causally related to stuttering
  - Demonstrated stimulus control of stuttering; stuttering varies under different stimulus conditions; stuttering frequency can be experimentally varied by manipulating the audience size and audience type; punishing stimuli; discriminative stimuli as in the Adjacency Effect, Consistency Effect, and Adaptation Effect; chorus reading and Shadowing; successful experimental manipulations of stuttering suggest that stuttering may be maintained by certain environmental factors, but such manipulations do not point out the original cause of stuttering
- Multiple factors and interactions of genetic and environmental factors; on the premise that most clinical conditions are a product of an interaction between genetic/neurophysiological variables and environmental variables, some hypotheses suggest that stuttering is caused by multiple factors and their interactions; some hypotheses and their justifications include:
  - The causation must be multiple because there is no single, convincing etiologic factor; this hypothesis does not point out multiple causes of

stuttering; in fact, it points out the absence of more convincing evidence for a single causation theory

o One of the interactionist hypotheses is the *demands and capacities model*; it is suggested that a child is likely to stutter if the communication demands the child faces exceed the capacity to meet those demands; demands may come from others, or they may be self-generated; child's emotional, cognitive, phonological, syntactic (or other linguistic) capacity may fail to meet the demands of communication; the result is stuttering; normally, as children grow older, their capacity for fluency increases; as it happens, the demands for greater fluency and complex language production also increase; but if there is a mismatch between a child's capacity to produce phonologically, syntactically, or in other ways complex utterances and the demands made on the child, stuttering will be the consequence; a limitation of this hypothesis is that most children and adults who stutter may do so on many simple words that may place little or no demand (saying one's own name, for example); being hard to measure, capacity is assumed from stuttering or fluency the child produces, the very phenomena the theory seeks to explain

o Various hypotheses that stuttering is multiply caused and that both genetic/neurophysiologic and environmental factors are important in its etiology is probably correct and appealing to many investigators, but it is too general to be of explanatory value; to be a strong contender to explain stuttering, the roles, the relative contributions of all postulated variables, and their interactions must be established

Bloodstein, O. (1995). *A handbook on stuttering*. San Diego, CA: Singular Publishing Group.

Conture, E. G. (2001). *Stuttering: Its nature, diagnosis and treatment*. Boston, MA: Allyn and Bacon.

Culatta, R., & Goldberg, S. A. (1995). *Stuttering therapy: An integrated approach to theory and practice*. Needham Heights, MA: Allyn and Bacon.

Curlee, R. F. (1999). *Stuttering and related disorders of fluency* (2nd ed.). New York: Thieme.

Daly, D. A. (1986). The clutterer. In K. O. St. Louis (Ed.), *The atypical stutterer: Principles and practices of rehabilitation*. Orlando, FL: Academic Press.

Daly, D. A., & Burnett, M. L. (1999). *Cluttering: Traditional views and new perspectives*. In R. F. Curlee (Ed.), *Stuttering and related disorders of fluency* (2nd ed.), pp. 222–254. New York: Thieme.

Duffy, J. R. (2005). *Motor speech disorders: Substrates, differential diagnosis, and management* (2nd ed.). New York: Elsevier Mosby.

Gregory, H. (2003). *Stuttering therapy: Rationale and procedures*. Boston, MA: Allyn and Bacon.

Guitar, B. (2006). *Stuttering: An integrated approach to its nature and treatment* (3rd ed.). Baltimore, MD: Williams & Wilkins.

Helm-Estabrooks, N. (1986). *Diagnosis and management of neurogenic stuttering*. In K. O. St. Louis, (Ed.). *The atypical stutterer* (pp. 193–217). New York: Academic Press.

Journal of Fluency Disorders, Volume 21, Issues 3–4, September–December 1996. [A special issue devoted to cluttering.]

Market, K. E. & associates (1990). Acquired stuttering: Descriptive data and treatment outcome. *Journal of Fluency Disorders, 15,* 21–31.

Myers, F. L., & St. Louis, K. O. (1992). *Cluttering: A clinical perspective*. Kibworth, England: Far Communications.

Rosenbek, J. C. (1984). *Stuttering secondary to nervous damage*. In R. F. Curlee & W. H. Perkins (Eds.), *Nature and treatment of stuttering* (pp. 31–48). Austin, TX: Pro-Ed.

Silverman, F. H. (2004). *Stuttering and other fluency disorders* (3rd ed.). Long Grove, IL: Waveland Press.

Van Riper, C. (1982). *The nature of stuttering* (2nd ed.). Englewood Cliffs, NJ: Prentice Hall.

Yairi, E., & Ambrose, N. G. (2005). *Early childhood stuttering*. Austin, TX: Pro-Ed.

Fluent Aphasias.   Several types of aphasia characterized by normal or even excessive fluency with impaired meaning; generally associated with posterior cerebral lesions; see Aphasia for a general description of etiology, symptoms, and assessment procedures; see Aphasia: Specific Types for a description of the following major fluent aphasias: anomic aphasia, conduction aphasia, transcortical sensory aphasia, and Wernicke's aphasia; contrasted with Nonfluent Aphasia.

Fluent Speech.   Speech that is smooth, flowing, effortless, and rapid within acceptable limits; negatively defined, it is speech that does not contain excessive amounts of pauses, repetitions, sound and silent prolongations, interjections, and other forms of dysfluencies; speech that is not produced with excessive effort, struggle, and unusual associated motor behaviors, such as rapid eye blinks and hand and feet movements that are a part of stuttered (dysfluent) speech.

Foreign Accent Syndrome.   A controversial syndrome of speech characteristics that are alien to the native language of the clients; its existence as a separate syndrome is debated, although several reports describe a constellation of symptoms; some consider the characteristics of foreign accent syndrome a feature of aphasia or apraxia of speech in a small number of clients; others consider it a separate syndrome; the basic feature is the inclusion of features of other natural languages the client does not speak; the speech is not thought of as disordered, but different, an essential feature of any *foreign accent*; monotone, for instance, is a characteristic of apraxia or dysarthria, but it is perceived as pathological because there is no natural language that totally lacks intonation contours; emergence of a foreign accent in a client who did speak a different language during childhood is not considered a genuine case of the syndrome; psychiatric clients who may exhibit a foreign accent are not considered to illustrate the syndrome because it is thought to be neurogenic, not psychiatric; the term *foreign accent syndrome* may be a misnomer because it is not a dialectal variation of a particular language; a monolingual British English speaking client's foreign accent may sound Italian, Polish, or Czech, although a careful analysis of the client's speech may reveal no particular features of the foreign language or languages.

Speech Characteristics of Foreign Accent Syndrome
- Foreign-sounding patterns of intonation
- Rising pitch at the end of sentences
- Excessively steep falls in pitch
- Inverted pitch contours
- Large pitch variations
- Distortions of vowels
- Insertions of epenthetic vowels
- Production of tense vowels instead of tense/lax vowels
- Various prosodic problems
- Atypical stress patterns (that give the impression of a foreign accent)
- Changes in timing and rhythm of speech

Neuropathology of Foreign Accent Syndrome
- Left hemisphere anterior lesions
- Smaller lesions than those found in clients with aphasia
- Lesions in Broca's area, the adjacent inferior motor strip, and the middle frontal gyrus
- Lesions in the basal ganglia in a few clients
- A few cases with the right hemisphere lesions and parietal lobe lesions have been reported, although the diagnosis of a true foreign accent syndrome in these clients is questionable

Blumstein, S. E., & Kurowski, K. (2006). The foreign accent syndrome: A perspective. *Journal of Neurolinguistics, 19*(5), 346–355.

Moen, I. (2000). Foreign accent syndrome: A review of contemporary explanations. *Aphasiology, 14,* 5–15.

Scott, S. K., Clegg. F., Rudge, P., & Burgess, P. (2006). Foreign accent syndrome, speech rhythm and the functional neuronatomy of speech production. *Journal of Neurolinguistics, 19*(5), 370–384.

Free Morpheme.   Morpheme that can stand alone and mean something; all words are free morphemes, although not all morphemes are words; grammatical morphemes are small elements of grammar that include the present progressive *ing*, the regular plural and the possessive inflections, prepositions, auxiliary and copula, pronouns, regular past tense inflections, and so forth; some of the grammatical morphemes are not *free*; they are called *bound* (e.g., the present progressive *ing* or the plural or past tense inflections that do not convey meaning by themselves); see also Bound Morphemes.

Fricatives.   Class of speech sounds produced by severely constricting the oral cavity and forcing the air through the point of constriction; English fricatives include /s/, /z/, /f/, /v/, /θ/, /ð/, /ʃ/, /ʒ/, and /dʒ/.

Friedreich's Ataxia. Rare, inherited neurodegenerative disease; affects 1 in about 50,000 individuals; involves the cerebellum, brainstem, and spinal cord; unsteadiness, clumsiness, ataxia, and mild dysarthria may be the early symptoms; progressive muscle atrophy follows; may lead to Dementia; begins before age 20 and causes death in about 20 years; associated with Ataxic Dysarthria and Mixed Dysarthria.

Fronting. Phonological process or pattern of articulation; the sounds produced in the back of the mouth are substituted with sounds produced in the front of the mouth, as in /t/ for /k/, /d/ for /g/, and /n/ for /ŋ/; see Articulation and Phonological Disorders.

Frontotemporal Dementia (FTD). Syndrome of neurodegenerative diseases that includes Pick's disease; form of cortical dementia with degeneration in the frontal and temporal regions; the expanded diagnostic category of frontotemporal dementia may occur in about 12% of persons younger than 65 in whom dementia is diagnosed, although the classic Pick's diseases may be somewhat uncommon; men may be more prone to this form of dementia than women; frontotemporal syndrome is a major form of non-Alzheimer dementia; significant changes in behavior and social conduct are a marked feature of FTD; the diagnostic category of FTD is still evolving and clinicians need to keep abreast of the research literature on this syndrome.

Etiologic Factors
- The major etiologic factor associated with behavioral change in FTD is the neuronal cell loss in the left and right frontal and temporal regions
- Cell loss may be more pronounced in the temporal lobe in about 25% of clients, and frontal lobe in another 25%; the rest will have cell loss in both the temporal and frontal lobes
- Degeneration may be predominant in either the left or right side of the brain
- In the classic form of Pick's disease
  - Focal atrophy in the anterior temporal and frontal lobes
  - Presence of Pick bodies (dense intracellular formations in the neuronal cytoplasm, especially in the nonpyramidal cells of the cortical layers 2, 3, and 6)
  - Presence of Pick cells (ballooned, inflated, or enlarged neurons, especially in the lower and middle cortical layers)
  - More pronounced atrophy in the dominant (left) hemisphere

Neurological and Behavioral Symptoms
- Onset of FTD is slow and the time of onset is difficult to establish
- Behavioral changes are the initial symptoms, especially in clients with predominantly right-sided brain cell atrophy; language problems are the initial symptoms in those with left-dominant atrophy
- Inappropriate and uninhibited social behavior (including sexual jokes)
- Other symptoms include excessive eating and weight gain with a craving for carbohydrates and a lack of insight into one's own condition
- Psychiatric symptoms are significant and include:
  - Apathy, depression, and irritability

- o Unusual mood fluctuations, including euphoria, excessive jocularity, and exaggerated self-esteem that alternate and contrast with their depressed states
- o Delusions without feelings of persecution
- Symptoms of dementia eventually emerge and include:
- o Significant intellectual deterioration
- o Impaired judgment, thinking, constructional skill, planning, and abstraction
- o Repetitive, ritualistic, and meaningless behavior (e.g., repeatedly folding napkins, constantly counting and hoarding food items)
- o Difficulty recognizing familiar faces and voices associated with predominantly right-sided atrophy
- Communication disorders associated with FTD are significant and include:
- o Reduced speech output often as a fairly early sign
- o Anomia and impaired confrontation naming, associated with left temporal lobe lesions
- o Nonfluent speech with verbal paraphasia, circumlocution, and use of general versus specific words—all due to a progressive loss of expressive vocabulary
- o Reduced spontaneous conversation, echolalia, and verbal stereotypes (meaningless repetitions of certain phrases)
- o Muteness in the final stages of the disease

Dickson, D. W. (2001). Neuropathology of Pick's disease. *Neurology, 56*(Suppl 4), S16–S18.

Hodges, J. R. (2001). Frontotemporal dementia (Pick's disease): Clinical features and assessment. *Neurology, 56*(Suppl 4), S6–S9.

Rossor, M. N. (2001). Pick's disease: A clinical overview. *Neurology, 56*(Suppl 4), S3–S5.

Functional Articulation Disorders. Disorders of speech production that are not organic; presumed to be of environmental origin although this is usually not confirmed with independent evidence of environmental causation; it only means that a neuroanatomic basis has not been demonstrated for the articulation disorder; children who exhibit them may be normal in most other respects.

Functional Communication. Effective and meaningful communication in natural (social) environments; includes any mode of communication (e.g., verbal, nonverbal, aided, nonaided); communication that helps achieve results and effects; need not be grammatically correct or complex; contrasted with responses given to arbitrary stimuli some clinicians may present during assessment and treatment; however, responses given to the same or similar stimuli in natural settings in the context of everyday communication are functional.

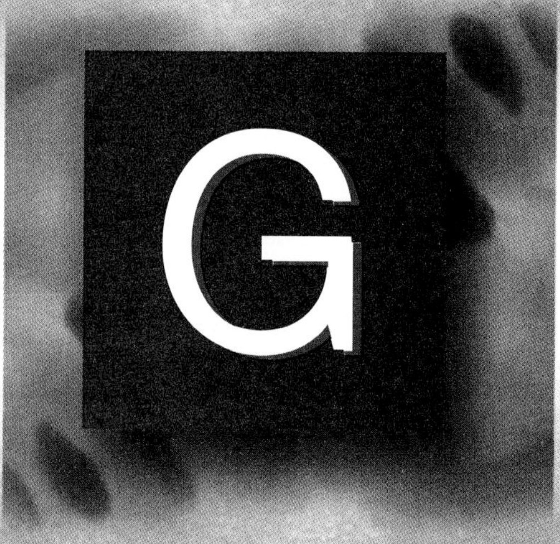
G

GABA. Gamma-amino butyric acid; an inhibitory neurotransmitter; reduced in some neurodegenerative diseases, including Huntington's Disease; its reduction is associated with intellectual impairments found in Dementia.

Galactosemia. Group of genetic disorders caused by defective galactose metabolism; children with these disorders are at risk for developmental and communication delay; see Language Disorders in Infants and Toddlers.

Gastroesophageal Reflux. Backflow of gastric contents into the esophagus, causing damage; associated with esophageal phase of swallowing; may affect the health of the laryngeal structures; may be associated with Voice Disorders.

Genetic Syndromes. See Syndromes Associated With Communication Disorders.

Gestural Communication. Method of communication that supplements oral communication with smiles and a variety of other facial expressions, body movements including shoulder shrugging, hand movements, pantomime, pointing, and head nodding or shaking; when used by people with limited oral language skills, gestural communication plays a crucial role of communicating the speaker's messages; gestural communication may be unaided as in smiling or hand movements, or aided, as in gestures combined with a communication board; procedures described under Augmentative and Alternation Communication (AAC).

Glides. Speech sounds that are produced by gradually changing the shape of the articulators; the only two English glides are /w/ and /j/.

Global Aphasia. Type of aphasia in which speech production and comprehension are severely affected; see Aphasia: Specific Types.

Glossectomy. Surgical removal of the tongue; the floor of the mouth also may be removed.

Glossopharyngeal Nerve. Cranial nerve that supplies the tongue and the pharynx.

Glossoptosis. Downward displacement of the tongue; found in some genetic syndromes including Pierre-Robin syndrome (see Syndromes Associated With Communication Disorders).

Glottal Sounds. Sounds produced at the level of the glottis; the only English glottal is /h/ although a glottal stop /?/ may be an allophonic variation of some stop sounds (as in bʌ?n for button).

Glycogen Storage Disease. Various types of inborn metabolic disorders characterized by defects in certain enzymes or transporters resulting in impaired metabolism of glycogen; children with this disease are at risk for developmental and communication delay; see Language Disorders in Infants and Toddlers.

Goiter. Enlarged thyroid gland.

Grammatical Morphemes of Language. Morphemes that change or modulate meaning; include such inflections as the regular plural or possessive and such grammatical elements as articles and conjunctions that modulate meaning; a significant aspect of language acquisition; an element that is usually omitted or misused by children who have language disorders; selected English grammatical morphemes are as follows:

Morpheme	Example
Present progressive *ing*	wal*king*, run*ning*, ea*ting*, wor*king*
Prepositions: in on under behind	 the ball is *in* the box the book is *on* the table the doll is *under* the blanket the car is *behind* the house
Regular plurals plural *s* plural *z* plural *əz*	 cat*s*, bat*s*, book*s* bag*s*, bear*s*, bed*s*, web*s* dishe*s*, matche*s*, watche*s*
Irregular plurals	men, women, children, feet
zero morpheme (the same plural and singular forms)	sheep, fish, deer
Past tense irregular verbs	went, came, ate, fell, meant, knew, sat, swam, sank, threw, wrote
Past tense regular verbs past *d* past *t* past *ted* past *ded*	 kill*ed*, turn*ed*, burn*ed* chas*ed*, walk*ed*, bak*ed*, mel*ted*, pain*ted*, ska*ted* board*ed*, hoard*ed*, load*ed*
Possessive nouns possessive *s* possessive *z* possessive *əz*	 bat*'s*, cat*'s*, Matt*'s*, goat*'s* boy*'s*, dad*'s*, dog*'s*, Joan*'s* mouse*'s*, judge*'s*, horse*'s*
Pronouns	I, you, he, she, it, we, they
Conjunctions coordinating correlative (used in pairs) subordinating	 and, but, or, nor, so, and yet either . . . or; neither . . . nor; not only; but also; whether . . . or although, because, since, if, until, when, where, while
Uncontractible copula	here I *am*; *is* she coming?; she *was* here
Contractible copula	she*'s* nice, she *is* nice; boy*'s* good, boy *is* good
Articles	the, a
Regular third person singular	he *works*, she *smiles*, Tom *hits*
Irregular third person singular	he *does*, she *has*
Uncontractible auxiliary	she *is* (in response to a question like *who is coming?*); he *was*, she *was*, it *was*

(continues)

(continued)

Morpheme	Example
Contractible auxiliary	she's running, she is running; mommy's coming, mommy is coming, it's eating, it is eating
Negation	*no* and *not*; *un*happy, *un*likely
Reflexive pronouns	them*selves*, my*self*
Comparatives/Superlatives	better, biggest best (irregular)

G

Granulovacuolar Degeneration. A buildup of fluid-filled vacuoles and granular remains within nerve cells; basic neuropathology of <u>Alzheimer's Disease</u> and found in some normal elderly people with low density.

H

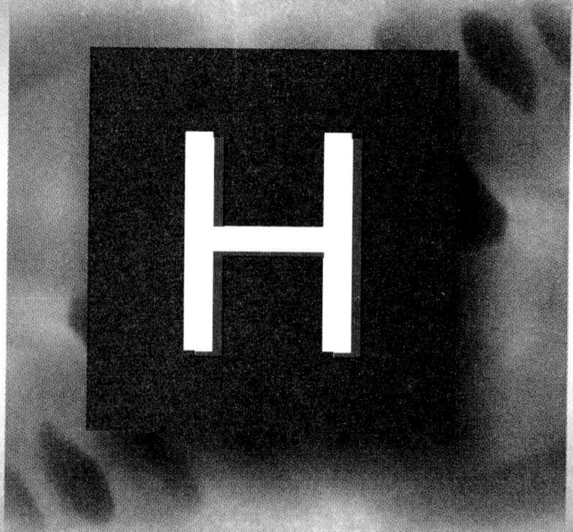

Hard of Hearing. Reduced hearing acuity; persons who are hard of hearing acquire, produce, and comprehend language primarily with the help of audition; may use amplification and visual cues to understand speech.

Hearing Impairment. Reduced hearing acuity; a hearing level that is greater than 25 dB HL in adults and 15 dB HL in young children who still are learning language; includes the Hard of Hearing and the Deaf; classified as shown under Hearing Loss; may be organic or nonorganic; nonorganic hearing loss may be malingering or psychogenic; may be peripheral or central; may be conductive (normal bone conduction and much worse air conduction), sensory (cochlear pathology), peripheral neural (involvement of the auditory branch of the cranial nerve VIII), or mixed (better bone conduction than air conduction); oral speech and language disorders are a common concomitant of hearing impairment, especially deafness; oral speech skills vary across children with the same degree of hearing impairment; communication disorders depend on a variety of factors including the age of onset, degree of loss, kind and quality of intervention, the child's age at which intervention is initiated, family support, presence of other physical and sensory problems, and so forth; it is claimed that even a mild loss of 15 dB HL during infancy and early childhood may cause delay in speech and language learning, although the evidence is not strong.

Epidemiology and Ethnocultural Variables

- Prevalence of hearing loss has been difficult to establish mainly because of the large number of variables that affect it; mainly the age of onset, the degree of hearing loss, and methods by which the loss is measured (how many frequencies are tested or whether the loss is self-reported) will affect the figures
- The number of individuals estimated to have a hearing loss in the United States varies from 14 to 40 million; such a wide range is not especially useful for educational and clinical service planning
- Recent evidence suggests that a permanent and significant hearing loss is evident in at least 10% of the population; this would mean 28 million or more people (depending on the census data) with hearing impairment
- It is estimated that 1% of the population is deaf (included in the 10% general prevalence)
- It is estimated that roughly 3 million U.S. children have a hearing impairment (deaf and hard of hearing combined); 50,000 school-age children may be deaf
- Age is a significant factor in the prevalence of hearing loss; under age 18, the prevalence is less than 2%; in the age group of 65 to 74, the prevalence may be as high as 23%; in the group aged 75 or more, the prevalence is over 30%
- Most children and adults with a hearing impairment are classified as *hard of hearing*
- Reliable figures on hearing impairments in all U.S. minority groups are scarce; available information suggests that a disproportionately greater number of minority group children may have hearing impairment
- It is estimated that about 45% of hard of hearing and deaf children belong to minority groups; of these, 20.4% are Hispanic, 17% are African American,

4.2% are Asian or Pacific Islander, 0.8% are American Indian, and about 3% are of other ethnicity or multiethnic

- National Center for Health Statistics surveys show a lower percentage of African Americans with hearing loss (4.2%) compared to whites (9.4%); it is not clear whether this is due to such methodological differences as undersampling or limited access to hearing health professions of the former group

Classification of Individuals with Hearing Loss

- Individuals with hearing loss may be classified into several subgroups, depending on the time of onset and the degree of loss
- Prelingually deaf: Most prelingually deaf are congenitally deaf; but this group also includes those who sustained hearing loss before age 5, a time period that is critical for speech and language development; oral language skills tend to be limited in this group; nonverbal communication modes (sign language, finger spelling, extensive use of gestures) may be common in this group
- Postlingually deaf: Individuals with onset of deafness between the ages of 5 and 10 years are classified as postlingually deaf; children in this group have better oral language skills than those who are prelingually deaf; nonverbal communication may still be common in this group
- Deafened: Individuals who are in their late teens or older age groups and sustain hearing loss are classified as *deafened*. Oral language skills may be intact, although they may need amplification or speech reading to understand spoken language; some loss in speech production skills may be evident
- Hard of hearing: Persons with reduced hearing acuity, congenital or acquired, but with a good potential to learn oral language skills are classified as hard of hearing; although they may use a hearing aid and may have some oral speech and language problems, their residual hearing is functional
- Sickle cell disease: Affects mainly Africans and African Americans, is associated with a high incidence of hearing loss; about 41% of adults with this diseases may have a hearing loss, often the sensorineural type of loss
- Auditory sensitivity (not hearing loss) is different in African Americans and whites for whom some data are available; generally, African Americans have better hearing sensitivity than whites; threshold of response to all frequencies is lower for African Americans than for whites; African American women have better auditory sensitivity than white women
- Generally, women of all ethnocultural backgrounds have better auditory sensitivity than men; at frequencies higher than 1,000 Hz, men show greater loss than women; at frequencies lower than 1,000 Hz, women show greater loss than men
- Hearing loss due to the normal aging process, called *presbycusis*, affects people differently; generally, women are less vulnerable to the effect than men, and African Americans are less vulnerable than whites

Etiology of Hearing Impairment

- Etiologic factors and types of hearing loss are interdependent; generally, genetic factors account for about 50% of infants with congenital hearing loss (severe to profound); of these 50%, inheritance of hearing loss is recessive in 38%, dominant in 11%, and 1% is sex-linked; the loss is nongenetic in 25%, unknown in another 25%

- Conductive hearing loss: This type of hearing loss is caused by factors that prevent the conduction of sound to the cochlea (relatively common); neural transmission of sound to the auditory centers in the brain is normal; problems lie in the outer ear, auditory canal, or middle ear; what is impaired is the air conduction of sound to the inner ear; the bone conduction of sound is normal in pure conductive hearing loss; conductive hearing loss may be congenital or acquired sometime after the birth; common causes of conductive hearing loss include:
  o Atresia or aplasia of the external ear canal, which are often due to genetic or congenital diseases or disorders that reduce or block sound transmission
  o Viral, bacterial, and fungal infections or diseases of the external auditory canal that causes swelling and consequently the sound transmission is attenuated; external otitis, for instance, is a common inflammatory disease of the auditory canal
  o Neoplastic tumors of the external auditory canal that block sound transmission or reduce it to a significant extent; for instance, osteomas (benign bony tumors of the ear canal) can cause conductive hearing loss
  o Collapsed ear canal, which is more common in elderly females and young children, is another condition that can block the air conduction of sound; the ear canal may collapse because its cartilages have lost their elasticity
  o Impacted cerumen, a common cause of temporary conductive hearing loss; treated effectively
  o Foreign objects in the ear canal; accidental insertion of various foreign objects into the ear canal (especially by children), blocking sound transmission
  o Stenosis or narrowing of the external ear may block sound transmission; congenital or due to various other diseases, including inflammation and tumor growth; normal aging also can cause stenosis
  o Disarticulation of the auditory ossicular chain, causing blocked sound transmission because of the broken interconnection between the auditory bones
  o Trauma to the middle ear, resulting in a torn tympanic membrane or damaged ossicular chain
  o Various middle ear infections, including acute suppurative otitis media (bacterial infection with puss formation) and recurrent otitis media (in combination with such other infections as sinusitis and rhinitis), causing conductive hearing loss in children
  o Tumors of the middle ear, both benign (e.g., polyps in the external auditory canal that bulge into the middle ear) or malignant (e.g., squamous cell carcinoma) that inhibit sound transmission
  o Ossicular fixation: Fixation of the small bones in the middle ear to each other or to the temporal bone, limiting their vibratory capacity
  o Otosclerosis: Spongifying growth on the footplate of the stapes, which dampens its vibration, causing conductive hearing loss

- Sensory hearing loss: This type of hearing loss is caused by interference with the normal functioning of the hair cells of the cochlea (relatively common) or the auditory nerve (cranial nerve VIII); in sensorineural hearing loss, the sound transmission from the inner ear to the brain is impaired; both the air and bone conduction of sound is impaired in sensorineural hearing loss; sensorineural loss may be congenital (genetic or acquired in utero) or acquired after birth; common causes of sensorineural hearing loss include:
  - Fetal alcohol syndrome: Maternal alcoholism during pregnancy affecting the fetal growth; causes inner ear or auditory nerve damage; may be associated with central nervous system damage
  - Ototoxicity: Toxic effects of certain drugs on the inner ear structures; may be due to maternal addiction during pregnancy or a person's own addiction; also may be due to ototoxicity from antibiotics, aspirin, diuretics, and chemotherapy given to treat cancer
  - Low birth weight: Fetal hypoxia (reduced oxygen supply to the fetus) and meningitis or encephalitis
  - Mechanical injury to the cochlea: Reduces effectiveness in transmitting sound to the auditory nerve
  - Maternal viral and bacterial infections: Maternal syphilis, cytomegalovirus infection, and congenital rubella that affect the fetal hearing mechanism
  - Vascular accidents that restrict the cochlear blood supply and cause cochlear cell damage
  - Noise exposure: Especially intense and prolonged
  - Such inner ear diseases as Meniere's disease: Can cause vertigo as well
  - Normal aging process: Can affect the health of the inner ear
  - Various genetic syndromes: See Syndromes Associated With Communication Disorders
- Peripheral neural hearing loss: This type of loss is caused by the involvement of the auditory branch of cranial nerve VIII; it is relatively rare and often caused by:
  - Tumors of cranial nerve VIII; the most common of the cranial tumors
  - Demyelinating diseases of cranial nerve VIII
- Mixed hearing loss: This type of hearing loss is caused by several factors that affect the neural conduction of sound to the cochlea through cranial nerve VIII; common causes include:
  - All of the factors that cause conductive loss also are involved in mixed loss
  - All of the factors that cause sensorineural loss also are involved in mixed loss
- Nonorganic peripheral hearing loss: Caused by psychological/behavioral factors
  - Malingering to gain advantages by knowingly faking a hearing impairment; a malingerer claims a disability that has some payoff
  - Psychogenic hearing loss, which suggests a lack of awareness of motivating factors on the part of the individual; unconscious motivation and Freudian mechanisms of conversion reaction (hysterical reaction) are invoked to explain this kind of a hearing loss; hard to verify this etiology; may be due to maladaptive reactions to difficult life situations

- Central auditory problems: These problems are presumably caused by abnormal central auditory processing of auditory stimuli; no discernible organic cause in most cases; pure tone thresholds may be normal; difficulty mostly in speech discrimination and in understanding filtered or altered speech stimuli; suggested common causes include:
  - Neoplasms and tumors in brain regions concerned with hearing, damaging those areas of the brain that process auditory stimuli
  - Such demyelinating diseases as multiple sclerosis; may cause generalized damage and damage to the auditory areas of the brain
  - Cerebrovascular diseases; may damage the auditory areas of the brain
  - Such neurodegenerative diseases as Alzheimer's disease; may cause widespread damage to the cortical regions, including the auditory areas
  - Various genetic disorders; many genetic syndromes are associated with hearing loss, although it may not always be central in origin
  - Asphyxia during birth; may cause injury to the auditory areas of the brain
  - Such infections as HIV
  - Traumatic brain injury; may affect the auditory areas of the brain

Communication Disorders

- Extent and severity of communication disorders associated with hearing impairment depends on a number of factors, including the severity of the hearing loss, age of onset of the loss (congenital or acquired sometime after birth), quality of aural rehabilitation and oral language training received, time at which rehabilitative services were initiated, family support, and special education services; the same level of hearing loss may produce widely differing effects on communication skills in different individuals
- Individuals who are congenitally deaf may more easily acquire nonverbal means of communication (e.g., American Sign Language—ASL) than verbal means, because individuals who master a comprehensive nonverbal language (especially ASL) are not considered communicatively handicapped, regardless of their oral language skills
- Children with cochlear implants may eventually master better oral language skills than those without such implants
- Parental interactions, and especially verbal interactions with their children who are either deaf or hard of hearing, may affect oral language skills in those children
- Individuals with hearing impairment may have various speech, oral language, fluency, voice and resonance, and reading and writing problems
- Speech problems
  - Neutralization of vowels, which results in all vowels sounding more like the neutral schwa
  - Confusion between diphthongs and vowels (e.g., /ai/ for /a/ or /a/ for /ai/)
  - Nasalized production of vowels and consonants
  - Vowel substitutions
  - Increased duration of vowels
  - Imprecise production of vowels
  - Omission of final consonants in words and omission of consonants in blends

- o Omission of /s/ in almost all positions
- o Omission of initial consonants
- o Substitution of voiced consonants for voiceless consonants
- o Substitution of nasal consonants for oral consonants
- o Distortion of sounds, especially of stops and fricatives
- o Addition of sounds (sʌtop for *stop*)
- o Breathiness before the production of vowels
- o Inappropriate release of final stops (cap^h)
- o Generally, reduced speech intelligibility
- o Production of only a few words per breath, resulting in wasted air
- o Generally slower than the normal speech rate, although slower rate may be associated with improved intelligibility
- Oral language problems
  - o Delayed onset of babbling
  - o Generally limited vocabulary; vocabulary may be limited to simpler words
  - o Poor comprehension of word meanings, especially complex or infrequently used words
  - o Lack of understanding of multiple meanings of words
  - o Difficulty understanding abstract, metaphoric, and proverbial phrases
  - o Slower acquisition of grammatical morphemes; overuse of nouns and verbs and omission of function words; omission or inconsistent production of many grammatical morphemes, including the articles, adverbs, prepositions, conjunctions, past tense inflections, plural inflections, present progressive *ing,* indefinite pronouns, quantifiers, and third person singular
  - o Incorrect production of the irregular plural and past tense forms
  - o Slower acquisition of verb forms
  - o Difficulty understanding and producing complex, compound, and embedded sentences
  - o Shorter sentences; non-English word order
  - o Limited syntactic variety (fewer types of sentences); speech may consist mostly of subject-verb-object constructions
  - o Pragmatic language problems including reluctance to speak
  - o Limited oral communication (saying very little)
  - o Lack of elaborated of speech
  - o Insufficient background information
  - o Occasional irrelevance of speech
  - o Improper linguistic stress patterns
  - o Difficulty with conversational repair strategies
  - o Inadequate or inappropriate conversational skills including topic initiation, topic maintenance, and conversation closing conventions
  - o Minimal language growth after age 12 or 13
- Fluency problems
  - o Generally limited fluency, due to limited oral language skills
  - o Increased rate of dysfluencies
  - o Slow rate of speech
  - o Inappropriate pauses during continuous speech production

- o Abnormal flow of speech
- o Abnormal rhythm of speech
- Voice and resonance problems
  - o Voice quality deviations, especially in the deaf
  - o Generally, high-pitched voice, harshness, and hoarseness
  - o Breathy voice due to inadequate vocal fold closure
  - o Lack of normal intonation, resulting in monotone
  - o Hyponasal resonance on nasal sounds
  - o Hypernasal resonance on nonnasal sounds
  - o Reduced vocal intensity or reduced variations in vocal intensity
- Reading and writing problems of the hearing impaired include the following:
  - o Poor reading comprehension
  - o Writing that reflects the language problems listed (poor syntax, omission of grammatical morphemes, limited variety of sentences, minimal information offered)

Bernthal, J. E., & Bankson, N. W. (2004). *Articulation and phonological disorders* (5th ed.). Boston, MA: Allyn and Bacon.

Carney, A. E., & Moeller, M. P. (1998). Treatment efficacy: Hearing loss in children. *Journal of Speech-Language-Hearing Research, 41,* S61–S84.

Elfenbein, J. L., Hardin-Jones, M. A., & Davis, J. M. (1994). Oral communication skills of children who are hard of hearing. *Journal of Speech-Language-Hearing Research, 37,* 216–226.

Hegde, M. N., & Maul, C. A. (2006). *Language disorders in children.* Boston, MA: Allyn and Bacon.

Martin, F. N., & Clark, J. G. (2003). *Introduction to audiology* (8th ed.). Boston, MA: Allyn and Bacon.

National Center for Health Statistics. (1994). *National Health Interview Survey,* Series 10, No. 188. Hyattsville, MD: National Center for Health Statistics.

Northern, J. L. (1996). *Hearing disorders.* Boston, MA: Allyn and Bacon.

Paul, R. (1995). *Language disorders from infancy through adolescence.* St. Louis, MO: Mosby.

Peña-Brooks, A., & Hegde, M. N. (2007). *Assessment and treatment of articulation and phonological disorders in children* (2nd ed.). Austin, TX: Pro-Ed.

Schow, R. L., & Nerbonne, M. A. (2002). *Introduction to audiologic rehabilitation* (4th ed.). Boston, MA: Allyn and Bacon.

Scott, D. M. (2002). Multicultural aspects of hearing disorders and audiology. In D. E. Battle (Ed.), *Communication disorders in multicultural populations* (pp. 335–360) (3rd ed.). Boston, MA: Butterworth-Heinemann.

Yoshinaga-Itano, C., & Downey, D. M. (1996). Development of school-aged deaf, hard of hearing, and normally hearing students' written language. *Votla Review, 98,* 3–7.

Hearing Loss. Roughly the same as <u>Hearing Impairment</u>; hearing loss may be conductive or sensorineural; generally, the greater the hearing loss, the higher the prevalence of oral language deficits although the deaf may be competent communicators through the American Sign Language; hearing loss is classified as follows:

- Mild hearing loss: 16–40 dB HL
- Moderate hearing loss: 41–70 dB HL
- Severe hearing loss: 71–90 dB HL
- Profound hearing loss: 90 dB and higher

Hemifacial Microsomia. Underdevelopment of one side of the face; associated with severe genetic syndromes; see Syndromes Associated With Communication Disorders.

Hemiparesis. Weakness of one side of the body; contrasted with hemiplegia, which is paralysis of one side of the body; due to various neurological diseases.

Hemorrhage. Bleeding within an organ because of blood vessel defects.

H

Hemorrhagic Stroke. A form of stroke caused by bleeding within the brain due to a ruptured artery; a cause of Aphasia; contrasted with Ischemic Stroke.

Heterochromia. Pigmentary disorder; part that should have the same color has multiple colors; in heterochromia irides, for example, the two irides are of different colors; a part of some genetic syndromes including Waardenburg Syndrome; see Syndromes Associated With Communication Disorders.

Human Immunodeficiency Syndrome (AIDS). A complex degenerative disorder due to HIV infection; may be associated with Dysphagia and Dementia; see also AIDS Dementia Complex.

Human Immunodeficiency Virus (HIV). Retrovirus that causes the acquired immunodeficiency syndrome; may be associated with Dysphagia and Dementia.

Hunter Syndrome. A variety of mucopolysaccharidosis syndromes; see Syndromes Associated With Communication Disorders.

Huntington's Disease (HD). Neurodegenerative disease with a genetic basis characterized by chorea, psychiatric problems, and intellectual decline; also called *Huntington's chorea*, although chorea may not always be present; results in a type of subcortical dementia; affects men and women equally; the typical age of onset is between 35 and 40 years; has a juvenile form with an onset as early as age 4; late onset in the 80s; incidence is estimated to be 40 to 70 persons per million; caused by neuronal loss in the caudate nucleus and putamen along with diffuse neuronal loss in the cortex; symptoms include chorea and Dementia; associated with motor speech disorders and language impairment; please see Dementia; also see hyperkinetic dysarthria under Dysarthria: Specific Types.

Etiology of Huntington's Disease

- Autosomal dominant inheritance is the main genetic basis
- Half the offspring of an affected person may have the disease (a 50% transmission probability)
- Mutation on the short arm of chromosome 4, thought to have been originated in Britain and spread to other parts of the world

- Formation of a destructive protein called *huntingtin*, which destroys the brain cells that control movement and memory
- Drug toxicity, postencephalopathy, and arteriosclerotic diseases

Neuropathology of Huntington's Disease
- Loss of neurons primarily in the basal ganglia, especially in the caudate nucleus and the putamen
- Some atrophy in the prefrontal and parietal lobes
- Reduced levels of such inhibitory neurotransmitters as GABA (gamma-amino butyric acid) acetylcholine

Early Symptoms
- Gradual changes in behavior and personality, including depression, irritability, anxiety, suspicious, complaining, and nagging personality; a false sense of superiority; emotional outbursts
- Neurological symptoms including abnormalities of movement (resembling fidgeting); early signs of chorea; seizure, motor problems, confusion, or disorientation
- Beginning problems of memory, judgment, and executive functions

Advanced Symptoms
- Intensified behavioral or psychiatric symptoms found in the early stages, and emergence of hostility, physical and verbal abuse, serious mood swings, paranoia, hallucinations, delusions; typically followed by chorea
- Neurological symptoms including generalized chorea (irregular, spasmodic, jerky, complex, rapid, and involuntary movements of the limb and facial muscles); may not be evident to the same severe extent in all clients; tic-like movements in the face; gait disturbances; rigidity in some clients; slow movement of all kinds terminating in little or no movement
- Attempted suicide in many cases; suicide in some 8% of the cases
- Further deterioration in intellectual skills, including memory, judgment, attention, and executive disturbances; confusion and disorientation
- Dysarthric speech, mostly affected by the choreiform movements of the articulators, respiratory muscles, and the larynx; results more often in Hyperkinetic Dysarthria
- Language impairment associated with Dementia; include impaired word-list generation, naming difficulties, shorter and simpler utterances, grammatically impaired sentences, speech comprehension deficits; muteness in the final stage of the illness
- The final stage is characterized by incontinence, sleep disturbances, dysphagia, extreme violence and confusion, heart disease, lung disease, and infections of various sorts
- Profound dementia and death within 10 to 20 years of onset

American Psychiatric Association (1994). *Diagnostic and statistical manual of mental disorders* (4th ed.). Washington, DC: Author.

Clark, C. M., & Trojanowski, J. Q. (2000). *Neurodegenerative dementias*. New York: McGraw-Hill.

Cummings, J. L., & Benson, D. F. (1983). *Dementia: A clinical approach.* Boston, MA: Butterworth.

Hegde, M. N. (2006). *A coursebook on aphasia and other neurogenic language disorders* (3rd ed.). Clifton Park, NY: Thomson Delmar Learning.

Jaques, A., & Jackson, G. A. (2000). *Understanding dementia* (3rd ed.). New York: Churchill Livingstone.

Simon, R. P., Aminoff, M. J., & Greenberg, D. A. (1999). *Clinical neurology* (4th ed.). Stamford, CT: Appleton & Lange.

Weiner, M. F. (1996). *The dementias: diagnosis, management, and research* (2nd ed.). Washington, DC: American Psychiatric Press.

Hurler Syndrome.   A variety of mucopolysaccharidosis syndrome; see Syndromes Associated With Communication Disorders.

Hydrocephalus.   Accumulation of the cerebrospinal fluid; causes dilation of the central ventricles and may cause brain atrophy and intellectual disabilities; may be a congenital condition.

Hydrophthalmos.   Variety of glaucoma in which the fibrous coats of the eye are enlarged and distended; associated with some genetic syndromes; see Waardenburg Syndrome under Syndromes Associated With Communication Disorders.

Hyperfluency.   Better-than-normal fluency of speech but may be essentially meaningless; found in some clients with fluent Aphasia.

Hyperkinesia.   Excessive and involuntary movement of the muscles due to damage to the basal ganglia; neurotransmitter imbalances in basal ganglia or other neurochemical problems may cause hyperkinetic movements; a main characteristic of Huntington's Disease; associated with Hyperkinetic Dysarthria (see Dysarthria: Specific Types).

Hyperkinetic Agraphia.   Disorder of handwriting associated with tics, chorea, and dystonia; disorganized writing.

Hyperkinetic Dysarthria.   Type of motor speech disorder caused by damage to the basal ganglia, resulting in involuntary tics, chorea, myoclonus, tremor, and dystonia; speech is characterized by impaired loudness, rate variations, and phonetic breaks; see Dysarthria: Specific Types.

Hypernasality.   Excessive nasal resonance on nonnasal sounds; may be due to a variety of causes including velopharyngeal insufficiency or incompetence, too deep a pharynx, short soft palate, and neural damage; see Velopharyngeal Dysfunction for conditions that cause hypernasality; associated with Dysarthria, Cleft Palate, and Cerebral Palsy; a form of resonance disorder; see Voice Disorders.

Hypertelorsim.   Abnormal distance between two organs (such as the eyes); part of several genetic Syndromes Associated With Communication Disorders.

Hypodontia.   Absence of one or more teeth.

Hypokinesia.   Reduced movement and decreased range of motion due to increased muscle tone; often a result of basal ganglia lesions; increased muscle rigidity, causing a reduced range of movement; not to be confused with Hypotonia, which is reduced muscle tone; a motor control problem associated with Hypokinetic Dysarthria; (see Dysarthria: Specific Types).

Hypokinetic Agraphia. Also known as micrographia, a disorder of handwriting characterized by unusually small letters that are progressively smaller in the same sample of writing.

Hyperkinetic Dysarthria. Type of motor speech disorder caused by damage to the basal ganglia, causing restricted range of movement and affecting respiratory, phonatory, articulatory, and prosodic aspects of speech; see Dysarthria: Specific Types.

Hyponasality. Reduced or absent nasal resonance in the production of nasal sounds; the same as denasality; due to nasal obstructions caused by inflammation of the nasal tissue, tumors or other kinds of growth, and foreign bodies; see Voice Disorders.

Hypoplasia. Underdevelopment or incomplete development of an organ; typically due to genetic or congenital causes; see Syndromes Associated With Communication Disorders.

Hypoplastic Philtrum. Genetic or congenital defect; underdevelopment of the vertical groove of the middle part of the upper lip; a part of several genetic Syndromes Associated With Communication Disorders.

Hypotension. Blood pressure that is too low.

Hypotonia. Neuromuscular disorder, characterized by reduced muscle tone or tension leading to flaccidity; found in cerebellar diseases; may be due to peripheral nervous system damage; may be congenital or acquired; various spinal cord disorders may cause it; associated with Ataxic Dysarthria and Flaccid Dysarthria.

Hypoxia. Reduced oxygen; due to anemia in adults and abnormal delivery of babies; a general cause is a vascular disorder that limits blood flow, resulting in tissue damage, including brain damage; associated with Aphasia.

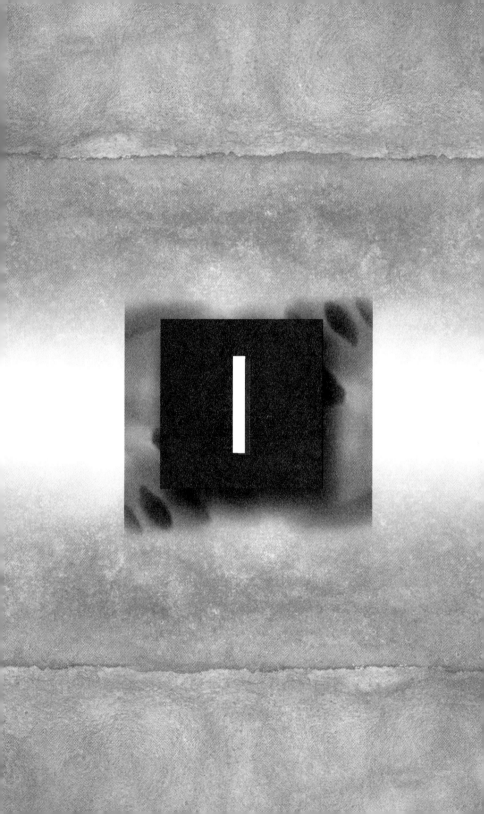

Iatrogenic.   A disease or problem due to a treatment or procedure.

Idiopathic.   Of unknown origin.

Idiosyncratic Processes.   Phonological processes; patterns of misarticulations that are unique to a given child; not found in normally developing children; see Articulation and Phonological Disorders.

Impression Trauma.   Trauma or injury to the head (or any other structure) at the point of contact with a striking object; see Traumatic Brain Injury.

Incidence.   The number of new cases of a disorder or a disorder observed in a specified time duration (e.g., one year) in a specified population; requires a longitudinal method of study; need to start with a healthy population (e.g., healthy babies) and follow them for a relatively long duration to find out how many of them begin to exhibit a disease or disorder; a term often misused because incidence of disorders is more poorly understood than Prevalence.

Incontinence.   Loss of voluntary control over excretory functions; may be urinary incontinence or fecal incontinence; associated with various medical conditions and neurodegenerative diseases that result in Dementia.

Initial Consonant Deletion.   Phonological process or articulation disorder in which the consonants in the initial word positions are omitted; see Articulation and Phonological Disorders.

Integument.   All of the covering layers of the body, including the layers of the skin and its derivates (e.g., nails and hair); disorders of integument are commonly associated with various genetic syndromes that may also affect communication skills.

Intellectual Disabilities.   A term that is preferred to *mental retardation*; some prefer the term *developmental disabilities*; the condition includes deficiencies in intellectual, social, and adaptive behaviors that are significantly below normal during the developmental period which extends up to age 18 or 22; communicative problems are a significant aspect of these deficiencies; causes are varied as well as their effects; individuals with profound disabilities need institutional care; intellectual disabilities may be associated with physical disabilities (e.g., neuromuscular disorders) or other clinical conditions (e.g., autism); individuals with mild disabilities may hold jobs and function in society; children with intellectual disabilities often are in need of special educational services.

Definitions and Terms
- The American Association on Mental Retardation (AAMR), whose name is being changed to the American Association on Intellectual and Developmental Disabilities, defines intellectual disabilities in terms of limitations in intellectual functioning and in adaptive behavior; disabilities are evident in conceptual, social, and practical adaptive skills and begins before age 18; intellectual limitations are measured through IQ tests—the scores should fall below 70 for the diagnosis; deficiencies in conceptual skills include limited language, reading, and writing skills; social skill deficiencies include limited interpersonal behaviors; practical skills refer to daily living activities

(dressing oneself, self-feeding, using money, holding a job, cooking a meal); a child or an individual with disabilities needs various kinds of support, a concept inherent to the definition
- Administration on Developmental Disabilities of the U.S. Department of Health and Human Services defines intellectual disabilities as a chronic disability in individuals 5 years or older, attributable to sustained mental or physical impairment, noticed before age 22, and results in functional limitations of at least three skill areas; the areas listed are similar to the deficiencies AAMR specifies; in this definition, the term *mental impairment* is probably the most troublesome.
- The American Psychiatric Association (APA) defines intellectual disabilities as below average intellectual level as measured by IQ tests with onset before age 18 and limitations in at least three adaptive skills (communication, self-care, home living, social/interpersonal skills, use of community resources, self-direction, functional academic skills, work, leisure, health, and safety).

Classification of Intellectual Disabilities
- Intellectual disabilities are classified in various ways; APA's classification, based primarily on IQ scores, is commonly used
  - Mild intellectual disabilities: individuals with an IQ range of 50–55 to 70 fall into this classification; majority of individuals with intellectual disabilities fall into this category; they may complete sixth grade in school, hold a job, but need sustained supervision and support
  - Moderate intellectual disabilities: evident in about 10% of children with the diagnosis of intellectual disabilities, it is characterized by an IQ range of 35–40 to 50–55; the children may be trained in certain skills, but they may complete only a second grade education; they need constant supervision and support
  - Severe intellectual disabilities: about 3% to 4% children with intellectual disabilities fall into this category; the IQ range of children in this category is 20–25 to 30–35; literacy and language skills will are extremely limited; need constant supervision and support

Epidemiology and Ethnocultural Variables
- Prevalence of intellectual disabilities is difficult to establish because of the varied clinical conditions that are associated, varied definitions, and varied levels; studies that include mild intellectual disabilities or those below IQs 100 but above 75 may report a much higher prevalence than studies that exclude such children; if intellectual disabilities that are associated with such other abnormalities as genetic syndromes or autism are excluded, a lower prevalence would be reported than if intellectual disabilities, when they exist, are also considered; children who are institutionalized may be typically excluded, also resulting in lower prevalence
- According to the National Dissemination Center for Children with Disabilities (NICHCY at http://www.nichcy.org), the prevalence of intellectual disabilities is about 3% in the general population (which means 3 out of every 100 individuals); the U.S. Center for Disease Control, which monitors intellectual disabilities in greater metropolitan Atlanta, Georgia, reports only a

1% prevalence (9.7 children in 1,0000); other reports suggest a national prevalence of 2.32%

- Roughly 10% of all children who receive special education services have intellectual disabilities
- Mild forms of intellectual disabilities are more common than severe forms
- More boys than girls are diagnosed with intellectual disabilities
- Prevalence is higher in older children (ages 6 to 10 years) than in younger children (3 to 5 years), but this differential may partly be due to difficulty diagnosing milder forms of intellectual disabilities in young children
- Reliable information on the prevalence of intellectual disabilities in various ethnocultural groups is limited; however, according to Harvard University's Civil Rights Project (http://www.civilrightsproject.harvard.edu):
  o About 1.5 million minority children are diagnosed with intellectual disabilities, emotional disturbance, or learning disability
  o Native American and African American children are one and a half to four times more likely than white children to be diagnosed with intellectual disabilities or emotional disturbances; the implication is that this outcome is due to overdiagnosis and does not suggest a higher prevalence of intellectual disabilities and emotional disturbances in minority children
  o Compared to whites, Asian and Hispanic children are underdiagnosed with intellectual disabilities, thus potentially denying them the needed special educational services and support
  o In some states, Hispanic children also may be overdiagnosed with intellectual disabilities
  o In many southern states, overdiagnosis of intellectual disabilities in African American children is more common than in the northern or western states; although the national prevalence rate is less than 3%, the prevalence of intellectual disabilities among African American children as diagnosed in southern school districts is as high as 5.41%
  o Once diagnosed, minority children are more likely than white children to be placed in restrictive, separated, or limited educational programs
  o Generally, the wealthier the school district, the more likely an African male is diagnosed with intellectual disabilities

Speech and Language Skills of Children with Intellectual Disabilities

- Communication skills of children with intellectual disabilities vary; two children with the same or similar IQ may have differing communication skills
- The level of communication skills depends on the degree of intellectual disabilities, the presence or absence of other limiting factors (e.g., hearing loss, vision problems, genetic syndromes, neurological deficits, craniofacial anomalies including cleft palate, emotional disorders, autism, or other pervasive developmental disorders), quality and timing of initiation of special education or other clinical services, and family support
- Phonological problems
  o Articulation problems are common in children with intellectual deficits; up to 70% of children with intellectual disabilities may have speech disorders

196

- o Children whose intellectual disabilities are also associated with craniofacial abnormalities (e.g., cleft palate or serious malocclusion) may have more serious articulation disorders
- o Articulation disorders of children with and without intellectual disabilities are similar and include:
  - Deletion of consonants in final positions (most frequent errors)
  - Simplification of consonant clusters; deletion of one or more phonemes in a cluster
  - Distortions of consonants
  - Substitution of consonants
  - See Articulation of Phonological Disorders for details
- Semantic problems
  - o Children with intellectual disabilities are generally slow in acquiring language; however, the sequence of acquisition is not deviant; the children follow the same general sequence of learning the different aspects of language, but at a slower rate
  - o Slowness of acquisition does not mean that the children will eventually achieve normal language skills, even with intervention; most retain some deficits
  - o The general characteristics of semantic language skills of children with intellectual disabilities are as follows:
    - Later than the usual babbling; fewer sounds in babbling
    - Later and slower acquisition of first few words
    - Relatively faster acquisition of single words than syntactic features
    - Slower acquisition of new words
    - Acquisition of fewer words at any given unit of time
    - Smaller and limited vocabulary
    - Less varied and more concrete vocabulary (e.g., mostly nouns)
    - Fewer adjectives and adverbs
    - Generally similar to the semantic problems described under Language Disorders in Children
- Morphological problems
  - o Deficiencies in morphologic productions are a hallmark of language disorders in all children, including those with intellectual disabilities
  - o Deficiencies in morphological skills may exceed limitations in vocabulary
  - o Morphological problems include:
    - Omission of many morphological features including the regular plural, possessive, present progressive *ing,* past tense inflections, prepositions, auxiliary, copula, irregular plural and past tense morphemes, third person singular, prepositions, pronouns, and so forth
    - Generally similar to the morphological problems described under Language Disorders in Children
- Syntactic problems
  - o Syntactic skills that lag behind vocabulary
  - o Telegraphic language productions
  - o Syntactic problems include:
    - Generally simplified and shorter sentence structures

- Fewer sentence types; lack of transformational variety
- Lack of complex, compound, and passive sentence forms
- Fewer relative clause usage
- Generally, less elaborated language
- Generally similar to the syntactic problems described under Language Disorders in Children

- Pragmatic problems
  o Moderate to severe intellectual disabilities are associated with significant difficulties in social communication (pragmatic language skills), although much of what we know about these skills is from research involving children with Down syndrome
  o Pragmatic language skills of children with intellectual disabilities are similar to those who are otherwise normal but have a language disorder
  o Pragmatic or social communication skills may include the following:
    - Reluctance to talk in social situations
    - Difficulty in initiating conversation
    - Abrupt and short answers to questions
    - Responses that are inappropriate to time, place, person, and topic of conversation
    - Difficulty in topic maintenance
    - Difficulty in adding new information during conversation
    - Deficient narrative skills
    - Problems in using conversational repair strategies (e.g., lack of appropriate responses to request for clarification and lack of requests for clarification when utterances are unclear)
    - Limited generalization of learned language and other skills
    - Generally similar to the pragmatic problems described under Language Disorders in Children

- Fluency problems
  o Stuttering is more frequent in children with Down syndrome than in the general population
  o Even without a diagnosis of stuttering, the fluency of children with intellectual disabilities is limited
  o The limited fluency of children with intellectual disabilities may be a function of their deficient language skills and may be characterized by:
    - Repetitions, of various kinds, including sound, syllable, word, and phrase repetitions
    - Interjections of sounds and syllables and extraneous comments
    - Pauses at inappropriate junctures and of unusually long durations
    - Revisions and incomplete phrases

- Hearing problems
  o Auditory disorders are frequent
  o Children with Down syndrome are especially vulnerable to middle ear infections and the resulting conductive hearing loss
  o Auditory problems associated with intellectual disabilities include the following:
    - Buildup of ear wax due to poor self-care skills

- History of middle ear infections and conductive hearing loss
- Sensorineural hearing loss
- Language comprehension problems
  - The degree of language comprehension deficits may be complicated by such other factors as hearing impairment
  - The lower the intellectual level, the poorer the language comprehension skill
  - Language comprehension deficits include:
    - Difficulty in understanding syntactic constructions that are complex, long, or both
    - Difficulty in comprehending the meaning of abstract words
    - Problems in understanding proverbs, metaphors, similes, and such other complex and abstract elements of language

Etiologic Factors of Intellectual Disabilities

- Various prenatal factors including maternal rubella, prenatal lead poisoning, mercury poisoning, prenatal immunization, maternal anoxia, prenatal trauma, X-ray and radiation, prematurity and low birth weight, fetal alcohol syndrome, and maternal drug abuse
- Natal factors including fetal anoxia and brain injury during birth due to such factors as birth canal compression and malpositioning of the baby
- Postnatal factors including post-immunization encephalitis, rabies vaccine, lead poisoning, mercury poisoning, or other kinds of toxicity can damage the growing brain
- Head trauma due to vehicular and other kinds of accidents, child abuse, and gunshot wounds can cause brain injury
- Metabolic disorders including phenylketonuria (PKU) and lipid metabolic errors (e.g., Tay-Sachs disease)
- Endocrine disorders including hypothyroidism can limit the growth and affect intellectual functions
- Cranial abnormalities including anencephaly (absence of cranial bones), microcephaly (extremely small head), hydrocephaly (enlargement of the head due to excessive collection of spinal fluids within the cranial vault), and macrocephaly (enlargement of the head due to abnormal increase in the brain size) are associated with genetic syndromes that limit intellectual skills
- Genetic factors resulting in such syndromes as Down syndrome, fragile X syndrome, fetal alcohol syndrome, Prader-Willi syndrome, cri du chat syndrome, and Williams syndrome (see Syndromes Associated With Communication Disorders) are among the many genetic syndromes associated with intellectual disabilities; 25% to 50% of cases of intellectual disabilities may be due to genetic factors; in excess of 280 genes are known to play a role in the causation of intellectual disabilities; many more are yet to be mapped
- Familial inheritance or prevalence may be a factor, although no specific gene has been identified; familial prevalence of intellectual disabilities is thought to be due to multiple genes each with minor defects; higher familial prevalence may be due to other factors, not necessarily genetic, that have not been identified

American Association on Mental Retardation. See the website http://www.aamr.org for the definition and classification of intellectual disabilities and for various kinds of resources.

American Psychiatric Association. (2000). *Diagnostic and statistical manual of mental disorders, Fourth Edition, text revision.* Washington, DC: Author.

Hegde, M. N., & Maul, C. A. (2006). *Language disorders in children: An evidence-based approach to assessment and treatment.* Boston, MA: Allyn and Bacon.

Nelson, N. W. (1998). *Childhood language disorders in context* (2nd ed.). Boston, MA: Allyn and Bacon.

Paul, R. (2001). *Language disorders from infancy through adolescence* (2nd ed.). St. Louis, MO: C. V. Mosby.

Reed, V. (2005). *An introduction to children with language disorders* (3rd ed.). Boston, MA: Allyn and Bacon.

Intention Tremor.   A neurological disorder, also known as kinetic tremor; absent during periods of rest but present during such voluntary movements as reaching for an object; due to cerebellar damage; among other neurological disorders, found in Ataxic Dysarthria.

Intracerebral Hematoma.   Accumulation of blood within the brain; often a result of hemorrhage due to damaged or burst blood vessels.

Intracranial Hematoma.   Accumulation of blood within the skull or the brain; due to damaged or burst vessels.

Intracranial Neoplasms.   See Brain Tumors.

Intubation Granuloma.   Lesion of the larynx that occurs at or near the vocal process of the arytenoid because of trauma caused by the insertion, positioning, or removal of an endotracheal tube; treatment is surgical; voice therapy except for vocal rest is not recommended.

Ischemia.   Interrupted or reduced blood supply to an organ or tissue, causing tissue death; cerebral ischemia is associated with Aphasia; often a result of occluded arteries in the brain; leads to a form of stroke.

Ischemic Strokes.   Cerebrovascular accidents in which specific or widespread areas of the brain may be damaged; caused by blocked arteries; a frequent cause of Aphasia; contrasted with Hemorrhagic Strokes.

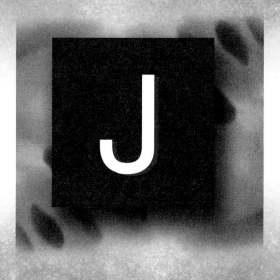

Jargon. Fluent but meaningless speech; characteristic of aphasia; often a result of word finding problems associated with brain injury; clients who cannot find the right word may invent meaningless words and substitute them for real words; also may mean the technical vocabulary of sciences and professions.

Jejunostomy. Surgical opening in the external abdominal wall to create a passage into the jejunum so a client with dysphagia can be fed nonorally.

Jejunum. A portion of the small intestine that extends from the duodenum to the ileum; may be a site to surgically manage Dysphagia.

Joint Attention. An adult and child interaction pattern involved in social communication; also called *joint reference*; the adult and the child looking at the same physical stimulus or event and talking about it; lack of joint attention is a sign of pragmatic language difficulty.

J

K

Keratosis.   Lesions marked by an overgrowth of the horny layer of the epidermis; see Voice Disorders for hyperkeratosis as a cause of voice disorder.

Kinesthesia.   Sensation of movement; impaired in certain neuromuscular disorders; may be associated with certain speech disorders.

Kyphoscoliosis.   Backward and lateral curvature of the spinal column; eventually affects lung and heart function; see Refsum Syndrome under Syndromes Associated With Communication Disorders.

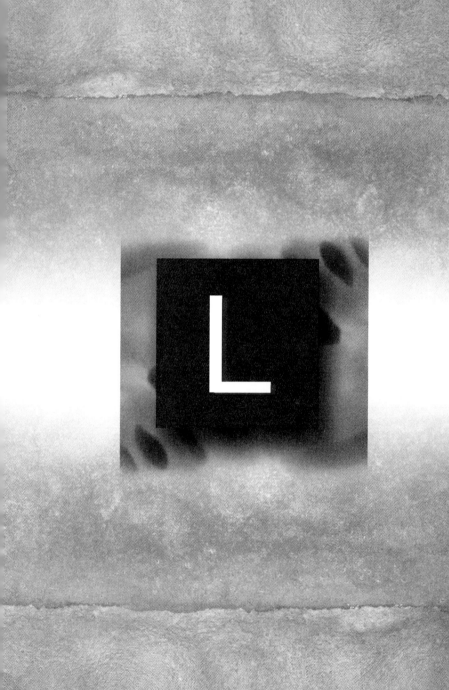

Lacuna. A hollow space, cavity, or gap in anatomic structures; characteristic of neurodegenerative diseases that are associated with Dementia.

Language Disorders in Adults. Difficulty in comprehending, formulating, and producing language; language disorders in adults often refer to loss or impairment of previously acquired language skills due to physical diseases, especially neurological diseases, and trauma; includes Aphasia, Dementia, and language disorders associated with Right-Hemisphere Injury and Traumatic Brain Injury.

Language Disorders in Children. Difficulty in learning to comprehend and/or produce semantic, phonological, syntactic, morphological, and pragmatic aspects of language; may be defined as deficient and/or inappropriate verbal behaviors in children; also known as *language delay, language deviance,* or *language impairment,* though *language disorders* is a preferred term; found in varied groups of children; some children with language disorders may have such associated conditions as autism, intellectual disability, neurological deficits, or hearing impairment; other children who have language disorders may have no other clinical condition that explains these disorders; somewhat controversially, significant expressive and/or receptive language disorders not explainable by impaired hearing, intelligence, or oral structures is called Specific Language Impairment (SLI), and is the main thrust of this entry; language disorders may be subtle in some children and may be residual problems in some treated children; some school-age children with language disorders may be classified as learning disabled; found in many genetic syndromes in children that affect communication; see Syndromes Associated With Communication Disorders; see Intellectual Disabilities, Autism Spectrum Disorders, and Hearing Impairment for language disorders associated with these conditions; see also Language Disorders in Infants and Toddlers and Language Disorders in Older Students and Adolescents; for phonological problems, see Articulation and Phonological Disorders; this section describes language disorders in children with no other significant intellectual, behavioral, or psychiatric conditions (specific language impairment).

Epidemiology and Ethnocultural Considerations
- Estimates of the prevalence of language disorders in children vary; this variability is due to methodological and definitional variability across studies; some investigators report only on children with specific language impairment, whereas others report on children with different kinds of language disorders; the former estimates will be lower than the latter estimates
- Prevalence of language disorders in children is often reported to be 12% to 15%, but the number will vary for different age groups and for language disorders in particular diagnostic categories (with or without other complicating conditions)
- Among kindergarten children, 7% to 8% may exhibit specific language impairment (limited language skills with no other concomitant problems)
- More boys than girls have language disorders; roughly, 8% of boys and 6% of girls may exhibit language disorders
- Less than 8% of 5-year-olds may have a language disorder

- If all children with language disorders, including those with autism spectrum disorders, hearing impairment, intellectual disabilities, neurological disorders, and so forth are included, the prevalence will be higher than 15%
- Familial prevalence of language disorders (especially SLI) is higher than that in the general population; the familial prevalence of SLI is estimated at 20% to 40% (much higher than the 7% to 8% for the general population)
- Some evidence suggests that the concordance rates of SLI among identical twins may be higher than that for fraternal twins or ordinary siblings
- Some molecular genetic studies have suggested that genetic susceptibility to language disorders may involve chromosomes 16 and 19
- Language disorders may be slightly more common among children of lower socioeconomic levels than upper socioeconomic levels; poverty may affect language acquisition in some children, although most families in all socioeconomic levels can provide the minimum conditions necessary for acquiring oral language
- Language disorders in children of varied ethnocultural backgrounds should be viewed within their cultural and linguistic contexts; disorders cannot be defined for children of one ethnocultural/linguistic background with standards that apply to another group
- Language disorders in ethnic and linguistic minority children are similar to those found in majority children: delayed language onset and deficient semantic, syntactic, and pragmatic language skills—all viewed from the unique ethnic, linguistic, and cultural perspective of a given child
- A bilingual child may have a language disorder in his or her primary language, secondary language, or both languages; a disorder in the secondary language needs to be justified in the context of the child's primary language
- An African American child may have a language disorder in his or her own Black English dialect, standard American English, or both; a disorder in the standard American English should be justified in the context of the Black English dialect, not in the context of the mainstream English

Risk Factors for Childhood Language Disorders

- Several risk factors increase the likelihood that a child will fail to learn language skills normally a variety of prenatal, perinatal, and neonatal risk factors are known, although not all apply to SLI:
- Prenatal risk factors: Factors that affect the normal development of a fetus are risk factors for language disorders and include:
  - Lack of good prenatal care for pregnant women; a general risk factor for language (and other) deficiencies in children
  - Maternal drug abuse including alcoholism, illicit and prescription drug abuse; babies may be congenitally drug addicted and may have intellectual or sensory deficits that increase the chances of later language disorders
  - Maternal infectious diseases, including chronic kidney or bladder infections, the TORCH group of infections (abbreviation for *toxo*plasmosis, *o*ther infections, *r*ubella virus, *c*ytomegalovirus, and *h*erpes simplex virus)
  - Premature birth and low birth weight are risks for later language disorders; factors that cause prematurity and low birth weight include infections of

the amniotic fluid or membrane, maternal drug or alcohol abuse, fetal distress, maternal age under 16 or over 36, maternal infections, multiple gestation, and uterine abnormalities

- Perinatal risk factors: Factors associated with labor and delivery that affect the health and development of the baby include:
  o Prolonged labor (more than 22–24 hours for the firstborn)
  o Precipitated or uncontrolled delivery
  o Abnormal fetal presentation
  o Cesarean delivery
  o Fetal distress causing abnormal heart rate
  o Factors that induce fetal brain injury
- Neonatal risk factors: Factors that occur during the neonatal developmental period and affect normal child development include:
  o Very low or very high birth weight
  o Hyperbilirubinemia (jaundice)
- Genetic syndromes: Various genetic syndromes are associated with language disorders in children, although such disorders would not be classified as specific language impairment; children with Down syndrome and other syndromes that affect the intellectual development of the child are likely to affect language development; language disorders are phenotypic of many genetic syndromes
- General intellectual deficiency: Below normal intelligence is a risk for language disorders; the greater the intellectual deficiency, the more severe the language disorder
- Sensory deficiencies: Hearing loss poses risks for normal oral language learning; the greater the loss, the higher the effect on oral language learning
- Neurological diseases or disorders: Cerebral palsy, encephalitis, brain tumors, severe epilepsy, strokes (though uncommon in children, they do occur), and traumatic brain injury are risk factors
- Psychiatric disorders: Various psychiatric or behavioral disorders, including childhood schizophrenia and autism spectrum disorders are risk factors
- Environmental risk factors: Severe child abuse, child neglect to the point of prolonged social isolation, and extreme poverty resulting in severely impoverished home environment (including critical nutritional deficiencies) have been suspected environmental risk factors

Characteristics of Language Disorders in Children

- Early communication deficits: Generally slower or delayed onset and development of language that results in restricted language skills; although SLI is not diagnosed until age 4, signs of language disorders are usually apparent long before age 4; infants and toddlers who are likely to have a clinically diagnosed language disorder are likely to exhibit
  o Avoidance of eye contact; babies may fail to look at the mother's face
  o Delayed onset of babbling and cooing that characterize normal infant vocalizations; the babies may babble rarely, or remain silent
  o Lack of response to whispered speech; this is one of the early signs of lack of response to speech

o Failure to imitate gestures; the baby may not imitate "bye-bye"
o Frequent crying with a relatively constant pitch and loudness
o Lack of emotional responses or flat affect
o Delayed onset of the first few words; the child may not learn to say "Mama" or "Dada" between 12 and 18 months
o Failure to respond to body parts when commanded; may not respond to such requests as "Show me your nose"
o Inability to follow simple one-step commands; the child may perform the action if gestures accompany the command (e.g., *hand me that pen* while pointing to the pen)
o Lack of smiling or reduced frequency of smiling
o Lack of play activities and diminished interest in socialization
o Either a reduced expression of gestures or an excessive reliance on gestures at the expense of verbal expressions
o Slower acquisition of language milestones; all milestones of language may be delayed; the extent of delay may vary greatly across children
o Beginning signs of phonological difficulties

• Phonological disorders: Language disorders often are associated with articulation and phonological disorders
o Continued production of Phonological Processes beyond the age limits by which time the processes disappear in children who are normally mastering speech and language skills; see Articulation and Phonological Disorders
o Prevocalic voicing (e.g., saying *dap* for *tap*) and deletion of word-initial weak syllables (e.g., saying *manda* for *Amanda*) may be prominent in children who are likely to have language disorders
o Some unusual phonological processes not frequently found in children developing language normally; children with language disorders may exhibit stopping of liquids (as in /t/ for /r/ substitutions) or substitution of liquids for glides (as in /l/ for /w/ substitutions)
o Children whose primary diagnosis is articulation and phonological disorders are likely to have language disorders as well
o Difficulties with certain speech sounds may be a reason why a child does not produce certain grammatical morphemes; a child who cannot produce /s/, /t/, /d/, or /z/ will not correctly produce the regular plural words (e.g., *cups* or *bags*), past tense words (e.g., *walked* or *painted*), possessive morphemes (e.g., *Mommy's* or *Man's*), or irregular third person words (e.g., *has*)

• Semantic problems: Impaired semantic skills (meanings, word knowledge, and relations between words and concepts) in children with language disorders include:
o Initial delay in saying the first few words; slow acquisition of new words
o Persistence of word Overextensions and Underextensions beyond age 3; overgeneralization (overextension) of words (e.g., calling all vehicles *cars*) or overly discriminated (underextended) words (e.g., saying *dog* only for the family dog, but not for any other dog)
o Late-appearing word combinations; slowness in combining individual words to form phrases and simple sentences
o Errors in naming common pictures, evident by the school age

- o Retarded acquisition of words that have abstract meanings; delayed understanding of popular sayings, proverbs, and slang; even more delayed production of such abstract phrases and sentences
- o Difficulty understanding terms that refer to the shape, size, quantity, color, dimension, and quality of objects or other stimuli; language skills may be mostly limited to concrete events and things
- o Generally limited verbal repertoire; limited social exchanges
- o Lack of complex or longer word productions; production of simpler and shorter words
- Deficient grammatical morphemes: A major diagnostic characteristic is difficulty with Grammatical Morphemes of Language and syntactic structures; omission of grammatical morphemes is especially diagnostic of SLI in children; children with SLI may be slow in learning grammatical morphemes or may never learn them without systematic intervention; specific difficulties may include:
  - o Omission of allomorphic variations of the regular plural in words, phrases, and sentences; omission of the plural /s/ (e.g., *cups*), /z/ (e.g., *bags*), and *ez* (e.g., *dishes*)
  - o Difficulty with irregular plural words; overgeneralization of regular plural inflections to irregular words (e.g., say *womans* for *women*)
  - o Omission of the present progressive morpheme in words, phrases, and sentences (e.g., saying *The boy walk* to describe a present progressive action)
  - o Omission of the allomorphic variations of the possessive morphemes; the possessive /s/, /z/, and the *ez* morphemes may all be missing in words, phrases, and conversational speech; production of such utterances as *cat bowl* for *cat's bowl* (missing possessive /s/), *baby bottle* for *baby's bottle* (missing possessive /z/), and *horse tail* for *horse's tail* (missing possessive *ez* morpheme)
  - o Omission of regular past tense allomorphic inflections /d/, /t/, and *ed* (e.g., the child might say *pull* for *pulled*, *walk* for *walked*, and *paint* for *painted*)
  - o Difficulty with irregular past tense words; overgeneralization of regular past tense inflections to irregular past tense words (e.g., *broked* for *broke*)
  - o Omission of the articles *the* and *a*, two English grammatical morphemes that are especially difficult to master
  - o Omission of the verbal auxiliary, including the present (auxiliary *is*) and past forms (auxiliary *was*); typical omission of both the present progressive and the auxiliary (e.g., *Boy ea* for *[the] boy is eating;* the article in such productions is also typically missing)
  - o Omission of the copula; (e.g., *Car nice* for *Car is nice*)
  - o Omission or misuse of the prepositions *in, on, under, behind, besides*, and so forth (e.g., *doll table* for *doll on table*); one or two pronouns already mastered may be substituted for other pronouns (e.g., *doll on table* for *doll under table*)
  - o Omission or misuse of pronouns; the pronouns *he, she, it,* and *they* may be either missing altogether or misused because of wrong substitutions

o Omission or misuse of the conjunctions *and, but,* and *because*; conse-quently, speech is full of short phrases, not longer sentences that contain conjunctions

o Incorrect use of learned grammatical morphemes, including overgeneral-izations (e.g., *womans* for *women, goed* for *went)*

o Difficulty with comparatives and superlatives (e.g., *big, bigger, biggest*); because the comparative and superlatives involve relation and relative properties of stimulus situations, they are especially affected in language disorders

o Missing adjectives and adverbs; may be misused

- Deficient syntactic skills: Telegraphic utterances (short utterances lacking in complex syntactic structures); deficiencies in grammatical morphemes further complicate the following kinds of syntactic deficiencies:

o Extremely limited use of syntactic structures or absence of many complex forms of syntactic constructions

o Production of single words or phrases instead of sentences

o Production of shorter sentences instead of longer sentences

o Production of simpler sentences instead of more complex sentences; embedded sentences, subordinate clauses, passive forms, and complex and compound sentences are likely to be missing

o Limited variety of syntactic structures (use of only a few types of sentences, mostly active declarative sentence forms); difficulty with various forms of questions (e.g., *what, why, when, where, who, how, which, yes,* and *no*), mands (requests and commands), negative sentence forms, and other varied syntactic structures

- Deficient or inappropriate social language: Significant pragmatic language disorders may or may not be found; to be sure, clinicians should assess them; the following kinds of pragmatic language problems may be evident:

o Difficulty in using clinically or spontaneously acquired language in social situations

o Failure to maintain Joint Attention with a caregiver (difficulty concen-trating on the stimulus being talked about)

o Difficulty in initiating conversation, especially with peers; a greater incli-nation to initiate conversation with adults than with peers (an opposite trend is seen in typically developing children); initiation of conversation at inappropriate times; shouting or interrupting to initiate speech

o Difficulty in talking with same-age peers; may offer more speech to younger children (similar language age)

o Difficulty in maintaining a topic of conversation; may partly be due to the small vocabulary, limited language experience, and generally restricted language skills

o Difficulty in conversational turn taking; interrupting the speaker or failing to take turns to speak

o Difficulty in using Conversational Repair Strategies; failure to request clarification when a speaker is not understood; may just repeat, not modify, language productions when a listener requests clarification

o Difficulty in maintaining eye contact during conversation

211

- o Deficient narrative skills; personal narratives with little information; abrupt termination of narratives; confused chronological sequence, misidentified characters, missed story details in storytelling or retelling; generally limited word output; these impairments may be more consistent than other problems (e.g., lack of eye contact, difficulty initiating conversation)
- o Difficulty in describing pictures or events presented; poor descriptions with only a few descriptive words
- o Verbal interactions limited to answering questions asked; lack of elaborate conversational skills
- o Limited use of gestures; lack of appropriate nonverbal behaviors (gestures, facial expressions) that typically accompany verbal behaviors
- o General passivity in social situations; silent or just passive listeners in the company of socially more active children
- o Language that may be irrelevant to time, space, and the conversational partners; seen less commonly in specific language impairment than in autism or intellectual disabilities
- Difficulty in spoken speech and language comprehension
  - o Difficulty in comprehending the meaning of complex words, phrases, and sentences, although language comprehension skills may be better than production skills; may comprehend the meaning of words not spontaneously produced
  - o Difficulty in comprehending abstract terms; comprehension may be limited to concrete terms and descriptions of events that are *here and now*
  - o Difficulty in comprehending syntactically longer productions; generally, the longer and more complex the syntactic productions, the greater the difficulty in comprehension

Effects of Childhood Language Disorders

- Problems of socialization; awkward social behaviors; limited peer interactions
- Aggressive, emotional, uncooperative, or otherwise socially inappropriate behaviors; inability to express personal needs may lead to such behaviors as snatching a toy from another child, throwing temper tantrums when in need of something, and whining instead of requesting; uncooperative in play and other social situations
- Academic difficulties, including:
  - o Difficulties with abstract and complex language in the upper elementary grades (and beyond); may have problems understanding or producing metaphors, proverbs, similes, and slang
  - o Difficulty understanding various academic subjects that are discussed in complex syntactic structures
  - o Difficulty in sophisticated and academic conversational exchanges because of basic deficiencies in conversational and narrative speech skills
  - o Below grade-level reading skills, possibly because of limited language; oral language problems reflected in oral reading; limited comprehension of what is read
  - o Writing difficulties, including telegraphic writing with omission of grammatical morphemes, spelling errors, short phrases, and wrong syntax; writing problems that parallel oral language problems

Etiologic Factors and Theories of Childhood Language Disorders

- Although there is no full-fledged and generally accepted genetic theory of language disorders, specific language impairment may have a genetic basis
  - Susceptibility to such disorders may be genetically based
  - Familial prevalence and concordance rates in twins suggest the importance of genetic factors
  - No genes have been identified for language impairments, but promising lines of research are being pursued
- Neuroanatomical theories point to brain morphologic anomalies
  - Smaller or same-size left perisylvian language areas (PLAs) compared to the corresponding regions on the right side; normally, the left PLAs are slightly larger than the comparable regions on the right side
  - Extra sulcus in Broca's area
  - Brain morphologic anomalies are not found in all children with language disorders; such anomalies may be an effect, not a cause, of limited language skills
  - Some children who have brain morphologic anomalies may still acquire language normally and some who do exhibit language disorders may not have such anomalies
- Decreased activation level in the temporal and frontal lobes; not clear whether this is a cause or consequence of language disorders
- Some theories suggest that language disorders are due to other, underlying deficits, although by definition children with SLI do not have them; underlying deficits may be part of the language disorder that needs to be explained, not the cause that explains it; some of the suggested underlying disorders include
  - Information processing deficits (e.g., slower reaction time on verbal and nonverbal tasks), temporal processing deficits, and limited memory skills
  - Attentional deficits and hyperactivity
  - Impaired symbolic play activity
- Environmental factors that may cause language development are not clear; there is no well-supported and generally accepted environmental theory of language disorders; some divergent maternal interactional patterns have been suggested as potential causes; the possibility that those maternal reactions are a consequence of child's limited communication skills cannot be ruled out; limited evidence suggests that mothers of children who have SLI
  - Interacted less with their children and asked fewer questions
  - Shouted more at them
  - Did not reason enough with them
  - Were more directive
  - Spoke in shorter and simpler utterances
- The role of the environment in maintaining impaired language or abnormal patterns of communication is well established; whatever the cause of the initial failure to learn appropriate language skills, the maintenance of impaired or limited language skills is mostly due to environmental contingencies
  - Children who whine or use undifferentiated gestures to make requests tend to stop these behaviors when taught verbal requests

- o Children who grab things or lead people to things they want will stop these behaviors when taught appropriate verbal behaviors
  - o Systematically reinforcing more appropriate verbal behaviors decreases inappropriate verbal behaviors
  - o Corrective feedback for inappropriate language productions will decrease their frequency
- Interaction between multiple genes and multiple environmental factors is the most likely explanation of language disorders in children; when multiple genes are involved, the effects are diffuse across genes, and no single gene abnormality may be evident
- Regardless of the initial etiology, language disorders are environmentally modifiable; all language treatment procedures are environmentally based

Carr, E. G., Levin, L., McConnachie, G., Carlson, J. I., Kemp. D. C., & Smith C. E. (1994). *Communication-based intervention for problem behavior.* Baltimore, MD: Paul H. Brookes.

Gauger, L. M., Lombardino, L. J., & Leonard, C. M. (1997). Brain morphology in children with specific language impairment. *Journal of Speech, Language, and Hearing Research, 40,* 1272–1284.

Hart, B., & Risley, T. R. (1995). *The social world of children learning to talk.* Baltimore, MD: Paul H. Brookes.

Hegde, M. N., & Maul, C. A. (2006). *Language disorders in children: An evidence-based approach to assessment and treatment.* Boston, MA: Allyn and Bacon.

Leonard, L. B. (1998). *Children with specific language impairment.* Cambridge, MA: MIT Press.

McCauley, R. J., & Fey, M. E. (2006) (Eds.). *Treatment of language disorders in children.* Baltimore, MD: Paul H. Brookes.

Nelson, N. W. (1998). *Childhood language disorders in context: Infancy through adolescence.* New York: McMillan.

Newbury, D. F., & Monoco, A. P. (2002). Talking genes: The molecular basis of language impairment. *Biologist, 49*(6), 255–260.

Owens, R. E., Jr. (2004). *Language Disorders: A functional approach to assessment and treatment* (4th ed.). Boston, MA: Allyn and Bacon.

Paul, R. (2001). *Language disorders from infancy through adolescence* (2nd ed.). St. Louis, MO: C. V. Mosby.

Planter, E., Swisher, L., Vance, R., & Rapcsak, S. (1991). MRI findings in boys with specific language impairment. *Brain and Language, 41,* 52–56.

Reed, V. (2005). *An introduction to children with language disorders* (3rd ed.). Boston, MA: Allyn and Bacon.

Language Disorders in Infants and Toddlers. Delayed language acquisition or limited language production in infants and toddlers; various types of communication deficits apparent as the infant grows older; not only oral language, but all aspects of communication, including nonverbal communication, may be deficient; communication delay may be associated with developmental disabilities; generally seen in two groups of children: those with *established risk* and those who are *at risk* for developing communication problems (often along with other developmental delays or disabilities); children with established risk have conditions known to be associated with overall developmental delay including language delay or disorders (e.g., children with genetic syndromes, neurological diseases, hearing loss, intellectual disabilities); children who are at risk experience variables that are likely to produce language problems, especially if early and effective intervention is not provided; both biological and environmental variables place children in a risk category; any variable that interrupts or impedes the normal interaction between children and their verbal environment is a risk factor; depending on the age of the children in this group, there may be no language disorder yet, only some initial signs of impending delay or disorder, delayed onset of preverbal behaviors, or delayed onset of early communicative behaviors; language disorders may continue throughout the school years and beyond unless effective intervention is offered early and consistently; some children, especially those with genetic anomalies, severe sensory deficits (e.g., hearing impairment), and intellectual disabilities may have residual oral language problems in spite of best intervention efforts.

Epidemiology and Ethnocultural Variables
- Prevalence rate may be as high as 10% of children under age 3
- Specific epidemiological and ethnocultural variables related to infants and toddlers is limited
- Epidemiological and ethnocultural variables described under Language Disorders in Children would apply to infants and toddlers as well

Etiology of Established Risk
- Most of the established risk factors are biological or disease-related
- Genetic syndromes, identified at birth or soon thereafter; see Syndromes Associated With Communication Disorders
- Congenital or acquired neurological disorders including cerebral palsy, progressive muscular dystrophy, Wilson's disease, intracranial hemorrhage, intracranial tumors, neurofibromatosis, seizure disorders, and head and spinal cord injury
- Various congenital malformations of the speech mechanism and such craniofacial conditions as cleft palate, hypoplastic mandible, microcephaly, and macrocephaly
- Metabolic disorders including mucopolysaccharidoses syndromes (including Hunter, Hurler, and Sanfilippo syndromes), galactosemia, pituitary diseases, glycogen storage disease, phenylketonuria (PKU), and Tay-Sachs disease
- Sensory disorders including hearing loss, visual impairment and blindness, and congenital cataract
- Atypical developmental disorders, including autism spectrum disorders and failure to thrive
- Severe toxic exposure including maternal PKU, cocaine and other drugs, fetal alcohol syndrome, lead poisoning, and mercury poisoning
- Chronic illnesses including chronic hepatitis, diabetes, renal disorders, cancer, cystic fibrosis, and heart problems that limit social interactions

- Severe infectious diseases including HIV, bacterial and viral meningitis, herpes, rubella, and encephalitis

Etiology of At-Risk Conditions

- Etiological factors of at-risk conditions include environmental factors, genetic background, and some disease-related conditions; however, many are environmental
- Some of the suggested at-risk factors need more rigorous research to confirm them
- Prenatal factors (associated with maternal health or behavior)
  - Maternal drug and alcohol abuse that can cause fetal growth problems, resulting in such conditions as <u>Fetal Alcohol Syndrome</u>
  - Excessive maternal smoking during pregnancy
  - Infections of the amniotic fluid
  - Maternal age that is below 16 or above 36
  - Maternal kidney infections
  - Multiple gestation
  - Placental bleeding
  - Excessive or insufficient amniotic fluid
  - Premature rupture of the membrane
  - Maternal preeclampsia, characterized by high blood pressure, proteinuria (high amounts of protein in the urine), and edema
  - Abnormal uterus
- Perinatal factors (that affect the baby in the process of birth)
  - Prolonged labor
  - Precipitated or uncontrolled delivery
  - Breach birth and other abnormal presentation of the infant
  - Cesarean delivery
  - Fetal distress due to various reasons
  - Abnormalities of the placenta
  - Conditions that cause fetal brain injury
- Neonatal factors (that operate during the first 28 days of the infant)
  - Low birth weight or very high birth weight
  - Yellow bile pigment (hyperbilirubinemia or jaundice) in the blood that can cause brain damage
  - Poor feeding or prolonged early feeding disorders
  - Various kinds of infections that can affect the brain
  - Collection of three or more anomalies (even in the absence of a genetic syndrome); these may include a webbed finger or toe, clefts of the lip or palate or both, eye or ear deformities, and so forth
- Mental illness, intellectual disabilities, and chronic or severe physical illness in one or both parents or in the primary caregiver can affect language acquisition in infants and toddlers
- Child abuse, especially social isolation
- Family history of language impairment and predisposing medical or genetic conditions (including intellectual disabilities)
- Chronically impaired social interaction among family members

- Adolescent mother or single parent
- Having four or more siblings, all preschool age
- Parental unemployment or parental education below 9th grade
- Physical or social isolation and separation of the child from the parent or primary caregiver for extended duration (e.g., prolonged periods of hospitalization)
- Bad, dangerous, or unstable living conditions or homelessness
- Poor family health care, inadequate prenatal care, lack of health insurance, and lack of access to pediatric health care
- Asphyxia, low birth weight (<1,500 g), and small for gestation age (<10th percentile)

Early Signs of Language Disorders in Infants and Toddlers

- Infants and toddlers who experience difficulty learning language are a diverse group with varied genetic, medical, behavioral, family, and environmental conditions that may adversely affect their interaction with the environment and parents/caregivers
- Some of the early signs of delayed language are nonverbal; others are verbal
- Nonverbal signs of potential language disorders include all of the prenatal, perinatal, and postnatal risk factors already listed; in addition, the following nonverbal signs suggest potential difficulty with language acquisition:
  - Early signs of behavior disorders including irritability and excessive crying may signal developmental problems
  - Chronic middle ear infections (otitis media), causing conductive hearing loss
  - Poor physical growth and health, often associated with other risk factors (potential genetic or hereditary conditions, intellectual deficits)
  - Poor motor skills, suggestive of potential neurological problems
  - Early feeding problems that may cause failure to thrive; suggestive of neuromuscular impairments (e.g., cerebral palsy or cleft palate)
  - Obvious neurological disorders, such as paresis or paralysis
  - Lack of socialization and poor interpersonal relations
  - Emotional problems, especially lack of emotional attachment; lack of normal play or abnormal play (both early signs of Autism)
  - Early signs of deficient intellectual development
  - Lack of waving, smiling, nodding, and such other nonverbal means of communication
  - Difficulty imitating simple motor actions (e.g., clapping)
- Early verbal signs of potential language disorders include:
  - Lack of response to mother's voice; general lack of interest in human voice, with a preference for mechanical noise (early signs of Autism)
  - Lack of response or inconsistent response to softer speech and nonspeech auditory stimuli but normal response to louder stimuli, suggestive of hearing loss
  - Delayed, limited, or no babbling; fewer speech-sound like vocalizations
  - Delayed discrimination of speech sounds and delayed onset of speech-sound production; production of fewer consonants than normal
  - Failure to associate objects with their typical sounds

o Difficulty in mutual gaze or joint attention (looking at the same object as the caregiver); difficulty shifting gaze from objects to people and back; difficulty in following a caregiver's gaze
o Delayed onset of the first few words
o Smaller vocabulary at each age level and slower expansion of the vocabulary
o Preference for gestures versus verbal responses
o Difficulty imitating speech sounds, syllables, or words when modeled by the caregiver

Billeaud, F. P. (2003). *Communication disorders in infants and toddlers* (3rd ed.). Boston, MA: Butterworth-Heinemann.

Hegde, M. N., & Maul, C. (2006). *Language disorders in children: An evidence-based approach to assessment and treatment.* Boston, MA: Allyn and Bacon.

Nelson, N. W. (1998). *Childhood language disorders in context* (2nd ed.). Boston, MA: Allyn and Bacon.

Paul, R. (2001). *Language disorders from infancy through adolescence* (2nd ed.). St. Louis, MO: C. V. Mosby.

Reed, V. (2005). *An introduction to children with language disorders* (2nd ed.). Boston, MA: Allyn and Bacon.

Rossetti, L. M. (2001). *Communication intervention birth to three* (2nd ed.). Clifton Park, NY: Thomson Delmar Learning.

Language Disorders in Older Students and Adolescents. Semantic, morphological, syntactic, and pragmatic language problems of older students and adolescents; may persist from early childhood or may be those that are due to a failure to acquire advanced skills of language and literacy; problems in reading and writing; deficiencies in advanced and academic discourse; limited capacity for critical, logical, and scientific reasoning; problems with abstract and figurative language.

Language Skills of Older Students and Adolescents

- Language learning continues during the adolescent years and even beyond; changes in language and literacy skills are more subtle and gradual (hence more difficult to track)
- Phonological and morphological changes are not significant during the adolescent years; typically, they are acquired by age 6 or 7
- Normative data on the language skills of older students and adolescents are limited; research shows that
  o There is a gradual but noticeable increase in sentence length during the preadolescent and adolescent years
  o Progressive changes may be measured in C-units (communication units) or T-units (terminable units); both contain an independent clause and subordinate clauses but the C-units also may be incomplete sentences produced in response to questions; the two units show a regular increase from 6th through 12th grade
  o Increases in language structures that occur at low frequency are still significant advances

- o Learning scientific, technical, literate, academic, logical, and discipline-specific terms and terms used in advanced reasoning and scholarly analysis also is a part of preadolescent and adolescent language acquisition
- o Skills in word retrieval, word definitions, word relations, and skills in the use of figurative language continue to improve during the adolescent years; in fact, such skills continue to improve throughout the life span, especially if the individuals (e.g., literary and scientific writers, scholars, professionals, journalists) face a constant need to increase such skills
- o Mastery of advanced syntactic structures and pragmatic features during the adolescent years

Epidemiology and Ethnocultural Variables

- Incidence and prevalence of language disorders in older students and adolescents have not been systematically researched
- In most states, public schools do not track older students (age 9 or 12 and higher) who are enrolled in speech-language services
- Very small number of older students (age 12 and higher) receive clinical speech-language services in public schools; reported figures are as low as 0.4% of children 12 years and older; one state (Florida) reported that 1.4% of students aged 13–20 years received speech-language services
- Based on the number of older students and adolescents who receive special education services (who also tend to have language disorders), the American Speech-Language-Hearing Association estimates that roughly 5% of older students and adolescents may have a language disorder
- It is difficult to assume that language problems of the early childhood years are fully remediated with or without treatment and that children 12 years and beyond have little or no need for services; prevalence of language disorders in older students may be underestimated and they may be underserved
- More than a quarter of adolescents in juvenile detention, a growing population in the United States, may have a language disorder
- Generally, difficulty in learning basic language skills in early preschool and early grade school years receives more research and clinical attention than difficulty mastering more advanced features of language during adolescent years
- Reliable information on ethnocultural variables as they affect language disorders in older students and adolescents is not available; nonetheless, language disorders in adolescents whose primary language is other than English or mainstream English (as in African American English) need to be analyzed in the context of primary language influences

Description of Language Disorders in Adolescents

- Semantic problems
  - o Difficulty understanding and correctly using literate lexicon necessary for thinking, logical reasoning, verbal analysis, and scholarly and scientific discourse is typical in older students (including adolescents) with language disorders; marked difficulty in understanding or correctly producing such

terms as *interpret, presume, assume, hypothesize, infer, summarize, define, compare, contrast, criticize, evaluate, support, reject, discriminate, explain, conclude, assert,* and *predict*
- Difficulty understanding and correctly using figurative language (e.g., proverbs, metaphors, and idioms) with or without verbal contexts
- Difficulty learning peer group slang; once learned, the older students may use it in inappropriate contexts (e.g., while talking to parents or teachers)
- Difficulty understanding and correctly using words with abstract and multiple meanings, proverbs, similes, and metaphors
- Word retrieval problems in conversational speech, resulting in false starts, pauses, revisions, repetitions, and other kinds of dysfluencies
- Deficient word definition skills; older students may find it especially difficult to define literate, technical, and scientific words
- Words that express relations may pose special problems; for example, difficulty understanding and correctly using words that are related by similar or contrastive meanings (e.g., synonyms and antonyms)
- Difficulty in using precise terms with clear referents; instead, excessive production of such terms as "this," "that," "you know what I mean," "this thing," and "that stuff"
• Syntactic problems
- Short sentences; limited sentence lengths, often measured in C-units or T-units and expressed in number of words per unit
- Limited use of low-frequency structures (e.g., passive sentences, such nonphrase postmodifications as "a tree *called the oak,*" or "Mr. Thomas *the history teacher*")
- Difficulty using complex sentences containing subordinate clauses (e.g., such nominal subordinate clauses as "Jane did not know *that she was the winner*"; such adverbial clauses as "*when you get your pilot's license,* you can start flying on your own"; and such adjectival clauses as "The man, *who was sleeping on the sidewalk,* had a sign that said *residentially challenged*")
- Failure to produce concise and precise grammatical constructions that suggest greater syntactic sophistication (e.g., *once licensed, you can start flying on your own* instead of the lengthier adverbial clause); note that sentence length does not always suggest greater syntactic skill
- Difficulty using cohesion devices or connectives (e.g., such expressions as *therefore, for example, similarly, moreover, consequently, furthermore, because, while, as well as, rather than, neither,* and *either*)
- Lack of grammatical agreement (e.g., noun-verb agreement)
- Incorrect pronoun usage, resulting in ambiguous use of pronouns (as referents)
- Persistence of syntactic errors from earlier language problems
• Pragmatic problems
- Difficulty using the correct register; for example, talking in slang register with teachers, instead of limiting it to conversation with peers
- Difficulty maintaining a topic of conversation for an extended period of time
- Failure to distinguish facts from opinions

- o Tactless expression of ideas or opinions
- o Difficulty managing conversational repair strategies; failure to respond to request for clarification, and inability to modify statements or add new information to help listener comprehension
- o Failure to request clarifications when speakers are not understood, leading to inappropriate or irrelevant responses
- o Difficulty sequencing events correctly; oral narratives may be out of sequence, and lack cohesion, logical progression, and story detail
- o Maze behavior (false starts and repeated attempts to express the same ideas)
- o Difficulty asking relevant questions and making relevant comments
- o Deficient listening skills
- Nonverbal communication problems
  - o Difficulty correctly interpreting facial expressions of speakers
  - o Misinterpretation of gestures that accompany speech
  - o Socially inappropriate gestures
  - o Misjudgment of spatial distance considered appropriate in social situations
- Reading and writing problems
  - o A quarter or more students in higher grades fail to read at grade level
  - o Reading and writing errors that reflect deficiencies in oral language, although oral language skills may be somewhat better than written skills
  - o Reading errors, including frequent revisions
  - o Difficulty understanding what is read
  - o Writing problems, including spelling errors, poor formation of letters, and errors of punctuation
  - o Especially difficult extended writing; poor organization of essays that contain sparse information and limited details, substance, background information, and logical sequence
  - o Deficient grammar; limited sentence varieties; incomplete or syntactically incorrect sentences; infrequent use of low-frequency (complex) syntactic structures
  - o Use of colloquial language instead of technical language in academic writing
  - o Lack of cohesion and temporal or chronological sequence

Hegde, M. N., & Maul, C. A. (2006). *Language disorders in children: An evidence-based approach to assessment and treatment.* Boston, MA: Allyn and Bacon.

Larson, V. L., & McKinley, N. L. (2003). *Communication solutions for older students: Assessment and intervention strategies.* Eau Claire, WI: Thinking Publications.

Nippold, M. A. (1993). Developmental markers in adolescent language: Syntax, semantics, and pragmatics. *Language, Speech, and Hearing Services in Schools, 24,* 21–28.

Nippold, M. A. (2007). *Later language development: School age children, adolescents, and young adults* (3rd ed.). Austin, TX: Pro-Ed.

Paul, R. (2001). *Language disorders from infancy through adolescence* (2nd ed.). St. Louis, MO: C. V. Mosby.

Reed, V. (2005). *An introduction to children with language disorders* (3rd ed.). Boston, MA: Allyn and Bacon.

Ripich, D. N., & Creaghead, N. A. (1994). *School discourse problems* (2nd ed.). San Diego, CA: Singular Publishing Group.

Language of Confusion. Confabulated and confused language associated with <u>Traumatic Brain Injury</u>; such psychoses as schizophrenia, state of intoxication, metabolic and chemical imbalances, and brain diseases.

Laryngectomee or Laryngectomized Person. A person who has had a partial or total <u>Laryngectomy</u>.

Laryngectomy. Surgical removal of all or part of the larynx because of disease or trauma; cancer of the laryngeal areas is the most common disease requiring surgical treatment; results in a loss of the natural source of sound to produce speech because of significant changes in the anatomy of the laryngeal area; creates a need to breathe through a surgically created stoma (hole) in the neck; creates a need to learn alternative modes of sound generation and speech production.

- Major types of laryngectomy
  - The type of surgery performed on an individual depends on the extent of the tumor that needs to be removed; generally varies from a removal of a small portion of the diseased larynx to the removal of the entire larynx because of an extensive tumor; each procedure has variations
  - Total laryngectomy: Most radical form of treatment in which the entire larynx, all membranes, cartilages and the hyoid bone, intrinsic muscles, and the upper tracheal rings are surgically removed; remaining portion of the trachea is brought forward, attached to the frontal part of the neck (just below the sternal notch) with an opening (*stoma*) created for permanent neck breathing
  - Near total laryngectomy: Less aggressive than the total laryngectomy, involves the removal of most of the structures except for a small, healthy portion of one vocal fold
  - Pharyngo-laryngectomy: Another radical form of treatment in which the larynx is totally removed (total laryngectomy) along with diseased portions of the pharynx when the cancer affects the pharyngeal area
  - Partial laryngectomy: Removal of diseased parts of the larynx
    - Hemilaryngectomy: Removal of one-half of the larynx; one vocal fold is removed along with some related structures and the other fold is saved
    - Supraglottic laryngectomy: Removal of structures above the vocal folds
  - Removal of other structures: Depending on the spread of cancer, removal of parts of the esophagus, tongue, and lymphatic system in the neck (radical *neck dissection*)

Reasons for Laryngectomy

- Carcinoma (cancer) of the larynx, the most common reason for laryngectomy; prevalence of laryngeal cancer is 11,000 to 13,000 cases a year in the United States; higher prevalence in older males than in females although the gender ratio has been shrinking; greatest prevalence rate is found among African American males
  - Supraglottal tumors (laryngeal cancer above the vocal folds): 24% to 42% of all cases of laryngeal cancer may have supraglottal tumors

- o Glottal tumors (cancerous growths on the vocal folds): The most frequent type, found in 55% to 75% of individuals undergoing laryngectomy
  - o Subglottal tumors (cancerous growths below the vocal folds): Rare, found in 1% to 6% of cases
- Laryngeal trauma; surgical removal of traumatized and severely damaged larynx that cannot be repaired; less frequently performed than surgery for laryngeal cancer; common causes of laryngeal trauma include:
  - o Blow to the larynx, gunshot wounds, neck stabbing, strangulation, and other kinds of violence
  - o Automobile, household, occupational, and other kinds of accidents
  - o Unsuccessful partial laryngectomy that necessitates a total laryngectomy
- Brainstem strokes that eliminate all control over the laryngeal structures; they may then be surgically removed

Potential Etiologic Factors of Laryngeal Cancer

- Smoking (cigarettes, pipes, cigars) is the most common cause; because not all smokers develop laryngeal cancer, genetic predisposition and smoking may interact to produce cancer
- Excessive alcohol intake; genetic predisposition may play a role because some individuals are more susceptible than others (with the same patterns of drinking)
- A combination of heavy smoking and drinking increases the risk of laryngeal cancer over and beyond the risk posed by each of these individual actions
- Laryngeal cancer risk is thought to increase when smoking is combined with occupational exposure to carcinogenic factors (e.g., exposure to asbestos)
- Possible link to diet (low consumption of vitamins A and C), in need of additional research
- Exposure to frequent or high-dose diagnostic or therapeutic radiation

Boone, D. R., McFarlane, S. C., & Von Berg, S. L. (2005). *The voice and voice therapy* (7th ed.). Boston, MA: Allyn and Bacon.

Case, J. L. (2002). *Clinical management of voice disorders* (4th ed.). Austin, TX: Pro-Ed.

Casper, J. K., & Colton, R. H. (1998). *Clinical manual for laryngectomy and head and neck cancer rehabilitation* (2nd ed.). Clifton Park, NY: Thomson Delmar Learning.

Doyle, P. C., & Keith, R. L. (2005). *Contemporary issues in the treatment and rehabilitation of head and neck cancer*. Austin, TX: Pro-Ed.

Laurence-Moon-Bardet-Biedl Syndrome. Same as Laurence-Moon syndrome (see Syndromes Associated With Communication Disorders).

Laurence-Moon-Biedl Syndrome. Same as Laurence-Moon syndrome (see Syndromes Associated With Communication Disorders).

LeFort III Osteotomy. Surgical procedure designed to correct or modify developmental deficiencies in the midface region.

Left Neglect. Lack of awareness of objects, people, and space on the left side of a person; a typical symptom of Right Hemisphere Syndrome; the person with left neglect may ignore to read aloud the left-half of a printed page, bump into things on the left side, ignore to use the left-sided pockets, and fail to draw the left side of a picture.

Levodopa. A neurotransmitter whose deficiency may cause movement disorders; most commonly prescribed drug treatment for clients with Parkinson's disease to control movement disorders.

Lewy Bodies. A type of brain pathology characterized by intraneural inclusion granules; often found in the basal ganglia, brainstem, spinal cord, and sympathetic ganglia of clients with Parkinson's disease; leads to a type of Dementia called the Lewy body dementia.

Linear Acceleration. The straight-line movement of the head when a force strikes it at midline; produces unique patterns of Traumatic Brain Injury.

Literacy and Literacy Problems. Reading and writing skills; part of language skills; correlated with language and literacy problems; children with language disorders are likely to experience academic difficulties, most notably, reading and writing problems; family literacy is a significant variable in promoting early (and subsequent) literacy skills in children; parents who read and write regularly, read often to their young children, and teach and reinforce the emergent literacy skills in them better promote later literacy skills than parents who do not engage in such activities.

- Literacy skills are described in terms of:
  - o Reading readiness: A concept used in the past that emphasized *reading readiness* as a prerequisite for teaching and learning literacy skills, especially reading skills; it was thought (with little or no experimental evidence) that only those children who had mastered certain visual, auditory, and linguistic skills and had attained a mental age of 6.5 years could be taught reading skills; unfortunately, not teaching reading and writing to children with a mental age lower than 6.5 ensured low skills in many children; currently, the concept of *emergent literacy* is considered more important than reading readiness in teaching and learning literacy skills
  - o Emergent literacy: Skills learned before entering first grade; related to literacy; include:
    - Awareness of printed material
    - Recognition of everyday signs in the community (e.g., a stop sign or signs in supermarkets)
    - A general interest in books; holding a book and pretending to read
    - An early interest in printing the letters of the alphabet
    - "Reading" a storybook by looking at the pictures
    - An early interest in learning to count
    - Learning nursery rhymes, reciting the days of the week or names of the months
    - A beginning awareness of phonemes or sounds of language
    - Correctly pointing to a word or a sentence
    - Correctly showing the front or the back of a book
    - Pointing to the beginning and the end of a story
    - Pointing to the named letter of the alphabet

- Problems in literacy: Age of the child is an important factor in judging whether the absence of the following skills is of clinical or educational significance:
  o Lack of print knowledge: Lack of awareness of general meaning of printed letters of the alphabet, words, and sentences
  o Lack of mastery of the oral recitation of the alphabet
  o Lack of sounding out printed words
  o Lack of reading aloud; struggling while reading; reading with multiple errors of omission of words, substitution of words, mispronunciation of words, and a general lack of fluency in reading
  o Impaired comprehension of material read orally or silently
  o Impaired drawing or copying of simple items; difficulty printing letters of the alphabet
  o Impaired writing skills; poor letter formation, frequent spelling errors, disorganized writing, wrong syntactic structures, writing restricted to simple sentences, lack of transition between paragraphs, incorrect punctuation or capitalization, poor lack of cohesion, lack of story or essay sequencing, and lack of details (telegraphic writing)
  o Lack of understanding of figurative and abstract language; difficulty understanding proverbs, idioms, similes, slang, and other popular sayings
- Additional variables, often considered part of literacy problems, include lack of phonological awareness, impaired phonological memory, and deficient rapid automatized naming; the value of these variables in critical literacy skills has not been experimentally established

American Speech-Language-Hearing Association (2001). *Roles and responsibilities of speech-language pathologists with respect to reading and writing in children and adolescents: Practice guidelines.* Rockville Pike, MD: Author.

Catts, H. W., & Kamhi, A. (1999). *Language and reading disabilities.* Boston, MA: Allyn and Bacon.

Erickson, K. A. (2000). All children are ready to learn: An emergent versus readiness perspective in early literacy assessment. *Seminars in Speech and Language, 21*(2), 193–203.

Hegde, M. N., & Maul, C. A. (2006). *Language disorders in children: An evidence-based approach to assessment and treatment.* Boston, MA: Allyn and Bacon.

Kaminski, R. A., & Good, R. H. (1996). Toward a technology for assessing basic literacy skills. *School Psychology Review, 25,* 215–227.

Nippold, M. A. (2007). *Later language development: School age children, adolescents, and young adults* (3rd ed.). Austin, TX: Pro-Ed.

Snow, C. E., Burns, S., & Griffin, P. (Eds.) (1998). *Preventing reading difficulties in young children.* Washington, DC: National Academy Press.

Snow, C. E., Scarborough, H. S., & Burns, M. S. (1999). What speech-language pathologists need to know about early reading. *Topics in Language Disorders, 20*(1), 48–58.

Whitehurst, C. G., & Lonigan, C. J. (1998). Child development and emergent literacy. *Child Development, 69*(3), 848–872.

Literal Paraphasia. A language problem found in clients with aphasia; the same as Phonemic Paraphasia in which one phoneme is substituted for another (e.g., *loman* for *woman*); see Aphasia.

Localizationist. One who advocates the view that the control of specific behaviors is located in particular areas of the brain; one who suggests specific sites of brain injury for particular kinds of impairments.

Locked-in Syndrome. Severe neurological condition in which the person is alert, but has severe quadriplegia and the body is immobilized except for eye movements; the person communicates through intact eye movements; orally, the person is mute; vascular occlusion of the basilar artery and the resulting brain damage is the most frequent cause.

Logoclonia. Repetition of the final syllables of words; uncommon in stuttering of early childhood onset; may be a sign of brain injury.

Low-velocity Injuries. Brain injury caused by such agents as an arrow, nail gun, knife, and other projectiles that travel at low velocity; see Traumatic Brain Injury.

L

Malingering. A behavioral or psychological disorder in which the person consciously fakes the symptoms of a disease or clinical condition to gain certain advantages; see Psychiatric Problems Associated With Communication Disorders.

Malocclusions. Deviations in the shape and dimensions of the maxilla (upper jaw) and mandible (lower jaw) bones and the positioning of individual teeth; misalignment of the maxilla and mandible and the upper and the lower row of teeth; the degree of deviation varies; may affect articulation in extreme cases; include the following types:
- Class I malocclusion: Normally aligned arches but misaligned individual teeth
- Class II malocclusion: Protruded maxilla and receded mandible
- Class III malocclusion: Protruded mandible and receded maxilla

Mandibular Hypoplasia. Underdevelopment of the mandible (lower jaw); a congenital or acquired abnormality that can affect speech production; found in several genetic syndromes; see Syndromes Associated With Communication Disorders.

Maxillary Hypoplasia. Underdevelopment of the maxilla (upper jaw); part of many genetic syndromes; depending on the severity, speech production may be affected; see Syndromes Associated With Communication Disorders.

Maximum Phonation Duration. Duration for which a person can sustain phonated sounds; the duration may be lower than normal in people with Voice Disorders.

Mean Length of Utterance (MLU). Average length of utterances measured in morphemes; an index of language acquisition or performance in young children.

Meningiomas. Tumors within the meninges that cover the brain; also called extracerebral tumors; a potential cause of cerebral infarct affecting language skills.

Meninges. The three layers of membranes covering the brain and spinal cord: the outermost membrane (*dura mater*), the middle membrane (*arachnoid*), and the innermost membrane (*pia mater*).

Mental Retardation. A term that is being replaced by *intellectual disabilities*; for epidemiology, etiology, characteristics, and associated communication disorders, see Intellectual Disabilities.

Metastasis. Spreading or migration of cancerous cells within the body; associated with neurogenic language disorders (see Aphasia), neurogenic speech disorders (see Dysarthria), and Voice Disorders due to Laryngectomy.

Microcephaly. Abnormally small head associated with intellectual disabilities; often a symptom of a congenital condition or a genetic syndrome.

Microdontia. Abnormally placed tooth or teeth due to a genetic or congenital developmental disorder; a symptom of certain genetic syndromes; may be associated with speech disorder.

228

Micrognathia. Underdeveloped mandible; associated with certain genetic syndromes, including Fetal Alcohol syndrome (see Syndromes Associated With Communication Disorders); may be associated with speech disorders.

Microphthalmia. Smaller than the normal eye size due to developmental disorders; part of several genetic syndromes including Fetal Alcohol syndrome (see Syndromes Associated With Communication Disorders)

Microtia. Gross underdevelopment of the pinna and absent external auditory canal; associated with such syndromes as Goldenhar syndrome and Oro-Facial-Digital syndrome type II (see Syndromes Associated With Communication Disorders).

Mixed Dysarthria. Combination of two or more forms of dysarthria; any or all forms of dysarthria may be combined, although a combination of flaccid-spastic dysarthrias is the most common; see Dysarthria: Specific Types.

Mixed Transcortical Aphasia. Combination of transcortical motor aphasia and transcortical sensory aphasia; language impairment but good repetition skills; see Aphasia.

Mohr Syndrome. Same as Oro-Facial-Digital syndrome type II (see Syndromes Associated With Communication Disorders).

Motor Agraphia. Writing disorders of adults who had acquired normal writing skills; due to neurological disorders; see Agraphia.

Motor Aphasia. Same as Broca's aphasia (see Aphasia: Specific Types).

Motor Speech Disorders. A group of speech disorders associated with neuropathology affecting the motor control of speech muscles or motor programming of speech movements; include Apraxia of Speech in Adults, Childhood Apraxia of Speech, and Dysarthrias.

M

Multi-Infarct Dementia (MID). Vascular dementia due to multiple strokes; see Dementia and Vascular Dementia.

Multiple Bilateral Cortical Infarcts. Repeated strokes in both the right and left hemispheres causing extensive brain damage; causes dementia with both cortical and subcortical pathology (mixed dementia).

Multiple Sclerosis. A progressive neurological disease in which the white matter of the central nervous system is demyelinated; the most common demyelinating disease that affects 100 persons per 100,000; occurs more often in women than men; more common among those living in cold or temperate climates; less common among those living in tropical regions; may affect the brainstem, cerebellum, cerebral hemispheres, and spinal cord; demyelination may extend to gray matter; causes are unclear, but a viral infection and an immunological reaction triggered by it are suspected; initially, the myelin sheath around the nerves in the affected areas may degenerate, but eventually oligodendrocytes that produce the myelin may be destroyed; associated with weakness, incoordination, and visual disturbances; symptoms may be relapsing—remitting in some and progressive in others; associated with Dysarthria.

Muscular Dystrophy. Genetic disease of muscle degeneration in which the skeletal muscles lose contractibility; types include: *pseudohypertrophic,* which affects mostly male children and involves progressive dystrophy of muscles in the face, causing flaccid dysarthria; and *myotonic muscular dystrophy,* which results in the persistence of muscle contractions in the absence of stimulation.

Mutational Falsetto. Continuation of prepubertal, high-pitched voice after attaining puberty; see Voice Disorders.

Mutism. Failure to speak; lack of verbal expression; although complete lack of communication is rare, persons who are mute simply do not or cannot express themselves; may be a psychiatric disorder or a symptom in the acute stage of aphasia or terminal stages of neurodegenerative diseases that cause Dementia; may be classified as:

- Selective mutism: Psychiatric disorder in which the person is capable of talking, talks in certain situations, but does not talk at all in other situations when speech is expected; the client may communicate with gestures, facial expressions, pulling or pushing others, or limited verbalizations in a monotonous or altered voice; a psychiatric diagnostic category in the *Diagnostic and Statistical Manual of the American Psychiatric Association;* for details, see Psychiatric Problems Associated With Communication Disorders; to be so classified as selective mutism, the problem should:
  - Last at least 1 month, excluding the first month of school
  - Be situation specific (e.g., a child may be mute in school but talk at home or in other situations; may be mute with parents but talk to peers)
  - Cause impairment in social or personal communication with negative effects on academic performance
  - *Not* be a result of shyness, embarrassment in social situations, ethnocultural differences, bilingual status, gender differences, or lack of knowledge on topics of conversation
- Mutism associated with other disorders: Not an independent diagnostic category, but a symptom associated with various neurological and neurodegenerative disorders; not a selective form of mutism, because it is the consequence of a disease process; may be associated with:
  - The final stages of progressive neurological diseases that lead to Dementia; such clients who are mute lose all neuromotor control over the vocal mechanism; such mutism is involuntary (versus *selective mutism*).
  - The final stages of AIDS Dementia Complex
  - Flaccid Dysarthria, Hypokinetic Dysarthria, Hyperkinetic Dysarthria, Spastic Dysarthria, and severe Apraxia of Speech
  - Acute stage of Aphasia in adults; likely to be transient; more lasting mutism may be associated with severe neuromotor disorders, orofacial weakness, paralysis, rigidity, hypokinesia, or hyperkinetic movements; aphasia in children is more often associated with mutism
  - Diffuse cortical damage (as in persistent vegetative state)
  - Seizure disorders and surgical removal of corpus callosum to control otherwise uncontrollable epilepsy in children

M

- Bilateral lesions of the orbito-mesial frontal cortex, limbic system, and reticular formation; in this case, it is an extreme form of Abulia, characterized by an extreme lack of motivation to talk or do anything; also called *akinetic mutism*
- *Locked-in syndrome*; clients in this condition have spastic quadriplegia and are totally immobilized, except for eye movements; no intellectual impairment and clients communicate with eye movements; brain injury is extensive, often associated with diseases of the basilar artery
- Toxic drug influences (especially the drugs given after liver and heart transplant); may be controlled by reduced dosage
- Surgery to remove midline posterior fossa tumors; called *cerebellar mutism*

American Psychiatric Association. (2000). *Diagnostic and statistical manual of mental retardation*: Fourth Edition, text revision. Washington, DC: Author.

Duffy, J. R. (2005). *Motor speech disorders: Substrates, differential diagnosis, and management*. St. Louis, MO: Elsevier Mosby.

McInnes, A., & Manassis, K. (2005). When silence is not golden: An integrated approach to selective mutism. *Seminars in Speech and Language, 26*(3), 201–210.

Toppelberg, C. O., Tabors, P., Coggins, A., Lum, K., & Burger, C. (2005). Differential diagnosis of selective mutism in bilingual children. *Journal of the American Academy of Child and Adolescent Psychiatry, 44*(6), 592–595.

Wintgens, A. (2005). Selective mutism in children. *Child Language Teaching and Therapy, 21*(2), 214–216.

Myasthenia Gravis. Easily fatigued muscles associated with a neuromuscular junction (point of contact between the lower motor neurons and the muscle) disorder; reduction in the acetylcholine receptors at the neuromuscular junction; reduced contractibility of the muscles because of reduced quantity of neurotransmitters; Dysarthria, Dysphagia, and Voice Disorders may be associated with it.

Myoclonus. Disorder of the muscle or muscles characterized by brief, abrupt, and involuntary contractions of muscles; a part of a muscle, a whole muscle, or a group of muscles may be affected; a sudden jerk while falling asleep is myoclonus in otherwise neurologically normal persons; myoclonic contractions may be rhythmic or irregular; associated with varied medical conditions including epilepsy, stroke, cerebral anoxia, traumatic brain injury, and kidney failure; also associated with such neurodegenerative diseases as Alzheimer's disease and Creutzfeldt-Jakob disease; involvement of facial muscles, jaw, tongue, larynx, and pharynx may affect speech production; associated with Dysarthria.

Myotonic Muscular Dystrophy. A form of degenerative muscle disease associated with Dysarthria; see Muscular Dystrophy.

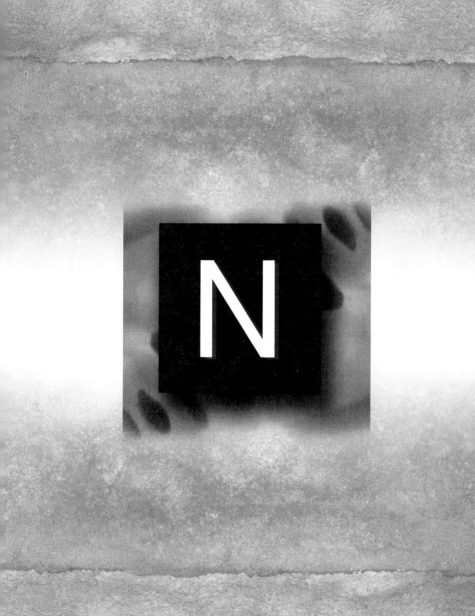

Narrative Skills. Language skills for describing events in a sequential, chronologically correct, and logically consistent manner; include storytelling or story retelling; skills that may be impaired in children or adults who have a language disorder; see Language Disorders in Children for details on narrative skills and impairments; include the following:

- Personal narratives: Descriptions of personal experiences in a logical and cohesive manner
- Script narratives: Descriptions of routine events in life; detailed and properly sequenced descriptions of how to make a sandwich or how to get to a certain place, for example, are script narrative
- Fictional narratives: Stories told with sufficient detail, logical sequence, and appropriate characterization; retelling a story that has just been told

Nasal Emission. Audible escape of air through the nose during speech, especially during the production of voiceless plosives and fricatives; associated with cleft palate or neuromuscular control problems related to the velopharyngeal mechanism (e.g., flaccid dysarthria); due to excessive efforts to close the velopharyngeal port that is inadequate or insufficient; see Cleft Palate and Velopharyngeal Dysfunction for additional information.

Neglect. Problem associated with brain injury, especially right brain injury in which one side of the visual field is ignored; the most common form is Left Neglect, associated with Right Hemisphere Syndrome.

Neologistic Paraphasia. Also known as Jargon, a language characteristic associated with aphasia; typically the result of word-finding problems; instead of meaningful and appropriate words that cannot be recalled at the moment, the client substitutes self-created syllables that are not words in the language; usually meaningless to listeners; see Aphasia.

N

Neonatal Risk Factors. Variables that predispose a newborn to developmental problems, including communication problems; a common neonatal factor that affects development is very low birth weight; see Language Disorders in Children and Language Disorders in Infants and Toddlers.

Nephritis. Disease of the kidneys due to various causes; prolonged kidney diseases and dialysis may be associated with *dialysis dementia*.

Neural Anastomosis. Connecting a branch of an undamaged nerve to a damaged nerve; a surgical treatment for certain dysarthric clients; to restore function and appearance, a branch of the intact cranial nerve XII (hypoglossal; tongue movement) may be connected to the damaged cranial nerve VII (facial; sensory to tongue, motor to face).

Neuritic (Senile) Plaques. Clumps of degenerating or degenerated neurons; associated with Alzheimer's Disease and normal aging; the amount of such plaques makes the difference; more extensively found in clients with dementia, especially dementia of the Alzheimer type.

Neurofibrillary Tangles. Twisted and tangled neurofibrils, which are filamentous structures in the cell body of nerves; basic neuropathology of Alzheimer's Disease.

Neurofibromatosis. A familial developmental neurological disorder involving muscles, bone, and skin; characterized by pedunculated soft tumors on the body; a condition that puts children at risk of developmental delay, including communication delay or disorder.

Neurogenic Fluency Disorders. Impaired fluency associated with neurological disorders; dysfluent speech in people with aphasia is especially noteworthy; a specific form of fluency disorder that is due to neurological impairment is called *neurogenic stuttering*; see Aphasia for information on neurogenic fluency problems; see Fluency Disorders for all other kinds of fluency problems, including neurogenic stuttering.

Neurogenic Stuttering. Fluency disorder of adult onset associated with neurological pathologies including strokes and brain tumors; see Fluency Disorders.

Neurotransmitters. Various chemical compounds within the axon terminal buttons that help transmit information across the synaptic space; include inhibitory and excitatory chemicals; depletion, associated with brain pathology, a frequent cause of impaired intellectual skills in Dementia.

Nonfluent Aphasias. Several types of aphasia, characterized by markedly reduced speech fluency; associated with more anterior cerebral lesions; see Aphasia for a general description of etiology, symptoms, and assessment procedures; see Aphasia: Specific Types for a description of major nonfluent aphasias; also see Fluent Aphasias.

Nonpenetrating (Closed-Head) Injury. A head injury in which the skull may or may not be fractured or lacerated and the meninges covering the brain remain intact.

Nonverbal Oral Apraxia. Difficulty in executing oral movements that are typically involved in speech when given commands; disturbed volitional movements of oral structures; due to lesions in various cerebral structures including the frontal and central opercula and anterior portions of the insula; may coexist with Apraxia of Speech.

Nuclear Agenesis (or Aplasia). The same as Moebius syndrome (see Syndromes Associated With Communication Disorders).

O

Occipital Alexia. The same as alexia without agraphia; see Alexia.

Oculo-Auriculo-Vertebral Dysplasia. The same as Goldenhar syndrome (see Syndromes Associated With Communication Disorders).

Odynophagia. Pain during swallowing.

Open-Head Injury. Head trauma in which the skull is fractured and the meninges are torn; the same as Penetrating Head Injury.

Oral Phase (Stage). A stage of swallowing in which the tongue action moves the bolus toward the pharynx; impaired oral stage swallowing is a part of Dysphagia.

Oral Preparatory Phase (Stage). The initial stage in swallowing, consisting of mixing food with saliva, mastication, and forming a bolus that is ready to be moved to the back of the tongue; impaired oral preparatory stage swallowing is a type of Dysphagia.

Orofacial Examination. Evaluation of the structural and functional integrity of oral and facial structures for speech production; a routine part of speech and language evaluation; see *Hegde's PocketGuide to Assessment in Speech-Language Pathology* (3rd ed.) for procedural details.

Orofacial Myofunctional Disorders. Group of disorders that include tongue thrust, lip incompetence, and deviant sucking habits (e.g., finger or thumb sucking); finger or thumb sucking may affect dental development and alignment and need to be eliminated before myofunctional therapy for tongue thrust; see Tongue Thrust.

Overextensions. A phenomenon of child language; inappropriately generalized word productions; a child who calls all adult females "Mommy" is overgeneralizing that word; suggests a failure to discriminate among stimuli; heard in children normally learning their language; a disorder if it persists beyond age 3 or so.

O

P

Palilalia. Compulsive and numerable repetition of words and phrases, sometimes with progressively faster rate and decreasing loudness; sound-syllable repetitions less common; more likely in spontaneous speech than in reading and automatic speech; more likely repetitions at the end of utterances, although might occur in the middle of utterances; most noticeable in conversational and narrative speech and least in oral reading and automatic speech (e.g., counting); repetitions may not show the Adaptation Effect in oral reading that characterizes repetitions associated with stuttering of early onset; no significant efforts at avoiding repetition of words and phrases; associated with many neurological diseases including Parkinson's disease, Pick's disease, Alzheimer's disease, traumatic lesions of the basal ganglia, multiple sclerosis, posttraumatic encephalopathy, progressive supranuclear palsy, strokes, tumors, Tourette's syndrome, seizures, and thalamotomy; may be associated with Hypokinetic Dysarthria.

Paraphasias. Unintended word or sound substitutions; possibly due to word-finding difficulties; a diagnostic feature of Aphasia.

Parietal-Temporal Alexia. The same as alexia with agraphia; see Alexia.

Parkinsonism. Generic term that suggests clinical signs and symptoms of Parkinson's disease without implying its etiology; vascular dementia and Alzheimer's disease may be associated with symptoms of Parkinson's disease without the typical etiology associated with the latter; see Parkinson's Disease for the symptoms and etiology.

Parkinson's Disease. A progressive neurological syndrome with depigmentation of the substantia nigra, a midbrain structure functionally related to the basal ganglia; typical age of onset is in the 50s and 60s; in the general population, the disease affects 106 persons in 100,000; but after age 50, it affects 1 in 100; relatively constant prevalence rate in all societies and around the world; more common in males than in females; dementia associated with approximately 35% to 55% of clients; survival up to 8 years after the initial diagnosis, longer if diagnosed early in life; associated with neurological, psychiatric, and communication problems, along with irregular and less legible handwriting; soft, monotonous, and rapid speech; crowded word productions without the usual pauses between phrases.

Etiologic Factors
- Historically, classified as idiopathic (of unknown origin); research over the years has suggested several potential causal factors
- Gene mutations on the long arm of chromosome 6; the protein the defective gene encodes is called *parkin*
- Exposure to pesticide, drug abuse, drinking well water, and rural living
- Encephalitis and arteriosclerotic conditions
- Degeneration of brainstem nuclei, widened sulci, loss of cells in substantia negra, neurofibrillary tangles and neuritic plaques, presence of Lewy bodies, and reduced dopamine levels

Early Neurological and Behavioral Symptoms
- Early symptoms include immobility or slow movement (bradykinesia), also called hypokinesia

- Tremors, often the pill-rolling type, are among the more obvious symptoms; they begin with a hand or leg, but spread to all limbs
- Rigidity or increased tone and resistance to movement; if these symptoms are severe, tremors may be absent
- A mask-like face, partly because of lack of emotional expression
- Problems of gait, posture, and equilibrium; difficulty standing up, small and shuffling steps, forward leaning, walking without hand swinging, and festinating gait
- Frequent falls, freezing during movement, and swallowing disorders

Advanced Neurological and Behavioral Symptoms

- Advanced symptoms, especially those that include dementia, found in some clients, especially in those who had the onset after age 60
- Intellectual impairments including deterioration in memory skills, reduced problem-solving skills, impaired visuospatial perception, and loss of reasoning skills
- Emotional disorders, including a flat affect, apathy, and depression
- Psychiatric symptoms, including sleep disturbances, confusion, hallucination, and delirium
- Loss of speech-language functions, related to the degree of cognitive loss (unlike in Alzheimer's disease)
- Generally better preserved language functions, compared to other forms of dementia; advanced stages associated with naming problems, difficulty generating word lists, and impaired discourse comprehension
- Motor speech disorders, most commonly, hypokinetic dysarthria; see Dysarthria: Specific Types.
- Voice problems, including a weak and breathy voice and abnormal pitch, rate, and loudness
- A unique writing problem (micrographia); handwriting in which letters become progressively smaller

Cummings, J. L., & Benson, D. F. (1983). *Dementia: A clinical approach.* Boston: Butterworth.

Hegde, M. N. (2006). *A coursebook on aphasia and other neurogenic communication disorders* (3rd ed.). Clifton Park, NY: Thomson Delmar Learning.

Murray, L. L. (2000). Spoken language production in Huntington's and Parkinson's diseases. *Journal of Speech, Language, and Hearing Research, 43*(6), 1350–1366.

Rajput, A. H. (2001). Epidemiology and clinical genetics of Parkinson's disease. In C. M. Clark & J. Q. Trojanowski (Eds.), *Neurodegenerative dementias* (pp. 177–192). New York: McGraw-Hill.

Simuni, T., & Hurtig, H. I. (2001). Parkinson's disease: Clinical picture. In C. M. Clark & J. Q. Trojanowski (Eds.), *Neurodegenerative dementias* (pp. 193–203). New York: McGraw-Hill.

Penetrating (Open-Head) Injury.   Injury where the skull is perforated or fractured; the Meninges torn or lacerated; see Traumatic Brain Injury.

Peristalsis. Constricting and relaxing movements of a tubular structure (such as the esophagus) to move its contents (such as food in the esophagus); esophageal peristaltic movements may be disordered in clients with Dysphagia.

Perseveration. Tendency to persist with the same response even though the stimulus has changed and the client is aware of it; associated with brain injury; see Aphasia.

Pervasive Developmental Disorder. Group of developmental disorders, including autism, Asperger disorder (syndrome), Rett disorder (syndrome), and the childhood disintegrative disorder, as classified by the American Psychiatric Association; the same group of disorders are also classified as Autism Spectrum Disorders.

Phonemic Paraphasia. A language problem associated with Aphasia; substitution of one phoneme in the intended word with another phoneme (e.g., saying *loman* for *woman*); an unnecessary phoneme may be added to a word (e.g., saying *wolman* for *woman*).

Phonological Awareness. A set of skills children are supposed to have about certain phonological properties of their language; knowledge that syllables and words are created from sounds and sound combinations; correlated with phonological disorders, reading skills, and reading problems; no convincing experimental evidence that teaching phonological awareness will help improve articulation or literacy skills; various subskills include:
- Rhyming: Identifying words that sound alike or rhyme, words that rhyme, or sort rhyming from nonrhyming words
- Alliteration: Identifying words that begin or end with a certain sound
- Phoneme isolation: Telling whether a specific sound occurs in the beginning, end, or middle of a word
- Sound blending: Blending two or more sounds that are temporally separated by a few seconds into a word
- Syllable identification: Identifying the number of syllables in a word through clapping, finger tapping, or by verbally stating
- Sound segmentation: Breaking down a word into its individual sounds; specifying the number of phonemes in a word; telling whether the same sound occurs in multiple words; changing a sound in a word by substituting it with a requested sound
- Invented spellings: Spelling words phonetically

Phonological Disorders. Errors of articulation, especially systematic errors on multiple phonemes that form patterns based on Phonological Processes; see Articulation and Phonological Disorders for a description of disorders; multiple errors of articulation found in the same individual viewed from the standpoint of phonological processes; presumably, not due to motoric problems but to phonological-linguistic rule-learning problems.

Phonological Processes. Multiple ways in which children who are still learning their speech sounds simplify their productions; simplifications compared to adult productions of the same speech sounds and result in a loss of phonemic contrast; based on the assumption that multiple errors reflect the operation of certain phonological rules and that the problem is essentially phonemic, not phonetic; originally proposed as psychologically real explanatory concepts in that processes explain error patterns; presumed psychological reality questioned by others; an alternative view is that the processes are ways of describing and categorizing errors without necessarily explaining them; assessed through a representative sample of conversational speech or through computerized software programs; see Articulation and Phonological Disorders; classified in varied ways, but the major processes include:

- Assimilation processes: Phonological patterns in which one sound in a word leads to a change in another sound in the same word; although in many cases, assimilative errors are similar to substitution errors; in assimilation, the influence of one sound on another is the main source of error; such an influence is not a factor in simple substitutions
  - Alveolar assimilation: Production of an alveolar in place of a velar
    - *dot* for *goat*
    - *tot* for *coat*
  - Coalescence: Production of a single sound in place of a two adjacent sounds
    - *fip* for *sweep*
    - *pip* for *beep*
  - Devoicing: Production of a voiceless consonant in place of a voiced consonant
    - *back* for *bag*
    - *sip* for *zip*
  - Diminutization: Addition of [i] or a consonant and [i]:
    - *eggi* for *egg*
    - *nodi* for *no*
  - Epenthesis: Insertion of a vowel (an error of addition); often between two consonants in a consonantal cluster
    - *bə lu* for *blue*
    - *sə mile* for *smile*
  - Labial assimilation: Production of a labial consonant in place of a nonlabial consonant in a word that contains another labial
    - *beab* for *bead*
    - *bop* for *top*
  - Metathesis: Production of sounds in a word in their reversed order
    - *peek* for *keep*
    - *likstip* for *lipstick*
  - Nasal assimilation: Production of a nasal consonant in place of an oral consonant in a word that contains a nasal
    - *nam* for *lamb*
    - *nun* for *fun*
  - Prevocalic voicing (voicing assimilation): Voiced production of voiceless consonants when they precede a vowel (prevocalic position)
    - *bea* for *pea*
    - *Dom* for *Tom*
  - Reduplication (doubling): Repetition of a syllable within a word
    - *wawa* for *water*
    - *kaka* for *cat*

P

- o Velar assimilation: Production of a velar consonant in place of a nonvelar in a word that contains a velar
  - *keak* for *teak*
  - *guck* for *duck*
- Substitution processes (simplification processes): Similar to *substitutions* in the traditional analysis, involve replacement of one sound for another sound
  - o Apicalization: Production of an apical (tongue tip) consonant in place of a labial consonant
    - *Dee* for *bee*
    - *Tee* for *pea*
  - o Backing: Production of more posteriorly placed consonants instead of more anteriorly placed consonants (velar consonants in place of alveolar consonants)
    - *boak* for *boat*
    - *hoop* for *soup*
  - o Affrication: Production of an affricate in place of a fricative or stop
    - *chun* for *sun*
    - *chu* for *shoe*
  - o Deaffrication: Production of a fricative in place of an affricate
    - *pez* for *page*
    - *ship* for *chip*
  - o Denasalization: Production of an oral sound with a similar place of articulation (homorganic sound) in place of a nasal
    - *by* for *my*
    - *dame* for *name*
  - o Depalatalization: Production of an alveolar fricative in place of a palatal fricative or affricate
    - *su* for *shoe*
    - *wats* for *watch* (diacritic under ts) ‿
  - o Final consonant devoicing: Production of an unvoiced final consonant in place of a voiced final consonant
    - *bet* for *bed*
    - *bik* for *big*
  - o Fronting: Production of more anteriorly placed consonants in place of more posteriorly placed consonants (e.g., alveolar consonants instead of velar consonants)
    - *tee* for *key*
    - *su* for *shoe*
  - o Gliding: Production of a glide (w, j) in place of a liquid (l, r)
    - *pwey* for *play*
    - *yewo* for *yellow*
  - o Glottal replacement: Production of a glottal stop () in place of other consonants (insert the phonetic symbol for the glottal stop)
    - *tuʔ* for *tooth*
    - *baʔ* for *bottle* (insert glottal stop and a schwa)
  - o Labialization: Production of a labial consonant in place of a lingual consonant
    - *fum* for *thumb*
    - *vase* for *days*

- o Stopping: Production of stop consonants in place of other sounds (often fricatives)
  - *teat* for *seat*
  - *doup* for *soup*
- o Vocalization (vowelization): Production of vowels in place of liquids or nasals
  - *fawo* for *flower*
  - *dippo* for *zipper*
- Deletion processes (structure processes): Similar to *deletions* in the traditional analysis, involve elimination of certain sounds in syllables and words
  - o Cluster reduction or cluster simplification: Omission (deletion) of one or more consonants in a cluster of consonants
    - *bes* for *best*
    - *seep* for *sleep*
  - o Consonant deletion: Omission of an intervocalic consonant
    - *mai* for *mommy*
    - *dai* for *Dotty*
  - o Initial consonant deletion. Omission of word-initial consonants
    - *at* for *pot*
    - *oop* for *soup*
  - o Final consonant deletion: Omission of a consonant at the end of a word or syllable
    - *kœ* for *cat*
    - *pu* for *pool*
  - o Unstressed (weak) syllable deletion: Omission of a syllable, usually an unstressed syllable
    - *nana* for *banana*
    - *tephone* for *telephone*

Bernthal, J. E., & Bankson, N. W. (2004). *Articulation and phonological disorders* (5th ed.). Englewood Cliffs, NJ: Prentice Hall.

Lowe, R. J. (1994). *Phonology: Assessment and intervention applications in speech pathology.* Baltimore, MD: Williams & Wilkins.

Peña-Brooks, A., & Hegde, M. N. (2007). *Assessment and treatment of articulation and phonological disorders in children* (2nd ed.). Austin, TX: Pro-Ed.

Smit, A. B. (2004). *Articulation and phonology: Resource guide for school-age children and adults.* Clifton Park, NY: Thomson Delmar Learning.

Stoel-Gammon, C., & Dunn, C. (1985). *Normal and disordered phonology in children.* Austin, TX: Pro-Ed.

Williams, A. L. (2003). *Speech disorders: Resource guide for preschool children.* Clifton Park, NY: Thomson Delmar Learning.

Phytanic Acid. Fatty acid concentrated in dairy products; excessively stored in tissue or plasma of clients with Refsum syndrome (see Syndromes Associated With Communication Disorders).

Pick Bodies. Dense intracellular formations in the neuronal cytoplasm, especially in nonpyramidal cells in the second, third, and sixth cerebral layers; neuropathological findings in frontotemporal Dementia, including Pick's Disease.

Pick Cells. Ballooned, inflated, or enlarged neurons, especially in the lower middle cortical layers; neuropathological findings in frontotemporal Dementia, including Pick's Disease.

Pick's Disease. Once considered a separate degenerative disorder; currently, a part of the frontotemporal dementia, characterized by atrophy in the frontal and temporal lobes, with Pick bodies (dense intracellular formations in the neuronal cytoplasm) and Pick cells (ballooned, inflated, or enlarged neurons); profound behavioral changes and eventual dementia; see Frontotemporal Dementia for details.

Pill Esophagitis. Inflammation of the esophagus due to medications getting lodged in it; damaging effects on the tissue; may be associated with esophageal phase swallowing problems.

Polydactyly. Genetic anomaly of supernumerary (extra) toes or fingers associated with several genetic syndromes; see Laurence-Moon syndrome and Oro-Facial-Digital syndrome type II under Syndromes Associated With Communication Disorders.

Polyneuritis. Simultaneous inflation of several peripheral nerves, associated with genetic syndromes including Refsum syndrome; see under Syndromes Associated With Communication Disorders.

Postanoxic Dementia. Dementia due to severe and chronic anoxia (oxygen deficiency); see Dementia.

Posterior Isolation Syndrome. Same as transcortical sensory aphasia (see Aphasia: Specific Types).

Posttraumatic Memory Loss (Amnesia). Loss of memory for events that follow brain injury; see Traumatic Brain Injury.

Pragmatic Language Skills. Appropriate language use in naturalistic communicative contexts; see Language Disorders in Children for disorders of pragmatic language skills; include conversational and narrative skills; major pragmatic language skills include:

- Topic initiation: Skill in introducing new topics during conversation at socially appropriate times and junctures
- Topic maintenance: Skill in maintaining conversation on the same or closely related topics for an extended but socially appropriate duration.
- Conversational turn taking: Skill in playing the role of a listener and speaker at appropriate times and junctures in conversational exchanges; not interrupting the speaker and taking turns when appropriate
- Eye contact: Appropriate durations for which a person maintains eye contact with his or her conversational partner or partners; may not be a typical pragmatic skill in some cultures
- Conversational repair strategies: Strategies to restore temporarily impaired communication; skill in changing wording or manner of speaking when listeners fail to understand and ask for clarification; skill in requesting and obtaining clarification when one does not understand a speaker

Preauricular Tags. Rudimentary appendage of auricular tissue on the face, often at the corner of the mouth and toward the ear; associated with certain genetic syndromes; see Goldenhar syndrome under Syndromes Associated With Communication Disorders.

Pretraumatic Memory Loss (Amnesia). Loss of memory for events preceding brain injury; see Traumatic Brain Injury.

Prevalence. The number of people who have a disorder at a given time; a head count of people who already have a condition; contrasted with Incidence.

Primary Focal Lesions. Localized brain lesions.

Primary Intracranial Tumors. Tumors originating in the brain or within the skull; versus metastatic tumors that migrate from their site of origin to other sites in the body.

Primary Progressive Aphasia. Atypical form of aphasia due to degenerative neurological disease of insidious onset and slow progression of symptoms leading eventually to dementia; also known as *slowly progressive aphasia*; possibly affecting the left perisylvian region of the brain; minimal or no generalized cognitive impairment in the early stages; dementia in the later stages; language symptoms resemble those of Broca's aphasia and may include apraxia of speech; see Aphasia and Aphasia: Specific Types.

Prognathism. Abnormally forward-projected jaw; determined in relation to the cranial base; may affect mandible, maxilla, or both; a feature of several genetic syndromes affecting the cranium.

Progressive Bulbar Palsy. Predominantly lower motor neuron disease that may result in Dysarthria, especially Flaccid Dysarthria.

Progressive Supranuclear Palsy (PSP). Degenerative disease of the brainstem, basal ganglia, and cerebellum; in its early stages, resembles Parkinson's disease; includes paralysis of the upward gaze (ophthalmoplegia); gait and balance problems; frequent falling; neck rigidity; mixed dysarthria and dysphagia in the early stages; cortical stuttering or palilalia associated with frontal atrophy; aphonia; slowly developing dementia.

Prosopagnosia. Difficulty recognizing familiar faces; voice may help recognize the face; difficulty matching known persons' pictures with names; possible symptom of Right Hemisphere Syndrome.

Pseudobulbar Palsy. Damage to the cortical regions and corticobulbar tracts causing upper motor neuron symptoms and Dysphagia, dysphonia, and Dysarthria.

Pseudodementia. Psychiatric symptoms that mimic dementia including slowness of movement, forgetfulness, disorientation, and impaired attention; rapid progression of symptoms; associated with severe depression and schizophrenia; see the next entry.

Psychiatric Problems Associated With Communication Disorders. Several communication disorders are psychiatric in nature and require unique strategies of assessment and treatment; some of them have a neurological component, whereas others are entirely psychiatric; dementia and neurodegenerative diseases may be associated with psychiatric as well as communication, behavioral, cognitive, and motor symptoms; communication disorders may be entirely psychiatric in nature, with no physical basis and include stuttering due to malingering or faking, certain forms of mutism, a type of aphonia, and a type of dementia; to assess psychiatric problems related to communication disorders, see the sources cited at the end of this main entry and the companion volume, *Hegde's PocketGuide to Assessment in Speech-Language Pathology* (3rd ed.); to treat or otherwise clinically manage psychiatric communication disorders, see the other companion volume, *Hegde's PocketGuide to Treatment in Speech-Language Pathology* (3rd ed.); the most commonly encountered psychiatric problems associated with communication disorders include the following.

Abulia. Extreme lack of motivation; may be associated with unwillingness to talk, leading to a form of mutism called *akinetic mutism*; a psychiatric disorder with a neurological basis with the following characteristics:

- Mutism and abulia may be associated with early stages of stroke or head trauma
- Does not affect consciousness; clients who are abulic and do not talk are alert and attentive
- No evidence of peripheral neuromotor disorder that causes mutism
- Frontal lobe damage is the most frequent cause of abulia
- Severe apathy and indifference
- Extremely limited or nonexistent speech; if present, speech is aphonic, whispered, or of very soft voice

Aphonia—Functional. Aphonia without a neurophysiological basis, is also called *functional aphonia* or *psychogenic aphonia*; it is not due to a neurophysiological problem that prevents vocal fold adduction and vibration (e.g., bilateral vocal fold paralysis with a wide-open glottis); functional aphonia is treated as a psychiatric or behavioral disorder

- No organic pathology leading to lack of voice (e.g., normal vocal folds with no neurological diseases)
- Sudden onset, often associated with stressful life events
- A history of psychiatric symptoms
- Presence of positive reinforcement of the problems (e.g., the client may be complimented on effective whispering and gesturing, with which he or she communicates well)
- Evidence of gain the client enjoys because of the disorder; aphonia may help avoid unpleasant or difficult academic, social, or occupational demands (e.g., an excuse from oral presentations in school or at work); maintained by negative reinforcement
- Normal voice during laughter or throat clearing, suggesting normal phonatory mechanism

Delusions and Hallucinations. Delusional speech may be an important feature of several types of communication disorders; although *delusional disorder* is a specific psychiatric problem, many clients with neurodegenerative diseases and dementia may exhibit coexisting delusional beliefs and persistently talk about them; other clients with neurodegenerative diseases may also have hallucinations

- Delusions: Pathologically false beliefs or thoughts that negatively affect the behavior; beliefs that are held against contradictory evidence; not easily persuaded otherwise by logic and explanations
- Delusions of persecution: Strong and baseless belief that other people, including family members, are conspiring to hurt or harm them in various ways; persons may believe (and accuse others) that they are conspiring to harm, cheat, or poison them; associated with Alzheimer's disease and dementia; when family members begin to assume the clients' prior responsibilities (e.g., paying the bills), the clients may grow increasingly suspicious of others
- Delusions without persecutory thoughts: Pathologically false beliefs or thoughts without a sense of being persecuted; associated with frontotemporal dementia; take various forms:
  o Grandiose delusions: Pathologically false beliefs that the person has accomplished great things, made important discoveries, is very wealthy, possesses exceptional talent, or in other ways is outstanding
  o Jealous delusions: Pathologically false beliefs that one's spouse is unfaithful, leading to meticulous collection of trivial and baseless "evidence" to justify and confront the spouse
  o Somatic delusions: False beliefs that one's own body's structures or functions are pathological or abnormal; belief that certain body parts are either missing or nonexistent
- Hallucinations: Pathological, and often bizarre, sensory experiences without objective sensory stimulation
  o Visual hallucinations: Pathological visual experiences, including a variety of abnormal perceptual phenomena; clients with dementia may see and talk about:
    ▪ Nonexistent, disturbing, threatening, or even frightening events, persons, and animals
    ▪ Swirling geometric shapes, movements in the peripheral visual fields, flashes of color, and halos around objects (these often drug-induced)
  o Auditory hallucinations: Pathological auditory experiences without objective auditory stimulation; clients may:
    ▪ Hear voices, commanding bizarre acts
    ▪ Hear annoying or frightening voices that do not necessarily command actions
    ▪ Hear constant running commentary about something
  o Speech-language pathologists may encounter delusions and hallucinations in:
    ▪ Parkinson's disease; visual hallucinations, which are more common than auditory hallucinations; aggravated by antiparkinsonian drugs
    ▪ Huntington's disease; persecutory delusions and hallucinations
    ▪ Progressive supranuclear palsy; frightening visual hallucinations and delusions
    ▪ AIDS dementia complex; hallucinations and delusions

P

- Creutzfeldt-Jakob disease; hallucinations and delusions
- Dementia caused by repeated head injury (as in professional boxers); delusions of persecution

Depression. Temporary or chronic feelings of sadness, hopelessness, loneliness, despair, and dejection; low self-esteem and self-reproach; verbalization of negative feelings; reduced motoric activity; loss of memory; lack of concentration; lack of pleasure in previously enjoyed activities; disinterest in everything; associated with dementia and neurodegenerative diseases; may resemble dementia (see Pseudodementia under this entry); although diagnosis and treatment of depression is not the responsibility of speech-language pathologists, it is essential to take note of depression because it will affect both assessment and treatment efforts:

- Speech-language pathologists are likely to encounter depression in:
  - o Dementia, including clients with AIDS Dementia Complex
  - o Early stages of neurodegenerative diseases with no serious signs of dementia (e.g., Alzheimer's disease, Creutzfeldt-Jakob disease, Huntington's disease, Parkinson's disease, vascular dementia, and dementia caused by repeated head injury)
- Note that the client's social and communication skills (or potential for them) may be vastly underrated because of depression

Euphoria and Mania. Exaggerated feeling of well-being (euphoria); hyperactivity, moving from one activity to another without completing any, incredible amount of physical energy, and exaggerated feeling of well-being (mania); no basis in reality; may alternate between feelings of hopelessness and depression.

- Speech-language pathologists may encounter euphoria (or mania) in:
  - o Frontotemporal dementia: Abnormally elevated mood, excessive jocularity, exaggerated self-esteem, which may alternate with depression
  - o Huntington's disease: Euphoric-like false sense of superiority
  - o AIDS dementia complex: Mania (as well as its opposite, depression)
  - o Creutzfeldt-Jakob disease: Euphoria (and depression)
  - o Vascular dementia: Frequent mood swings, including euphoria
  - o Dementia caused by repeated head injury (as in professional boxers); euphoria (and depression)

Factitious Disorders. Disorders invented by the client; typically take the form of physical diseases that require hospitalization and sometime serious and painful treatment, but may occasionally take the form of stuttering or a voice disorder; the characteristics include:

- An absence of motivation for the symptoms and an uncontrollable desire to play the role of a sick person (contrasted with malingering)
- Willingness to endure pain and making frequent and persistent demands for complicated and painful surgical or medical procedures; may convince some medical professionals to perform extensive and painful procedures
- Frequent travel to various hospitals and specialists in varied distant places to get treatment for never-cured illnesses that keep appearing
- Self-inflicted injuries or self-induced diseases (e.g., injecting harmful substances into oneself, ingesting anticoagulants to induce serious bleeding)

- Tendency to report problems with a dramatic flare, a sense of triumph at having a mysterious or difficult-to-treat disorder; showing off needlessly amputated limbs with a sense of pride and satisfaction, while still seeking treatment for some other factitious disease
- Psychological or psychiatric symptoms (e.g., memory loss, depression, anxiety) or symptoms of serious physical diseases; the latter is sometimes called the *Munchausen syndrome*, characterized by an intention to get hospitalized and stay in the hospital

Malingering. Motivated faking or feigning a disease or a disorder to gain a certain advantage from the problem (contrasted with factitious diseases); avoiding pain or treatment that is not aversive; conscious and well-planned symptoms resembling a variety of disorders; speech-language pathologists occasionally see malingered stuttering, voice disorders (especially mutism or aphonia), cognitive dysfunction (especially faked memory loss) that is disproportionate with the extent of traumatic brain injury, movement disorders with no neurological basis, and hearing loss; malingered chronic pain and various forms of physical and mental disability (related to auto accidents and occupations) more common in medical and psychiatric practice; also seen are functional visual loss (malingered blindness), epileptic-type seizures, and various simulated physical illnesses; the general characteristics include:

- A clear advantage the person gains from the problem; malingerers may:
  - Derive positive reinforcement from the disorder; a potential for monetary gain is the motive for many kinds of malingered physical pain and disability associated with auto accidents, industrial accidents, and employment; malingerers often are entangled with legal issues related to their feigned disorder; some gain or positive reinforcement is at least suspect when, for example, a factory worker who is suing his or her employer for a hearing loss that appears to be feigned
  - Derive negative reinforcement from the disorder; an army captain who needs to shout orders to soldiers, but has suddenly gone mute on the battleground, may quickly be removed from the dangerous battlefield and placed in a distant and safe hospital; thus, the avoidance of a stressful combat zone provides quick and effective negative reinforcement for the feigned disorder
- Symptoms or features that are at odds with the known characteristics of the disorder; for instance:
  - Malingered stuttering: A person who feigns stuttering may continue to stutter under DAF, masking noise, and slower speech; may show no adaptation effect; may stutter on medial or final syllables
  - Malingered hearing loss: A person who fakes a hearing loss may turn toward the direction of a sound that is suddenly presented; may carefully avoid dangerous sound signals in the environment that are not supposed to be heard (e.g., may carefully avoid traffic without seeing it); may follow a command quickly given at normal vocal intensity; pure tone audiogram may not fit any pattern of conductive, sensorineural, or mixed loss; an otologist will have ruled out auditory pathology

251

      o Malingered mutism: A person who feigns mutism or aphonia may very well articulate whispered speech all the time, thus avoiding most of the handicaps of not being able to speak; while whispering, a normal voice may be briefly heard; normal voice may be heard when the person coughs; family members may have heard the normal voice under an emergency (e.g., a client who shouts *fire!* and then remains voiceless); no vocal pathology to account for the disorder

- Noncompliant during clinical examination; generally, the client may:
  - o Be unwilling to be assessed (possibly because of the fear of detection)
  - o Refuse to participate in assessment tasks or participate reluctantly
  - o Claim inability to perform a requested task (a person who feigns stuttering may claim he or she cannot read aloud any more; a person who fakes mutism may claim inability to cough when requested, but may do so reflexively)
  - o Feign misunderstanding of instructions given during assessment, often to explain noncompliance or wrong responses
  - o Fail to follow through suggestions (e.g. a person who feigns stuttering may not comply with a request to bring a taped speech sample from home)
  - o May not keep assessment or treatment appointments
    - A history of other psychiatric disorders (e.g., personality disorder, hypochondria, pathological lying)
    - Traditionally, malingering is explained as a *conversion reaction,* a Freudian term that means that a repressed and unconscious sexual or other kind of socially unacceptable conflict has surfaced in disguise as the symptom the client presents; there is little or no experimental support for this *psychopathological, psychoanalytic,* or *psychodynamic* explanation of behavior disorders

Mutism—Selective. Psychiatric variety of mutism; not forced by physical diseases; nonpsychiatric mutism associated with the final stages of many neurodegenerative diseases and dementia; a transient form associated with stroke and other kinds of brain injury; see also Mutism; characteristics include:

- Mutism limited to specific situations
- Not due to shyness, embarrassment in social situations, ethnocultural differences, bilingual status, gender differences, or lack of knowledge on topics of conversation
- Lasts at least one month; in case of children, it should persist after the first month in school because some children may be naturally reluctant to speak in new situations
- Successful communication with gestures and facial expressions, although social, personal, or academic communication may be negatively affected
- Limited verbalizations that may be characterized by monotonous or altered voice

Pseudodementia. Dementia-like symptoms associated with depression; absence of responses or inappropriate responses suggesting true cognitive impairments (dementia); no true dementia; characteristics include:

- Apathy, lack of interest in anything, limited speech, low vocal intensity, and sad disposition

- Rapid progression of cognitive impairment (contrasted with generally slow progression of dementia associated with neurodegenerative diseases)
- Better visual memory and better performance on visual memory tasks than in dementia associated with neurodegenerative diseases
- Previous episodes of depression or other psychiatric problems

Psychogenic Stuttering. Controversial disorder of fluency with an adult onset and characterized by stuttering-like dysfluencies; may or may not be associated with neurological diseases; presumably caused by psychological problems; characteristics and explanations include:

- Adult onset; reported age range of 19 to 79 years (unlike early-onset stuttering)
- Prevalence is roughly the same in men and women (contrasted with higher prevalence in males of early-onset stuttering)
- Dysfluencies are similar to those found in stuttering of early childhood onset and include sound or syllable repetitions, prolongations, "hesitations," word repetitions, "blocking," tense pauses, phrase repetitions, and interjections
- Associated motor behaviors including facial grimacing and struggle
- Rate variations (both slow and fast speech rate)
- Constant dysfluency rate in some individuals and situation-specific variability in others
- Relatively unaffected by choral reading, masking, delayed auditory feedback, and singing (contrasted with early-onset stuttering), although variability across individuals prevents diagnostic rules based on these variables
- Psychiatric diagnoses associated with psychogenic stuttering include conversion reaction, depression, anxiety, personality disorder, posttraumatic neurosis, adjustment disorder, and drug dependence
- Stressful life conditions associated with psychogenic stuttering include illness, death, or other tragic events in the family; marital problems and divorce; negative feelings associated with unemployment; difficult work responsibilities or dissatisfaction with work; physical disability; childhood emotional trauma
- Complaints of weakness, fatigue, incoordination, or seizures, even in the absence of confirmed neurological diseases
- Confirmed neurological diseases associated with psychogenic stuttering in some individuals; include neurodegenerative diseases, convulsive disorders, traumatic brain injury, or stroke; lesions in either the left or right hemispheres of the brain, or the brainstem and cerebellum; no aphasia, dysarthria, or apraxia of speech in a majority of clients
- Diagnosis of "psychogenic stuttering" in individuals with confirmed neurological diseases is both troublesome and challenging
- Explanation of stuttering as a conversion reaction is Freudian; it means that a repressed and unconscious sexual or other kind of socially unacceptable conflict is *converted* into behavioral symptoms of stuttering; there is little or no experimental support for this *psychopathological, psychoanalytic,* or *psychodynamic* explanation of behavior disorders

Schizophrenia. Serious psychiatric disorder characterized by aberrant speech, a diagnostic marker; the most serious *psychotic* problem with delusions, hallucinations, disorganized speech, and disorganized or catatonic behavior; generally classified into paranoid, catatonic, disorganized, undifferentiated, and residual subtypes.

- General behavioral symptoms include:
  o Exaggerated or abnormal thinking and bizarre delusions (e.g., a client may believe that his or her brain, heart, or other internal organs have been replaced without any surgical wounds); persecutory delusions are more common than other forms
  o Hallucinations of various kinds; auditory hallucinations
  o Disorganized thinking, inferred from aberrant speech
  o Grossly disorganized behavior; childlike silliness or uncontrollably agitated or violent actions; socially inappropriate actions (and speech); incongruent or bizarre actions (e.g., wearing multiple overcoats on a hot day)
  o Catatonic behavior; extreme degree of apathy or unresponsiveness to environmental stimuli; lack of awareness of the surroundings; assuming rigid postures for long periods of time with resistance to be moved
  o Affective symptoms; emotional flattening, lack of initiative and motivation, and disinterest in social activities
  o Impaired personal care, failure to meet job responsibilities or academic demands
- Speech and language characteristics associated with schizophrenia include:
  o Empty, meaningless, brief, or irrelevant speech
  o Extremely limited fluency of speech, suggesting a poverty of thoughts
  o Frequent and abrupt changes in the topic of discussion or conversation; speaking on topics or ideas that are remotely or loosely related to the point of discussion
  o Irrelevant answers to questions and irrelevant comments
  o Meaningless repetition of words and phrases
  o *Word salad*, or meaningless, incoherent, and unusual word combinations
  o Incoherent, disorganized, illogical, and vague speech; alternatively, the speech may be excessively concrete
  o A general poverty of speech; little expressive speech with brief answers empty and devoid of content; conversely, excessively detailed verbosity
  o Inappropriate stress patterns
  o Rapidly deteriorating prosodic features of speech (abnormal melody and pitch of the voice)
  o Poor eye contact and impaired gestures and body language
  o Expression of delusional thoughts
  o Expression of speech that suggests hallucinations
  o Lack of affect and feelings associated with speech and its variable content
  o Markedly reduced emotional expressions in speech; alternatively, a tendency to express emotions that are incongruent with the situation, stimuli, questions asked, or one's own experiences (e.g., laughter while narrating a sad experience)
  o Memory and intellectual impairment, although schizophrenia is not associated with intellectual impairment

P

American Psychiatric Association (1994). *Diagnostic and statistical manual of mental disorders* (4th ed.). Washington, DC: Author.

Baumgartner, J. (1999). Acquired psychogenic stuttering. In R. F. Curlee (Ed.), *Stuttering and related disorders of fluency* (pp. 269–288). New York: Thieme.

Baumgartner, J., & Duffy, J. R. (1997). Psychogenic stuttering in adults with and without neurologic disease. *Journal of Medical Speech-Language Pathology, 5*, 75–95.

Bianchini, K. J., Greve, K. W., & Love, J. M. (2003). Definite malingered neurocognitive dysfunction in moderate/severe traumatic brain injury. *Clinical Neuropsychology, 17*(4), 574–580.

Duffy, J. R. (2005). *Motor speech disorders: Substrates, differential diagnosis, and management*. St. Louis, MO: Elsevier Mosby. [*see Chapter 14 on acquired psychogenic and neurogenic speech disorders*]

Gorman, W. F. (1982). Defining malingering. *Journal of Forensic Science, 27*(2), 401–407.

Hinson, V. K., & Haren, W. B. (2006). Psychogenic movement disorders. *Lancet Neurology, 5*(8), 695–700.

Lauter, H., & Dames, S. (1991). Depressive disorders and dementia: The clinical review. *Acta Psychiatrica Scandinavica Supplementum, 366*, 40–46.

Seery, C. H. (2005). Differential diagnosis of stuttering for forensic purposes. *American Journal of Speech-Language Pathology, 14*(4), 284–297.

Speedie, L., Rabins, P., Pearlson, G., & Moberg, P. (1990). Confrontation naming deficits in dementia of depression. *Journal of Neuropsychiatry and Clinical Neuroscience, 2*(1), 59–63.

Turner, M. (1999). Malingering, hysteria, and the factitious disorders. *Cognitive Neuropsychiatry, 4*(3), 193–201.

Vossler, D. G., Haltiner, A. M., Schepp, S. K., & associates (2004). Ictal stuttering: a sign suggestive of psychogenic nonepileptic seizures. *Neurology, 63*(3), 516–519.

Zapotocky, H. G. (1998). Problems of differential diagnosis between depressive pseudodementia and Alzheimer's disease. *Journal of Neurological Transmission Supplement, 53*, 91–95.

Ptosis.   Drooping or retrogression of an organ or part; drooping of the upper the eyelid as seen in Noonan syndrome (see Syndromes Associated With Communication Disorders).

Pulmonary Stenosis.   Narrowing of the opening between the pulmonary artery and the right ventricle.

Pure Agraphia.   Isolated writing disorder; loss of previously learned writing skills due to recent neurological problems; not the writing problem of children that may be due to a failure to acquire the skill; normal or near-normal oral language; see Agraphia.

Pure Alexia. Reading disorders without writing disorders; loss of previously learned reading skills due to recent neurological impairment; not *dyslexia,* which is a failure in learning to read during early childhood without neurological problems; pure alexia is also called *alexia without agraphia;* see Alexia.

P

R

Random Paraphasia. Word substitution problem associated with aphasia; the intended and substituted words have no apparent connection (e.g., substituting the word *window* for *banana*); see Aphasia.

Receptive Aphasia. Same as Wernicke's aphasia; see Aphasia: Specific Types.

Reduplicative Paramnesia. Belief in the existence of multiple and identical persons, places, and body parts; associated with Traumatic Brain Injury.

Reflux Esophagitis. Backflow of gastric contents into the esophagus, causing inflammation or possibly ulcers of the esophagus; heart burn, chest pain, and Dysphagia may be the consequences.

Retinitis Pigmentosa. Eye disease characterized by progressive retinal atrophy and migration of pigmentation; initial symptom is night blindness; progressive loss of vision; associated with several Syndromes Associated With Communication Disorders.

Retrograde Amnesia. Difficulty remembering events preceding Traumatic Brain Injury; the same as *pretraumatic memory loss.*

Reversible Ischemic Neurological Deficit. Also known as minor strokes; complete or nearly complete recovery of stroke symptoms, usually within 24 hours.

Right Hemisphere Syndrome. Syndrome of perceptual, attentional, emotional, and communication deficits associated with brain injury in the right cerebral hemisphere; often due to the same neurological diseases that cause left hemisphere injury and aphasia; varying degrees of functional involvement depending on the site, nature, and extent of damage; syndromes of right and left hemispheres produce different constellation of symptoms because of the hemispheric asymmetry; the right and the left hemispheres specialize in different kinds of functions; functions of the right hemisphere are less well understood than those of the left hemisphere; behavioral deficits other than communication deficits may be more prominent in a few individuals; associated with communication disorders in about 50% of cases; generally dominant perceptual and attentional problems; increased chances of communication disorders with lower level of education and cortical lesions (rather than subcortical lesions); the relationship between specific communication disorders and the right hemisphere is poorly understood.

Hemispheric Asymmetry
- The left hemisphere is slightly larger than the right hemisphere, even in fetuses
- The lateral sulcus in the left hemisphere (surrounding which are the areas important for language) is slightly larger than that in the right hemisphere
- The left planum temporale is significantly larger than that in the right hemisphere
- More folded left temporal operculum than the corresponding region in the right hemisphere

Right Hemisphere Functions
- Attention and orientation; in right-handed individuals, the right hemisphere is responsible for:
  - Readiness to respond to stimuli (*arousal*)

o Orienting (directing one's attention to stimuli); general spatial awareness and orientation
o Sustained attention, attention to selected stimuli in the context of changing stimuli (*vigilance*), and selective attention (ignoring certain stimuli while paying attention to others)
- Visual perception; the right hemisphere is responsible for:
  o Perception of holistic, gestalt-like stimuli (e.g., understanding the meaning of a total picture versus its parts)
  o Recognition of human faces
  o Maintenance of one's own body image
- Emotional experiences and expressions; the right hemisphere may control:
  o Emotional experiences (the posterior region of the right hemisphere may be more active during emotional experiences than the left hemisphere regions)
  o Expression of negative emotions (e.g., anger and fear)
- Certain aspects of communication, although the major speech and language functions are a specialty of the left hemisphere; the right hemisphere may be responsible for:
  o Discourse comprehension and production
  o Comprehension of nouns (may be less efficient in comprehending the meaning of verbs)
  o Understanding implied meanings of what others say
  o Understanding ambiguous and alternative meanings of what others say
  o Understanding emotional tones of what others say; expressing one's own emotional tone through language
  o Understanding and expressing prosodic features of speech
  o Understanding the context of what others say
  o Managing the pragmatic aspects of communication (e.g., turn taking, topic maintenance, and socially appropriate communication)

Epidemiology and Ethnocultural Variables

- Prevalence of right hemisphere syndrome in the general population has not been accurately determined; no reliable data exist on the prevalence of the syndrome in varied ethnocultural groups
- Prevalence of various disorders in clients with right hemisphere syndrome may vary, but generally (Blake et al., 2002):
  o Attention, left neglect, perception, memory, and reasoning problems in about 67% of clients
  o Problems in awareness and orientation along with hyperresponsiveness in about 40% of clients
  o Hyporesponsiveness, problems in calculation, and emotional experiences and expressions in 30% to 40% of clients
  o Purely linguistic problems in less than 30% of clients
  o Problems of interpersonal interactions and prosodic problems in 16% to 20% of clients; possibly higher
  o Hemiparesis on the left side in excess of 90% of clients
  o Dysarthria in 68% of clients
  o Dysphagia and homonymous hemianopsia in about 30% of clients

259

Perceptual, Attentional, and Other Behavioral Deficits

- Left-neglect, characterized by reduced sensitivity to stimuli on the left side, reduced awareness of space, or absence of previously learned responses to stimuli on the left visual field; due to damage in the right hemisphere; left hemisphere damage also may cause right-side neglect, but much less frequently; the client may:
  - Fail to respond to all kinds of sensory stimuli, including visual, auditory, and tactile stimuli present in the left visual field
  - Have a strong right focus; stimuli on the right side captures the client's attention; even when an array of stimuli are presented to only the right visual field, only the extreme right stimuli may be attended to
  - Need specific instruction to attend to stimuli on the left
  - Have difficulty shifting attention from right side stimuli to left side stimuli
  - Use only right-sided pockets or right-sided drawers
  - Fail to perceive left-sided tactile and perceptual stimuli in the absence of sensory deficits (e.g., may fail to perceive touch or pinprick applied to the left side of the body)
  - Copy only the right side of a geometric design (e.g., crowding all the numbers of a clock into the right half of the circle)
  - Paint only the right half of a face or other images (e.g., a painter may paint only the right side of his or her own face in creating a self-portrait)
  - Read only the right half of a printed page and complain that what is read does not make sense
  - Bump into things on the left side
  - Deny the existence of paralyzed left body part or claim that it belongs to someone else; may not recognize one's own ring or watch when worn on the left hand
  - Exhibit motor neglect; the client may behave as though his or her left side is paralyzed even though the left side is neurophysiologically normal
  - Fail to localize stimuli on the left side; less common than visual neglect, some clients may not perceive sounds coming from the left side
  - Fail to give a margin on the left side when writing
  - Have difficulty in recognizing faces (Prosopagnosia); voice may help recognition; difficulty in matching known persons' pictures with names; associated more often with posterior right hemisphere damage
  - Fail to recognize stimuli the client constantly dealt with (e.g., a carpenter may not recognize his hammer)
  - Recover from left-sided neglect a few weeks or months post-onset
- Disorientation: May be due to attentional and perceptual defects; the client may:
  - Be seriously disoriented immediately post-onset (acute stage)
  - Be confused about space (topographic disorientation); may get lost in finding one's own room; not understand maps
  - Be confused about geographic location; relatively rare, but some clients may believe that their home or hospital is in some other state or country
  - Experience reduplicative paramnesia, a belief in the existence of multiple and identical places or persons (e.g., a woman may think there are

R

two identical hospitals in town and a man may believe he has two identical wives at home)

- Constructional impairment: Form of visuospatial deficit more often associated with parieto-occipital damage; the client may:
  - Have difficulty constructing block designs
  - Have difficulty reproducing two-dimensional stick figures
  - Be unable to draw or copy geometric designs
  - Ignore components in constructing designs or copying figures
- Affective deficits: Significant problems related to emotional experiences; the client may:
  - Have difficulty in *experiencing* emotions only if the limbic system also is involved
  - More frequently have difficulty in *expressing* emotions
  - Not recognize emotional expressions of other people, including those in pictures and drawings
  - Be unable to state emotions expressed in isolated sentences
  - Have problems in expressing emotions through tone, prosody, facial expressions, and context
- Denial of illness: Clients with right hemisphere syndrome deny problems; the client may:
  - Deny the existence of physical problems (e.g., paralysis of an arm)
  - Be indifferent to problems that are acknowledged or minimize the consequences
- Impaired reasoning, planning, and making correct inferences: Problems with reasoning and logical deductions; the client may:
  - Have difficulty drawing inferences from logical premises or situations
  - Be impaired in reasoning, planning, organizing, and problem-solving skills
  - Have difficulty in planning such activities as shopping or vacationing
  - Find it difficult to organize such activities as parties
  - Be unable to plan a meal
  - Fail to identify absurd statements or may offer justification of absurd statements with bizarre reasons
- Other behavioral deficits: The client may be:
  - Depressed
  - Impulsive and uncharacteristically uninhibited in his or her behavior
  - Distractible
  - Delayed in responding to stimuli

R

Communication Disorders

- Communication deficits associated with right hemisphere syndrome are unlike those found in left brain injury; word-finding problems, commonly associated with left brain injury are not serious, although some clients may have difficulty naming categories (the client may name individual flowers, but not say *flower* to include all of them); paraphasia and circumlocution are not significant problems; right brain injury does not affect grammar to the extent left brain injury does

- Prosodic problems; evidence is conflicting; suggested prosodic impairments include:
  - Monotonous speech, lacking in intonation; may fail to signal meaning suggested by intonational variations (e.g., a rising intonation to suggest a yes/no question)
  - Emotionally flat speech; being aware of it, clients may use specific verbal expressions ("I am upset with you" or "I am sad about that")
  - Hypermelodic speech (high pitch and excessive pitch variability)
  - Impaired stress patterns; instead of changing pitch to stress words, the client may increase intensity (loudness)
  - Reduced speech rate; a slower rate may contribute to the monotonous speech quality
  - Impaired comprehension of prosodic features
- Inappropriate and anomalous speech; client may:
  - Confabulate
  - Be inappropriately humorous (uncharacteristic to the client)
  - Ramble; the speech may not make much sense
- Problems in distinguishing significant from irrelevant information; the client may:
  - Offer irrelevant details when telling a story
  - Offer unimportant details when talking
  - Miss the main point to be expressed
- Problems in comprehending implied and abstract meanings; the client may:
  - Be more concerned with literal meanings of messages than implied meanings
  - Be unable to interpret proverbs, idiomatic expressions, figures of speech, and metaphors
  - Fail to understand the overall meaning of situations, events, stories, or stories told through pictures
  - Fail to give the name of a category (e.g., *vegetables*) while being able to name individual items in the category (e.g., *carrots, cucumbers*)
  - Fail to understand the meaning of ironic, humorous, or sarcastic statements
  - Not detect logical absurdities in statements
- Problems in social communication (pragmatic skills); difficulty in maintaining conversation in social contexts; the client may:
  - Have difficulty recalling isolated and unimportant details of stories
  - Be unable to correctly sequence events in narration
  - Offer irrelevant comments while narrating an event
  - Not maintain eye contact with listeners
  - Fail to maintain topics during conversation
  - Fail to take turns or to yield to others in conversation because of excessive talk
  - Give impulsive responses
  - Fail to clarify statements when the listener does not understand or ask for clarification when a speaker's statements are unclear (conversational repair strategies)
- Auditory comprehension of language; clients may:
  - Have difficulty comprehending language

R

262

- Reading and writing problems; may be primarily due to left neglect and other attentional deficits; clients tend to exhibit:
  o Left neglect dyslexia (reading only the right portion of a printed page)
  o Reading comprehension problems
  o Motor writing problems (e.g., repetition of letters) and spatial agraphia (e.g., poor spacing, crowding of words)
- Dysarthria, a motor speech disorder due to brain injury, may be found in right hemisphere syndrome; dysarthric characteristics may include:
  o Weak production of consonants
  o Characteristics similar to hypokinetic dysarthria

Etiologic Factors and Neuropathology

- Generally, the same etiologic factors affect both the left and right hemispheres, and include:
  o Cerebrovascular accidents (strokes); ischemic and hemorrhagic strokes are the most common conditions that cause right hemisphere syndrome
  o Tumors; right hemisphere brain tumors, though less common than strokes, are also significant causes; tumors tend to produce more focal symptoms
  o Head trauma; also tend to produce more focal symptoms than strokes
  o Various neurological diseases; Alzheimer's disease may affect the right hemisphere, although the clinical picture will be more complex than what is found in straightforward right hemisphere syndrome; symptoms of dementia will be obvious
- Lesions may be located in either the posterior or anterior brain regions
- Posterior right hemisphere lesions are not associated with motor disabilities, requiring a shorter duration of hospitalization
- Anterior (frontal lobe) lesions are associated with motor disabilities, requiring longer periods of hospitalization

Blake, M. L., Duffy, J. R., Myers, P. S., & Tompkins, C. A. (2002). Prevalence and patterns of right hemisphere cognitive/communicative deficits: Retrospective data from an inclient rehabilitation unit. *Aphasiology, 16,* 537–547.

Hegde, M. N. (2006). *A coursebook on aphasia and other neurogenic language disorders* (3rd ed.). Clifton Park, NY: Thomson Delmar Learning.

Myers, P. S. (1999). *Right hemisphere damage.* Clifton Park, NY: Thomson Delmar Learning.

Tompkins, C. A. (1995). *Right hemisphere communication disorders: Theory and management.* Clifton Park, NY: Thomson Delmar Learning.

Rigidity. Stiffness of muscles and joints.

Robin Sequence. A genetic anomaly that includes micrognathia (unusually small mandible), cleft palate, and upper airway obstructions; some describe this sequence as Pierre-Robin syndrome; others consider it a genetic sequence that may be associated with many syndromes, including Stickler Syndrome, Velo-Cardio-Facial Syndrome, and Treacher-Collins Syndrome; see Syndromes Associated With Communication Disorders.

Dorland's Illustrated Medical Dictionary (1994, 28th ed.). Philadelphia, PA: W. B. Saunders.

Jones, K. L. (2005). *Smith's recognizable patterns of human malformations* (6th ed.). Philadelphia, PA: W. B. Saunders.

Jung, J. H. (1989). *Genetic syndromes in communication disorders*. Austin. TX: Pro-Ed.

Kahn, A. (2000). *Craniofacial anomalies*. San Diego, CA: Singular Publishing Group.

Shprintzen, J. R. (2000). *Syndrome identification for speech-language pathology*. San Diego, CA: Singular Publishing Group.

Shprintzen, J. R. (1997). *Genetics, syndromes, and communication disorders*. San Diego, CA: Singular Publishing Group.

Wiedemann, H. R., & Kunze, J. (1997). *Clinical syndromes* (3rd ed.). London: Mosby-Wolfe.

R

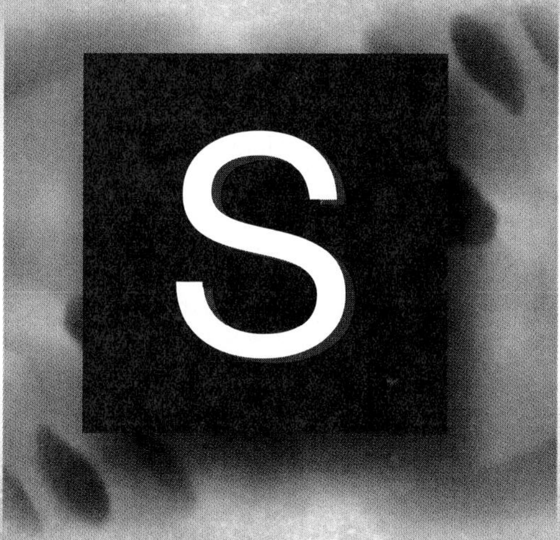
S

Sanfilippo Syndrome. Type of mucopolysaccharidosis syndrome (see Syndromes Associated With Communication Disorders).

Savant Syndrome. Presence of extraordinary skills in a person who has cognitive or behavioral disabilities; often associated with autism; extraordinary arithmetic, musical, or writing skills may coexist with extremely limited oral communication skills, aberrant behaviors, and limited social skills.

Scheie Syndrome. Type of mucopolysaccharidosis syndrome (see Syndromes Associated With Communication Disorders).

Secondary Intracranial Tumors. Metastatic intracranial tumors that had their origins elsewhere in the body, but have migrated to the brain where they attach themselves to brain tissue and begin to grow.

Seizures. Neurological disorder due to abnormal electrical discharges in the brain, causing loss of consciousness and convulsions; associated with epilepsy and other neurological diseases.

Semantic Aphasia. Another name for Wernicke's Aphasia; see Aphasia: Specific Types.

Semantics. The study of meaning in language; a branch of linguistics.

Semantic Paraphasia. Variety of word substitutions found in clients with Aphasia, substitution of a word that is related in meaning to the intended word (e.g., saying *son* for *daughter*).

Semantic Relations. Theoretical and abstract relational meanings attributed to word combinations; categories into which children's early productions may be assigned; usefulness questioned because of the argument that these abstract relations may not be empirical for children; include the following:
- Nomination: This car; that doll
- Agent-Object: Daddy hammer (Daddy is hammering); mommy cook (mommy is cooking)
- Agent-Action: Mommy run (mommy is running)
- Action-Object: Kick ball; hit nail
- Modifier-Head: Big ball; more juice
- X + Dative: Give Bobby (give it to Bobby); kiss mommy
- X + Locative: Ball box (ball is in the box)
- Nonexistence: No truck; no baby
- Recurrence: More juice; more jump
- Notice: See this; hi Kermit
- Instrumental: Cut scissors (cut it with scissors)
- Attribution: Red car; big ball
- Rejection: No milk (I don't want milk)
- Denial: Not hungry; not sleepy

Sensorineural Hearing Loss. Type of hearing loss due to damage to the cochlea or auditory nerve that carries sound impulses to the brain; may be congenital and profound; affects speech and language acquisition if congenital; see Hearing Impairment.

S

Sequential Bilingualism. Acquiring two languages, one after the other; acquisition of a second language after having mostly acquired the primary language.

Sequential Motion Rates (SMRs). A measure of rapidity and sequential correctness with which articulatory movements are executed; impairment in the correct sequenced movements of articulators is a diagnostic sign of Apraxia of Speech; see *Hegde's PocketGuide to Assessment in Speech-Language Pathology* (3rd ed.) for assessment procedures.

Shadowing. Repeating what another person reads orally; a technique that reduces stuttering; the clinician reads orally and asks the client to follow; the client does not see the text and is typically a few words behind in repeating what the clinician reads.

Sickle Cell Disease. An inherited blood disorder that is a risk factor for strokes in children and consequent language problems; the most common single gene blood disorder in African American children; affects one in every 375 African American children; more common in Africa, Arabia, South Asia, and Mediterranean regions; defective gene is located on chromosome 11; the gene involved controls a protein in red blood cells called *hemoglobin,* which binds oxygen in the lungs and carries it to peripheral tissue; the cells get hardened as they get distorted into sickle shapes; sickle-shaped cells then block the flow of blood in the arteries; symptoms include muscle pain; liver, kidney, and spleen damage; hearing loss and potential language difficulties; possibly causing strokes resulting in aphasia in children.

Silent Period. Time of silent observation during which children listen to a second language, but produce little of it; thought to be a stage in bilingualism.

Simultaneous Bilingualism. Acquisition of two language at the same time; a characteristic noted in children whose parents each speak a different language; being simultaneously exposed to two languages, the child may learn both at the same time.

Sly Syndrome. Type of mucopolysaccharidosis syndrome (see Syndromes Associated With Communication Disorders).

Spasmodic Dysphonia. Hyperfunctional voice disorder, classified as a form of dystonia of the larynx; may be classified into adductor and abductor spastic dysphonia, although some experts believe that the abductor type is not a form of spasmodic dysphonia because its symptoms are very different (see Abductor Spasms); the adductor type is more common and the abductor type is controversial because some consider it a separate disorder; characterized in most individuals by severe overadduction of the vocal folds and strained or choked-off voice quality; phonation may be impossible; in other individuals, characterized by sudden abduction of the folds and resulting aphonia; earlier, thought to be psychogenic; currently, most experts favor a neurological explanation although this, too, is debated; possibly of heterogeneous etiology because any evidence of neurological involvement may be present or absent across clients; affects mostly adults; typical onset in the late 30s; slightly more common in females (about 59%

S

of the cases) than males; diagnosis assisted by neurological examination though it may not offer definitive evidence; see Voice Disorders.

Etiologic Factors of Spasmodic Dysphonia

- Early theories suggested psychological variables, including conversion reaction as the cause; unconscious and socially unacceptable urges may be transformed into a voice disorder (meaning of a *conversion reaction*, a Freudian explanation of neurosis)
- Current thinking on etiology favors a neurological basis for the disorder although some psychological variables may play a role; neurological factors are not convincingly demonstrated, and may be completely absent in some individuals; neurological abnormalities found in some clients include:
  o Evidence of brain lesions on MRI; the lesions, found in a small number of individuals, are likely to be in the left frontal or temporal lobes or the white matter under these lobes; the medial prefrontal to frontal cortex and the right posterior temporal/posterior cortex are other possible sites of lesions
  o Metabolic or electrophysiological abnormalities
  o Abnormal brainstem auditory-evoked responses
  o Abnormal brain hypoperfusion
  o Possibility of the vagus nerve abnormalities
- The influence of psychological variables in maintaining the disorder is suggested because:
  o The vocal symptoms are inconsistent
  o The presence or absence of symptoms may be partly associated with certain emotional states of the speaker
  o The symptoms may be absent when the person is laughing and singing; the symptoms may dissipate when the speaker says "ee" in a high-pitched voice or exerts effort in speaking

Voice Problems of Spasmodic Dysphonia

- The problems associated with the adductor variety include:
  o A severely hyperfunctional voice with strained and strangled voice quality; voice may sound like the person is being choked
  o Tight closure of the vocal folds and even the false folds, observed through endoscopic examination; the lower pharyngeal airway closure also may be observed; the person may fight this tight closure and try to squeeze voice out of the tightly shut vocal folds
  o Vocal folds adduction with excessive force and effort
- The problems associated with the abductor variety, which is observed much less frequently than the adductor variety (and may even be a different kind of disorder), include:
  o Inappropriate opening of the vocal folds when they should be approximating to produce voice; opposite of what is found in the adductor type
  o Intermittently breathy voice because of poor adduction; aphonia (absence of voice); sudden abductions triggered by unvoiced consonants

Boone, D. R., McFarlane, S. C., & Von Berg, S. L. (2005). *The voice and voice therapy* (7th ed.). Boston, MA: Allyn and Bacon.

Case, J. L. (2002). *Clinical management of voice disorders* (4th ed.). Austin, TX: Pro-Ed.

Spastic Dysarthria. Motor speech disorder characterized by muscle rigidity; bilateral damage to pyramidal and extrapyramidal systems produce this type of dysarthria; see Dysarthria: Specific Types.

Spasticity. Neuromuscular impairment characterized by increased tone or rigidity of muscles; damage to the extrapyramidal system (also called *indirect activation system* or *indirect motor system*) causes muscle stiffness; stiff and spastic muscles resist movement; hyperactive reflexes (hyperflexia) also are effects of lesions in the extrapyramidal system; associated with Spastic Dysarthria.

Specific Language Impairment (SLI). Language disorders in children who are otherwise normal, although some children may have subtle cognitive deficits; the term suggests that the children have an impairment that is specific to language; the basic features of SLI include:

- SLI is typically diagnosed after age 4 to avoid diagnosing language disorders in late talkers, although many early signs of language impairment will be evident before age 4
- SLI is present in 7% to 8% of preschool and school-age children
- Many children who are in regular classrooms but receive language treatment have this kind of language disorder
- SLI may affect different language skills somewhat differentially
- Generally, pragmatic language skills may be better than syntactic and morphological skills; dominant language deficiency is omission or misuse of grammatical morphemes
- SLI is a diagnosis made on negative grounds (such other factors as intellectual disabilities or neurological deficits do not explain the disorder)
- Some experts believe that SLI suggests limited language skills with no pathology
- Others believe that SLI is not truly specific to language and that there are important, though subtle, cognitive deficits
- See Language Disorders in Children for details

Hegde, M. N., & Maul, C. A. (2006). *Language disorders in children: An evidence-based approach to assessment and treatment.* Boston, MA: Allyn and Bacon.

Leonard, L. B. (1998). *Children with specific language impairment.* Cambridge, MA: MIT Press.

Spinal Muscle Atrophy. Also called *progressive muscle atrophy*; a group of muscle disorders that results in progressive limb wasting and weakness; cranial nerve weakness may or may not be present; may be inherited or may occur sporadically; associated with Flaccid Dysarthria and Dysphagia.

Spondylitis. Inflammation of one or more of the vertebrae; associated with several genetic syndromes; see Syndromes Associated With Communication Disorders.

Stem Cells. Precursor cells that differentiate themselves into virtually any kind of body cells; fetal or embryonic stem cell implantation into the brain is potential future treatment of some neurodegenerative diseases, including Huntington's disease and Parkinson's disease.

Stickler Syndrome. See Syndromes Associated With Communication Disorders.

Stopping. A phonological process found in children who are learning language normally or in children who have an articulation (phonologic) disorder; a disorder if it persists beyond the normal age range; characterized by substitutions of stop consonants for fricatives and affricates.

Strabismus. Visual disorder in which the two eyes do not focus together; one eye deviates from the other either inwardly (convergent strabismus) or outwardly (divergent strabismus).

Stridency. Voice disorder characterized by an unpleasant, shrill, and metallic-sounding voice; caused by excessive pharyngeal constriction and an elevated larynx.

Strident. Consonants that are produced by forcing the airstream through a small opening, causing intense noise; English /f/, /v/, /s/, /z/, /ʃ/, /ʒ/, /tʃ/, and /dʒ/ are stridents.

Strokes. Same as cerebrovascular accidents or "brain attacks"; common causes of aphasia; may be ischemic or hemorrhagic; syndromes with an acute onset, causing focal brain damage and Aphasia.

Stupor. State of unresponsiveness; the client may be aroused briefly by strong stimuli, including pain; a neurological disorder; may be a symptom in the acute stage of Traumatic Brain Injury.

Stuttering. Disorder of fluency, with an onset in early childhood years; see Fluency Disorders.

Subacute Stage. Period following the acute stage of an illness; recovery from some of the initial and perhaps serious problems.

Subcortical Aphasia. Several atypical forms of aphasia that are due to damage to the left subcortical regions; see Aphasia: Specific Types.

Subdural Hematoma. Accumulation of blood between the dura (tough outer covering of the central nervous system) and arachnoid (the middle of the three membranes covering the central nervous system).

Substitution Processes. Phonological process in which one sound is substituted for multiple sounds or for sounds in an entire class; see Phonological Processes.

Suffix. Grammatical morpheme added at the end of a word (e.g., *ing* added to a verb, the regular plural *s* added to a noun, the regular past tense inflection added to a verb); often missing in the language production of children with language disorders and hearing impairment.

Suprasegmentals. Prosodic features of language that include stress, intonation, timing, duration of syllables, pausing, and so forth that give speech a certain rhythm; impaired in neurological disorders; see Dysarthria.

Supratentorial Level. Anatomical division of the brain that includes the externally visible frontal, temporal, and occipital lobes along with the basal ganglia, thalamus, hypothalamus, and olfactory (I) and optic (II) cranial nerves.

Swallowing Disorders. See Dysphagia.

Sydenham's Chorea. Neurological disease characterized by jerky, involuntary, and purposeless movements of body parts; affects children in the age range of 5 to 15 years; may follow such infectious diseases as strep throat, rheumatic fever, or scarlet fever; associated with Hyperkinetic Dysarthria in children, although the condition clears up in about 4 months.

Synchondroses. The union of two bones by cartridge; a characteristic of some genetic syndromes.

Syndactyly. Fusion of fingers or toes; a genetic defect; found in such syndromes as Apert syndrome and Oro-Facial-Digital syndrome (see Syndromes Associated With Communication Disorders).

Syndrome. Constellation of signs and symptoms that are associated with a morbid process.

Syndromes Associated With Communication Disorders. Various genetic or congenital syndromes that affect the normal acquisition of speech and language; most syndromes also affect physical and general behavioral development as well; varied etiology as specified under each syndrome, although some form of genetic abnormalities often underlie them; the following are among the more frequently described syndromes associated with communication disorders; most syndromes have multiple symptoms, communicative disorders being a part of the total symptom complex; description of communicative disorders associated with many syndromes are at best sketchy; detailed patterns of speech and language are often not described; some of the major syndromes are described in alphabetical order.

Aicardi Syndrome. Genetic syndrome with craniofacial anomalies including cleft lip and palate, central nervous system disorders; severely affected infants may not survive.

Etiology
- X-linked dominant pattern of inheritance; abnormalities on Xp22
- Most severe in male children

Physical and Behavioral Symptoms
- Brain and corpus callosum abnormalities
- Cleft lip and palate
- Abnormalities of the choroid coating of the eye and retina (chorioretinal lacunae) is an ocular feature
- Rib anomalies and other skeletal abnormalities
- Intellectual disabilities and the associated behavioral deficits

Speech, Language, and Hearing
- Possibility of conductive hearing loss due to middle ear infections associated with cleft palate; no significant hearing loss in most children

S

- Minimal or negligible speech and language skills, depending on the degree of intellectual disabilities
- Speech disorders comparable to those found in children with Cleft Palate

Alport Syndrome. Genetic syndrome that affects kidney functions and causes hearing loss and speech and language problems; also known as *hereditary nephritis*; more severe in males than females with a more rapidly progressing course.

Etiology
- Thought to have an autosomal dominant inheritance
- May be due to X-linked inheritance in some cases
- Suspected gene mutation
- It is estimated that 1 in 50,000 Americans carry the gene, although not always expressed

Physical Symptoms
- Nephritis (kidney disease) beginning in early childhood
- Kidney failure in some cases, requiring kidney transplant
- Ocular abnormalities (cataract and myopia)

Speech, Language, and Hearing
- Articulation disorders; progressive deterioration in articulatory skills, especially in males
- Bilateral, sensorineural, and progressive hearing loss, starting around age 10; more common in males than females

Angelman Syndrome. Genetic syndrome that affects more males than females; characterized by intellectual disabilities, unique facial features, and muscular disorders; genetically similar to Prader-Willi syndrome; common craniofacial and central nervous system abnormalities.

Etiology
- Deletion of DNA material on the long arm of chromosome 15 (15q11–q13), inherited from the mother; the same deletion of paternal origin causes Prader-Willi syndrome

Physical and Behavioral Symptoms
- Feeding disorders during infancy; failure to suck
- Open-mouth posture with a protruded tongue
- Cranial abnormalities, including microcephaly, brachycephaly (*brachy* means short), and large mouth and chin
- Neurological disorders including seizures, progressive ataxia, hyperactive reflexes, and hypotonia during infancy
- Behavioral deviations including uncontrolled outbursts of laughter, arm flapping, and severe intellectual disabilities with limited attention and social interaction
- Possible impaired sleep patterns

Speech, Language, and Hearing
- Severely impaired speech and language development; sometimes described as *no speech development*

- Severely limited speech and language comprehension
- No significant hearing loss
- Voice limited to random and limited vocalizations

Apert Syndrome. Genetic syndrome whose dysmorphology includes cranial Synostosis, Syndactyly of hands and feet, midfacial Hypoplasia, Strabismus, hearing loss, and speech problems; affects growth, nervous system, and craniofacial structures; also known as *acrocephalosyndactyly*.

Etiology

- Possibly, spontaneous autosomal dominant mutations; abnormalities on the long arm of chromosome 10
- Limited parent-to-child transmission because of low reproductive capacity

Physical and Behavioral Symptoms

- Syndactyly (fusing of fingers, toes, or both), typically of the second, third, and fourth digits
- Cranial synostosis resulting in smaller anterior-posterior skull diameter, flat frontal and occipital bones, and high forehead
- Increased intracranial pressure, causing compensatory growth in cranial structures
- Midfacial hypoplasia (incomplete development) with a small nose
- Forward carriage of the tongue in the mouth
- Arched and grooved hard palate
- Class III malocclusion, irregularly placed teeth, thickened alveolar process, long or thickened soft palate, and cleft of the hard palate (in 25% to 30% of cases)
- Low-set and posteriorly rotated ears
- Hydrocephalus and increased intracranial pressure
- Intellectual disabilities and attending behavioral deficits

Speech, Language, and Hearing

- Feeding disorders
- Tendency toward hyponasality, possibly because of the small nasal pharynx; both hyponasality and hypernasality associated with cleft palate
- Articulation disorders; mostly alveolar or anteriorly produced consonants (e.g., /s/ and /z/) and labial dental sounds (e.g., /f/ and /v/); hypoplastic maxilla minimizing tongue movement necessary for speech production
- Various levels of language deficiency, depending on intellectual and hearing levels; no significant oral communication skills in the most severely affected
- High incidence of conductive hearing loss associated with chronic middle ear infections and diseases

Asperger's Syndrome (Disorder). Also described as an autism spectrum disorder or a pervasive development disorder; see Asperger's Disorder under Autism Spectrum Disorders for details.

Ataxia-telangiectasia Syndrome. Neurodegenerative, autosomal recessive syndrome that results in death in the early 20s, although some survive into their early 40s; also known as *Louis-Bar syndrome*; prevalence is about

1 per 10,000 children, with no family history in many cases; degeneration begins after a period of normal development of the child.

Etiology
- Autosomal recessive inheritance
- Abnormality on chromosome 11 (11q22.3)

Physical and Behavioral Symptoms
- A thin, drawn, mask-like, and expressionless face
- Progressive cerebellar ataxia, beginning in early childhood and followed by dystonia
- Telangiectasia (dilation of small blood vessels), causing focal red lesions on the skin or on mucous membranes; may begin after the onset of ataxia
- Deficient immune system
- Frequent infections of the upper and lower respiratory systems, a cause of mortality
- Leukemia and Hodgkin's and non-Hodgkin's lymphoma, a cause of mortality
- Feeding disorders after the onset of ataxia; may be limited to disorders of mastication, drooling, and impaired oral-motor control

Speech, Language, and Hearing
- No significant hearing loss
- Normal acquisition of language
- No evidence of intellectual disabilities during infancy and early childhood years
- Expressive language development arrested by age 3; normal comprehension
- Combination of cerebellar ataxia and dystonia, causing dysarthria; increasingly unintelligible speech
- Significant voice disorders, comparable to those found in some forms of dysarthria; progressively worsening, tremulous, and weak voice
- Hypernasality

Beckwith-Wiedemann Syndrome. Includes multiple anomalies; most common syndrome characterized by overgrowth (hence, also called *gigantism syndrome*); prevalence is about 1 in 13,000 live births; speech and language impairments; craniofacial, gastrointestinal/abdominal, and central nervous system abnormalities.

Etiology
- Autosomal dominant inheritance
- A gene defect on chromosome 11 (11p15)

Physical and Behavioral Symptoms
- Hypotonia, possibly due to hypoglycemia during infancy
- Improved development with effective treatment for hypoglycemia
- Overgrowth of the body, causing childhood gigantism which plateaus; overgrowth of the genitalia; slower growth after puberty; possibly no adult gigantism
- Large mouth, mandible (mandibular prognathism), and tongue; cleft palate or submucous cleft

- Umbilical hernia and enlarged liver
- Seizures and hydrocephalus (infrequent)
- Wilms' tumor (rapidly developing malignant tumors of the kidneys)

Speech, Language, and Hearing

- Early feeding difficulties due to the large tongue (macroglossia) and hypotonia
- Chronic middle ear infections, leading to conductive hearing loss; more frequent with cleft palate
- Delayed speech onset and articulation disorders, possibly because of the macroglossia; distortions of speech sounds; production of the lingua-alveolar sounds at the mandibular arch and fronting errors because of the large tongue; compensatory articulation associated with clefts
- Normal intelligence in many, and mild disabilities in some, causing delayed language development and language disorders
- Hoarse voice; hypernasality associated with hypotonia and cleft palate; hyponasality associated with hypertrophic tonsils and adenoids

Binder Syndrome.   Genetic syndrome characterized by midfacial retrusion (backward positioning or movement of the mandible); also known as *maxillonasal* Dysplasia.

Etiology

- Possible multifactorial inheritance and autosomal dominant inheritance

Physical and Behavioral Symptoms

- Flat facial profile, a result of maxillonasal dysplasia (midface deficiency; no growth in the maxilla from the childhood years on)
- Mandibular Prognathism
- Normal mandibular growth, short nose, and short anterior cranial base
- Impaired chewing, but uncommon feeding disorders

Speech, Language, and Hearing

- Distortion of anteriorly produced speech sounds; lingua-alveolar and lingua-dental sounds most affected
- Compensatory bilabial sound production (contact between the upper teeth and lower lip)
- No significant language disorders
- Hyponasal speech
- Hearing loss or voice problems are not typical

Bronchio-Oto-Renal Syndrome.   Genetic syndrome characterized by malformations of the auricle, bronchial fistulas or cysts, and abnormalities of the kidneys; also known as *Melnick-Fraser syndrome*; a relatively common syndrome of multiple anomalies associated with hearing loss and speech-language problems.

Etiology

- Autosomal dominant inheritance
- Abnormalities on the long arm of chromosome 8 (8q13.3)
- Varied expression

Physical Symptoms
- Pulmonary abnormalities, including bronchial fistulas or cysts
- Renal abnormalities, including Hypoplasia of kidneys, anomalies of the collecting system, or both
- Outer ear anomalies, including preauricular pits
- Narrow or malformed external auditory canal, displaced or malformed auditory ossicles, fused or unconnected stapes, and hypoplastic apex of the cochlea
- Cleft palate (submucous variety)
- Varieties of malocclusion

Speech, Language, and Hearing
- Conductive, sensorineural, or mixed hearing loss
- Articulation disorders, mainly distortions and substitutions, typically associated with hearing loss, cleft palate (when present), and severe forms of malocclusions of the dental arches
- Possible language delay depending on the age of onset of hearing loss and its severity
- Resonance disorders associated with hearing loss and submucous cleft palate

Cat Eye Syndrome. Genetic syndrome so named because of the iris coloboma (any defect of the eye or iris); also known as *chromosome 22 partial tetrasomy* and *Schmid-Fraccaro syndrome.*

Etiology
- Genetic abnormality, consisting of extra chromosome material on chromosome 22 (q11)

Physical and Behavioral Symptoms
- Iris coloboma, the most distinguishing feature
- Small protuberant ears with preauricular tags or pits
- Cardiac abnormalities
- Kidney malformations, including hypoplastic or aplastic

Speech, Language, and Hearing
- Feeding disorders as a consequence of hypotonia
- Delayed speech development; compensatory articulation due to cleft palate, found in a quarter of the children
- Mild conductive hearing loss due to middle ear infection associated with cleft palate and ear anomalies
- Mild to severe language disorders, depending on the intellectual status of the child
- Hypernasality, associated with cleft palate; voice may be normal

CHARGE Association. Syndrome of multiple anomalies, CHARGE is an acronym for **C**oloboma, **H**eart anomalies, **A**tresia choanae, **R**etarded growth, **G**enital hypoplasia, and **E**ar anomalies; called an *association* instead of a syndrome mainly because of lack of etiologic specificity; features of this association may be found in Velo-Cardio-Facial syndrome and Wolf–Hirschhorn syndrome; no consistent pattern across individuals.

S

Etiology
- May be sporadic although autosomal dominant inheritance
- Varied genetic factors because of association with other syndromes

Physical and Behavioral Symptoms
- Feeding disorders that need to be treated for the child to thrive
- Choanal atresia (an abnormal opening of the nasal cavity into the nasopharynx on either side), a possible cause of feeding disorders
- Congenital heart anomalies
- Brain malformations and consequent behavioral and intellectual dysfunctions
- Craniofacial anomalies, including facial paresis; microcephaly; low-set, posteriorly rotated ears; protuberant eyes; cleft palate; cleft lip; and micrognathia
- Ocular abnormalities, including the iris, choroid, retina, and optic nerve coloboma
- Retarded physical growth, resulting in a short stature
- Underdevelopment of genitals
- Intellectual impairment

Speech, Language, and Hearing
- Feeding disorders complicated by craniofacial anomalies
- Articulation disorders due to the hearing loss and craniofacial anomalies
- Delayed language and language disorders; perhaps no significant language
- Hoarse voice and breathiness, possibly due to unilateral vocal fold paralysis
- Hearing impairment (conductive, sensorineural, and mixed types)

Cornelia de Lange Syndrome. Syndrome characterized by microcephaly, intellectual disabilities, and severe speech and language problems; also known as *de Lange syndrome* and *Brachman-de Lange syndrome*; skeletal and facial anomalies; males and females equally affected.

Etiology
- Thought to be due to heterogeneous factors; possibility of abnormalities on chromosome 3; autosomal dominant inheritance
- May be sporadic

Physical and Behavioral Symptoms
- Retarded physical growth
- Brachycephaly (shortness of the head); low-set ears and bushy eyebrows that meet at the midline; small nose, upward-tilted nares; down-turned upper lip
- Coarse, shaggy, and excessive hair growth low on the forehead and neck; webbed neck
- Flat hands with short, tapering fingers
- Severe intellectual disabilities and associated behavioral and cognitive deficits

Speech, Language, and Hearing
- Sensorineural hearing loss
- Severe articulation disorders

S

- Severe language disorders typically associated with intellectual disabilities
- Hoarse voice

Cri du Chat Syndrome. Autosomal chromosome disorder associated with intellectual disabilities and speech-language problems; the earliest and distinctive feature is the infant's cry resembling that of a cat, hence the name; the characteristic cry is not heard in all children with this syndrome; associated with cleft palate and speech, language, and hearing problems.

Etiology
- Absence of a part of the fifth chromosome's short arm (5p15.2)
- The short arm of chromosome 5 may be deleted

Physical and Behavioral Symptoms
- Failure to thrive, because of feeding difficulties associated with cleft palate
- Severe neurological and neuromuscular disorders, including hypotonia, during infancy; subsequently, hypertonia and hyperreflexia
- Low-set, posteriorly rotated ears, microcephaly, cerebral asymmetry, retrognathia, narrow oral cavity, laryngeal hypoplasia, cleft palate, and cleft lip
- Small hands and feet
- Intellectual disabilities

Speech, Language, and Hearing
- A high-pitched cry persisting throughout early childhood years
- Absence of significant speech or severe articulation disorders; compounded by cleft palate and cleft lip
- Severely affected language development; may be absent in cases of severe intellectual disabilities
- Absence of normal voice and resonance features

Crouzon Syndrome. Syndrome characterized by cranial and midface abnormalities, ocular hypertelorism, strabismus, hearing loss, and speech and language problems; also known as *craniofacial dysostosis* (defective cranial bone formation).

Etiology
- Autosomal dominant pattern of inheritance with varied expression
- Abnormality of a gene (FGFR2, fibroblast growth factor receptor 2) located on the long arm of chromosome 10

Physical and Behavioral Symptoms
- Craniofacial abnormalities due to craniosynostosis (fusion of the cranial suture, especially that of the coronal sutures)
- Hypoplasia of the midface, maxilla, or both; small maxillary structure (maxillary hypoplasia), facial asymmetry, malocclusion Class II, highly arched palate, shallow oropharynx, long and thick soft palate, short front-to-back cranial diameter (Brachycephaly), "parrot-like" nose
- Increased intracranial pressure, causing headaches and ataxia; hydrocephalus
- Ocular hypertelorsim (two eyes that are far apart) and bulging eyes

- Cognitive or intellectual disabilities, possibly due to the untreated cranial abnormalities and increased intracranial pressure

Speech, Language, and Hearing

- Conductive hearing loss in one-third to one-half of individuals, possibly due to abnormalities of the ear and chronic middle ear infections
- Articulation disorders associated with hearing loss and abnormalities of palatal and oral cavity structures
- Hyponasality
- Language disorders depending on the degree of hearing loss and cognitive deficits

Down Syndrome. Syndrome resulting from one of the most common chromosomal abnormalities; occurs in 1 per 1,000 births, one of the most frequently occurring genetic syndromes; associated with varying degrees of intellectual disabilities; severity of speech and language disorders depends on the degree of intellectual disabilities and severity of hearing loss.

Etiology

- Extra whole number chromosome 21, resulting in 47, rather than the normal 46, chromosomes; a segment of chromosome 21, 21q22.3 is the most abnormal part
- Increased risk with advanced maternal age
- Predisposition to <u>Alzheimer's Disease</u>

Physical and Behavioral Symptoms

- Brachycephaly and microcephaly; maxillary hypoplasia, midface dysplasia, flat facial profile, small ears, small nose, small chin, malocclusion, and <u>Epicanthal folds</u>
- Shortened oral and pharyngeal structures, narrow and high arched palate, relatively large and fissured tongue that tends to protrude, and dental anomalies
- Hyperflexible joints
- Cardiac malformations in about 40% of cases
- Neurological characteristics include a generalized hypotonia, cerebellar and cerebral hypoplasia, and a tendency to develop Alzheimer's disease
- Short neck with excess skin on back of it, obesity, small statue, short fingers and toes (brachydactyly), and permanently deflected fingers (clinodactyly)
- Early feeding difficulties, due mostly to hypotonia
- Intellectual disabilities; varying degree of limitation
- Cleft palate

S

Speech, Language, and Hearing

- Chronic middle ear infections and conductive hearing loss more common than sensorineural or mixed loss
- Articulation disorders; numerous distortions, a general slurring of speech, and an increased speech rate; the severity is affected by the degree of intellectual disability, oral and facial structural anomalies, and hearing loss

- Delayed language and language disorders; generally sociable, but below-normal language skills; relatively better vocabulary compared to highly deficient syntactic and morphological skills; concrete and telegraphic speech
- Fluency disorders, especially stuttering
- Impaired speech prosody and rhythm due to short phrases and sentences
- Hypernasality, nasal emission, hoarseness, breathier voice, and lower pitch

Dysautonomia. Also known as *Riley-Day syndrome*, limited to Ashkenazi Jews from Eastern Europe, in whom the incidence is between 1 and 3 in 10,000 births; characterized by an impaired autonomic nervous system.

Etiology

- Autosomal recessive inheritance
- Gene defect on chromosome 9 (9q31–q33)

Physical and Behavioral Symptoms

- Feeding problems and associated aspiration and vomiting; aspiration pneumonia
- Neurological problems, including hypotonia, hypothermia (low body temperature), syncopy (fainting episodes), absence of reflexes, ataxia, and low blood pressure

Speech, Language, and Hearing

- Onset of speech disorders, paralleling the onset of neurological symptoms; dysarthria and hypernasality; monotonous voice
- Language development normal until the onset of neurological problems
- No significant prevalence of hearing loss

Ectrodactyly-Ectodermal Dysplasia-Clefting Syndrome (EEC Syndrome). Syndrome of multiple anomalies that affects the development of ectodermal and mesodermal tissue; associated with clefts of the lip and palate; infrequent association of intellectual disabilities.

Etiology

- Autosomal dominant inheritance with variable and sometimes incomplete expression
- Abnormalities on chromosome 7 (7q11.2–q21.3)

Physical Symptoms

- Congenital absence of fingers and toes (Ectrodactyly)
- Ectodermal Dysplasia (sparse and brittle hair and scanty eyebrows, absence of lashes, and dystrophied nails)
- Cleft lip and palate, more common than cleft lip alone; cleft hands and feet
- Microcephaly, maxillary hypoplasia, choanal atresia, missing or malformed teeth
- Absent sweat glands that predispose the individual to heat strokes—a unique feature
- Intellectual disabilities, although not a common feature

Speech, Language, and Hearing

- Feeding problems associated with cleft palate

- Mild to moderate conductive hearing loss due to frequent middle ear infections
- Articulation disorders, characterized by distortions and lingual protrusions and related to oral structural anomalies and hearing loss; compensatory articulatory strategies associated with cleft palate
- Hoarseness of voice and hypernasality
- Delayed language acquisition; severity of language disorders related to the degree of hearing loss and intellectual disabilities

Fetal Alcohol Syndrome (FAS). Congenital syndrome (not genetically inherited) in which the prenatal and postnatal growth is affected due to the toxic effects maternal alcoholism during pregnancy had on the embryo; associated with physical abnormalities, intellectual disabilities, and speech and language problems.

Etiology

- Maternal alcoholism; embryonic exposure to a minimum of 1 or 2 ounces of absolute alcohol per day; more severe effects with more than two ounces a day
- Significant variables include the rate at which alcohol is metabolized (before it affects the embryo) in the mother's body, frequency and duration of drinking, and the embryonic stage at which the abuse is intensive

Physical and Behavioral Symptoms

- Low birth weight due to the negative effects of alcohol on the embryonic and fetal growth
- Feeding disorders, mainly due to hypotonia and micrognathia
- Craniofacial anomalies include Microcephaly, Maxillary Hypoplasia, posterior rotation of the ears, prominent forehead and mandible, short palpebral (eyelid) fissures, thin upper lip, Hypoplastic Philtrum, Epicanthal Folds, small eyes (Microphthalmia), small teeth with faulty enamel, and cleft palate, cleft lip, or both
- Severe growth retardation, which begins as disrupted embryonic and fetal growth
- Heart anomalies; kidney disorders, mainly due to anomalous kidney structures
- Nail growth problems and small hands and feet
- Intellectual and learning disabilities

Speech, Language, and Hearing

- Hearing loss not characteristic; conductive hearing loss in case of middle ear infections or external and middle ear anomalies
- Delayed speech acquisition and disorders of articulation; consistent with the extent of intellectual disabilities
- Aggravated speech and resonance problems associated with clefts; potential compensatory articulation
- Language disorders including deficits in syntactic, semantic, and pragmatic aspects of language, especially associated with intellectual disabilities; learning disabilities

S

- Limited fluency, partly because of limited language skills
- Voice problems, including hoarseness; may be due to persistent crying in early childhood
- Hypernasality associated with cleft palate

Fragile X Syndrome. X-linked genetic syndrome caused by a chromosomal abnormality; also known as *X-linked mental retardation* and *Martin-Bell syndrome*; so named because of a tendency for the affected chromosome to break easily, although that fragility may not be the causes of it; associated with more severe intellectual disabilities in males than females; thought to be one of the most common genetic syndromes with an estimated incidence of 1 in 3,000 or 4,000 children; in males alone, the incidence is 1 in 2,000 children.

Etiology
- X-linked inheritance of intellectual disabilities
- Abnormality on Xq27.3 (the so-called fragile site on the long arm of the X chromosome)

Physical and Behavioral Symptoms
- Large, long, and poorly formed pinna; a big jaw, high forehead, mandibular prognathism, thick lips, macrocephaly, dental abnormalities, and submucous cleft
- Intellectual disabilities

Speech, Language, and Hearing
- Hearing loss not a characteristic
- Language characterized by jargon, perseveration, echolalia, telegraphic utterances, inappropriate and irrelevant language, and self-talking in a low monotonous voice; may be more pronounced in males than in females; limited functional oral skills; similar to language of autism
- Lack of nonverbal communication that normally accompany speech
- Occasional hoarseness or a high-pitched voice
- Articulation disorders, especially in affected males, possibly due to the craniofacial anomalies; features of Cluttering; compensatory articulation may be associated with cleft palate; apraxia of speech and dysarthria.

Goldenhar Syndrome. Genetic syndrome characterized by oculo-auriculo-vertebral dysplasia; rarely associated with intellectual disabilities; also called *Facio-Auriculo-Vertebral syndrome, First and Second Bronchial Arch syndrome,* and *hemifacial microsomia*; a frequently occurring genetic anomaly in humans, affecting 1 in 5,000 children.

Etiology
- Etiologically heterogeneous, not technically a genetic syndrome; sporadic occurrence with no family history
- With an affected parent, suspected autosomal dominant inheritance; oculo-auriculo-vertebral anomalies found in other syndromes, including Treacher Collins Syndrome.

Physical and Behavioral Symptoms
- Craniofacial anomalies include Hemifacial Microsomia, mostly due to an underdeveloped mandible; hypoplastic or dysfunctional facial, masticatory,

and palatal muscles; cleft-like lateral extension of the mouth; high arched palate, cleft palate, cleft lip, and unilateral hypoplasia of the pharynx or palate; Microtia and Preauricular Tags
- Feeding disorders, possibly due to hypoplasia of the pharynx
- Cervical spine anomalies, spina bifida, club foot, and other limb anomalies
- Unilateral vocal cord paresis
- Ocular abnormalities, including clefts of the eyelids or orbits, microphthalmia, strabismus, and clefts of the eyelids or orbits
- Congenital heart and kidney diseases
- Cognitive impairments and resulting behavioral deficiencies

Speech, Language, and Hearing
- Hearing loss a significant feature; more common conductive hearing loss than sensorineural loss; typically unilateral loss due to middle and external ear malformations
- Delayed speech onset and disorders of articulation; distortions and substitutions possibly related to craniofacial abnormalities
- Resonance problems, including hypernasality
- Hoarse or breathy voice, partly due to the unilateral vocal fold paresis
- Delay in language acquisition in case of intellectual disabilities

Laurence-Moon Syndrome.   Genetic syndrome characterized by retinitis pigmentosa, hypogonadism, obesity, and intellectual disabilities; previously also known as *Laurence-Moon-Biedl syndrome, Bardet-Biedl syndrome*, and *Laurence-Moon-Bardet-Biedl syndrome*; four subtypes, each considered separate from Laurence-Moon syndrome; polydactyl, a feature of Bardet-Biedl syndromes, is absent in Laurence-Moon syndrome; the latter is associated with spastic paraplegia, which is absent in the former four types.

Etiology
- Suspected autosomal recessive inheritance
- No specific gene abnormality detected yet

Physical and Behavioral Symptoms
- Spastic paraplegia and hypotonia
- Retinitis pigmentosa and initial difficulty in night vision
- Retarded sexual development (hypogonadism)
- Obesity, due to endocrine disorders
- Intellectual disabilities and associated behavioral limitations
- Motor control problems due to neurological impairment

Speech, Language, and Hearing
- Infrequent sensorineural hearing loss
- Delayed onset of speech and articulation disorders associated with hypotonia and intellectual disabilities
- Delayed language and language disorders typically associated with intellectual deficits
- Infrequent hypernasality and breathy voice

Moebius Syndrome.   Also spelled *Möbius*, genetic syndrome characterized by congenital bilateral facial palsy; mild intellectual disabilities in 10% to 15%

of the affected individuals, occasional hearing loss, articulation disorders, and some language problems; a rare genetic disorder.

Etiology

* Heterogeneous causation; no specific gene abnormality identified
* Neuropathology includes Agenesis or Aplasia of the motor nuclei of the cranial nerves; underdeveloped cranial nerves VI (abducens, controlling eye movement) and VII (facial); potential involvement of cranial nerve V (trigeminal, eye, and jaw) and cranial nerve XII (hypoglossal, controlling tongue movement)
* Sporadic occurrence of the syndrome; may be due to autosomal dominant inheritance in some cases

Physical and Behavioral Symptoms

* Paralysis of the facial and eye muscles and tongue weakness
* Feeding problems during infancy; inability to keep the head tilted back to swallow; aspiration and chocking; drooling
* Bilabial paresis and weak tongue control for lateralization, elevation, depression, and protrusion; short or deformed tongue
* Ocular problems, including unilateral or bilateral paralysis of the abductors of the eye; eyelids that may not fully close; lack of blinking and lateral eye movements; strabismus that may be surgically corrected; eye sensitivity to light (due to lack of blinking)
* Greater involvement of the upper portion of the face than the lower; diminished strength, range, and speed of articulatory movements
* Mask-like face with diminished emotions and expressions
* Delayed or absent motor skills, mainly due to the upper body weakness
* High palate, submucous cleft, and abnormal dentition
* Intellectual disabilities in up to 15% of cases

Speech, Language, and Hearing

* Infrequent conductive hearing loss due to fluids in the ears
* Mild to severe Dysarthria; bilabial, linguadental, and lingua alveolar sounds more severely affected than sounds of other classes
* Delayed language and language disorders, especially in children with frequent hospitalization and intellectual disabilities

Mohr Syndrome. Genetic syndrome characterized by cranial, facial, lingual, palatal, and digital anomalies; a subtype of a large group of syndromes called *Oral-Facial-Digital syndromes* with differing etiologies; classified as *Oral-Facial-Digital syndrome type II*; affects craniofacial structures, limbs, and the central nervous system.

Etiology

* Autosomal recessive disorder
* No specific defective gene identified

Physical and Behavioral Symptoms

* Abnormalities of the extremities, including shortness of fingers and toes (Brachydactyly); deflected fingers (Clinodactyly); supernumerary toes

or fingers (Polydactyly), often a bilateral reduplication of the big toe (hallux); and fused finger or toes (Syndactyly)
- Cranial and orofacial abnormalities, including midline partial tongue cleft, lobate tongue with nodules, midline cleft lip, cleft palate, abnormal cranial sutures, and broad or bifid nasal tip; mandibular Hypoplasia; Microtia, external auditory canal atresia; and auditory ossicular malformations
- Intellectual disabilities and attendant behavioral deficits

Speech, Language, and Hearing
- Conductive hearing loss, due to auditory canal and auditory ossicular abnormalities
- Delayed speech and articulation disorders, aggravated by a combination of intellectual disabilities, hearing loss, lingual anomalies, and cleft lip and palate
- Language delay and disorders complicated by associated factors (e.g., intellectual disabilities and hearing loss)

Mucopolysaccharidoses (MPS) Syndromes.   Group of syndromes characterized by a metabolic disorder; excessive storage of complex carbohydrates in the body, due to a lack of enzymes that break down mucopolysaccharides (sugar molecules), leading to their excessive accumulation in the systems; causes progressive intellectual disabilities, clouding of the corneas, skeletal dysplasia, coarse hair and bushy eyebrows, hearing loss, large tongue, anomalies of the hand, flat nasal bridge, and Hypertelorism; varieties include Hunter syndrome, Hurler syndrome, Maroteau-Lamy syndrome, Morquio syndrome, Sanfilippo syndrome, and Scheie syndrome; known for its extremely variable expression.

Etiology
- Autosomal recessive inheritance in all varieties except for Hunter syndrome
- X-linked recessive inheritance in Hunter syndrome

Physical, Behavioral, and Communication Problems
- *Hunter Syndrome:* Also called *MPS Type II;* unlike all other varieties of MPS, the Hunter has an X-linked inheritance with gene abnormality located on Xq27.3–q28; symptoms similar to Hurler syndrome except for the following: less severe symptoms; absence of corneal clouding; slower progression of symptoms; higher survival rate; hearing loss in about 50% of cases; feeding and swallowing problems due to changes in the oral and cranial structures (described under the next entry) that occur later in childhood; speech disorders associated with oral and cranial abnormalities that emerge; initially normal language development, but arrested in later childhood; chronic wet hoarseness and hyponasality.
- *Hurler Syndrome:* Most severe of the MPS syndromes; also called *MPS Type I;* symptoms include coarse facial features, clouded corneas, skeletal dysplasia, thick coarse hair, enlargement of viscera, and bushy eyebrows; anomalies of the middle ear; thick lips, large tongue, thickened palate and alveolar ridge, and depressed nasal bridge; short fingers and short broad hands; short neck and trunk; thickened and stiff joints; severe

S

and progressive intellectual disabilities; conductive hearing loss; heart anomalies; enlarged liver and spleen; severely limited speech development; severe articulation disorders; extremely limited language skills; hoarseness of voice and hyponasality.

- *Maroteaux-Lamy Syndrome:* Also called *MPS Type VI;* similar to Hurler syndrome except for normal or near-normal intelligence; mild forms similar to Scheie syndrome; chronic otitis media and conductive or sensorineural hearing impairment associated with severe expression; articulation disorders due to tongue enlargement and alveolar ridge abnormalities; adequate language skills because of near-normal intelligence; hyponasality and hoarseness.

- *Morquio Syndrome:* Also called *MPS Type IV;* abnormalities on chromosome 16; dwarfism due to bone dysplasia; hip dysplasia, short neck and trunk; extremely mild corneal clouding; liver and heart anomalies, progressive mixed or sensorineural hearing loss; speech and language skills within normal limits; high-pitched hoarse voice and hyponasality.

- *Sanfilippo Syndrome:* Also called *MPS Type III;* genes on chromosomes 17, 14, and 12 may all be involved; similar to Hurler syndrome with milder somatic symptoms; characteristics include enlarged head, somewhat aggressive behavior, and rapid intellectual deterioration resulting in dementia; hearing impairment in 10% of cases; initially normal speech and language skills that deteriorate; death occurs usually before age 20.

- *Scheie Syndrome:* Milder form of Hurler syndrome; difficult to diagnose before age 6; no significant intellectual disabilities; normal physical stature and average life expectancy; hearing impairment in 20% of cases.

Noonan Syndrome.   Also known as *pterygium coli* syndrome with neck webbing; genetic syndrome characterized by congenital heart disease, facial and skeletal anomalies, cryptorchidism, and intellectual disabilities in 50% to 60% of cases; physical resemblance to etiologically different Turner syndrome (found only in females and due to chromosome X abnormalities); not related to sex chromosome abnormalities; occurs in both males and females.

Etiology

- Autosomal Dominant inheritance; the defective gene is 12q24.

Physical and Behavioral Symptoms

- Craniofacial abnormalities, including webbing of the neck (pterygium), triangular facial shape, deeply furrowed philtrum, generally narrow growth of the face, malocclusion, constricted maxillary arch, low-set and posteriorly rotated ears, down-slanting eyes, Epicanthal Folds, and open bite; occasional cleft palate
- Congenital heart problems, including Pulmonary Stenosis, pulmonary valve weakness, and cardiomyopathy
- Growth and genitourinary deficiencies, including short stature, shield-shaped chest, Hypertelorsim, Ptosis of the eyelids, cryptorchidism, and male infertility
- Early feeding problems

- Perceptual problems and learning disabilities
- Normal or above normal intelligence in some cases

Speech, Language, and Hearing

- Conductive or sensorineural hearing loss, though not characteristic of the syndrome
- Articulation problems that are typically associated with maxillary abnormalities; compensatory articulation with submucous cleft
- Delayed language development and limited expressive language skills associated with limited intelligence; better spoken language comprehension than expression
- Normal voice except for an occasional high pitch; hypernasality with submucous cleft

Oral-Facial-Digital Syndromes (OFD). Eight varieties (OFD1 through OFD8) of genetic disorders with different etiologic factors; all share certain common characteristics; characterized by cranial, facial, lingual, palatal, and digital anomalies; also called *Mohr syndrome.*

Etiology

- Sex-linked recessive inheritance in OFD1 and OFD8
- Autosomal recessive inheritance in OFD3, OFD4, OFD5, and OFD6
- Suspected autosomal dominant inheritance in OFD7
- Unknown pattern of inheritance in OFD2
- OFD1 associated with abnormalities on Xp22.3–p22.2; specific gene abnormality unclear for the others

Physical Symptoms

- Feeding disorders in all subtypes
- Polydactyly (limb abnormalities), associated with all OFD variations
- Corpus callosum and cognitive impairments in all subtypes except for OFD5
- Midline cleft of the upper lip, sometimes just a notch, in OFD1, OFD5, and OFD7
- Cleft palate with or without clef lip in OFD4, OFD6, and OFD7
- Kidney dysfunctions in OFD7
- Midline partial tongue cleft and lobate tongue with nodules in most subtypes

Speech, Language, and Hearing

- Conductive hearing loss in OFD1 and OFD4
- Delayed speech onset and acquisition in all subtypes; dysarthria in OFD1; articulation problems related to mandibular and lingual abnormalities and hearing loss when present
- Language delay, depending on the intellectual level; may be severe in all subtypes except for OFD5; limited functional communication skills
- Hypernasality if cleft palate is present; more likely in OFD1, OFD4, and OFD6
- No significant voice disorders

S

Otopalatodigital Syndromes. Genetic syndromes characterized by otologic, palatal, and digital anomalies; associated with cleft palate, hearing loss, and mild intellectual disabilities; two types with differing characteristics.

Etiology
- Otopalatodigital syndrome Type I, with X-linked recessive inheritance, with abnormalities on Xq28
- Otopalatodigital syndrome Type II, also with X-linked recessive inheritance; specific gene abnormality not known

Physical and Behavioral Symptoms
- Type I characterized by cleft palate, micrognathia, malocclusion, hypertelorism, broad nasal root, widely spaced toes, short fingers, short and broad finger tips, short fingernails, small stature, hypodontia; congenital malformations of the ossicular chain; early feeding disorders; intellectual disabilities and associated behavioral deficits
- Type II characterized by extremely small oral and pharyngeal cavities, cleft palate, maxillary and mandibular hypoplasia, hypertelorism, broad and high forehead; syndactyly, clinodactyly, bowed limbs, and narrow chest; early feeding disorders; hydrocephalus, intellectual disabilities, and associated behavioral deficits

Speech, Language, and Hearing
- Speech, language, and hearing characteristics of Type I include bilateral conductive hearing loss possibly due to otitis media; delayed speech and articulation disorders; compensatory articulation and hypernasality due to cleft palate; delayed language and language disorders associated with intellectual disabilities
- Speech, language, and hearing characteristics of Type II include conductive hearing loss; articulation disorders that are often more severe than those found in Type I; articulation shifted to the posterior parts of the mouth (due to small oral and pharyngeal cavities); hypernasality and muffled resonance; language disorders consistent with intellectual disabilities

Pendred Syndrome. Genetic syndrome due to thyroid deficiency; a major cause of congenital deafness; goiter in middle childhood; intellectual disabilities; males and females equally affected.

Etiology
- Genetic mechanism of the syndrome is autosomal recessive inheritance
- Gene abnormality on chromosome 7 (7q31)

Physical and Behavioral Symptoms
- Enlarged thyroid (goiter)
- Hypothyroidism in early years
- Delayed skeletal maturation as the child grows older

Speech, Language, and Hearing
- Bilateral, mild to profound sensorineural hearing loss; progressive deterioration in hearing
- Severe delay in language acquisition, consistent with the level of hearing loss
- Significant errors of articulation, due mostly to the hearing impairment

Pierre-Robin Syndrome. Controversial genetic syndrome characterized by Mandibular Hypoplasia, Glossoptosis, and cleft of the soft palate; may not be a separate syndrome, but the Robin Sequence; associated features may be found in several other syndromes, including Stickler Syndrome, Treacher Collins Syndrome, and Velo-Cardio-Facial Syndrome; much variability in its diagnosis.

Etiology

- Thought to be autosomal recessive inheritance
- Autosomal dominant inheritance is suspected if the features are a part of the Stickler syndrome
- Occurrence may be sporadic; maternal drug use may be an etiologic factor; suspected mechanical disruption of the embryonic growth

Physical and Behavioral Symptoms

- Craniofacial anomalies, including Mandibular Hypoplasia, Glossoptosis (downward displacement of the tongue); cleft of the soft palate; velopharyngeal incompetence due to the cleft; dental abnormalities, deformed pinna, low-set ears, and temporal bone and ossicular chain deformities
- Failure to thrive because of the tongue placement that may create breathing difficulties, apnea, and dysphagia; vomiting
- Intellectual disabilities associated with hypoxia due to breathing difficulties

Speech, Language, and Hearing

- Unilateral or bilateral conductive hearing loss associated with otitis media and cleft palate
- Delayed language and language disorders, mostly due to the hearing loss; more severe if accompanied by intellectual disabilities
- Hypernasality and nasal emission mainly due to the velopharyngeal incompetence
- Articulation disorders and compensatory articulation

Prader-Willi Syndrome. Genetic syndrome characterized by Hypotonia, slow motor development, small hands and feet, underdeveloped genitals, almond-shaped eyes, obesity due to insatiable appetite, and intellectual disabilities in most but not all cases; genetically, but not phenotypically, related to Angelman Syndrome.

Etiology

- Deletion in the region of the paternal long arm of chromosome 15 (15q11.2–15q12); absence of the maternal 15q11 in Angelman syndrome
- Maternal uniparental disomy of chromosome 15 is another cause

Physical Symptoms

- Low muscle tone and resulting early feeding difficulties
- Failure to thrive initially, mostly because of the early feeding difficulties
- Craniofacial abnormalities include a thin upper lip, upslanting almond-shaped eyes, strabismus, and myopia
- Neurological symptoms include hypotonia and a high threshold for pain
- Small hands, feet scoliosis, and osteopenia
- Underdeveloped genitals
- Intellectual disabilities

S

- Behavioral problems include excessive and compulsive eating because of an insatiable appetite, sleep disturbances, and self-destructive behavior
- Obesity after the first year, due to compulsive and excessive eating

Speech, Language, and Hearing

- Hearing loss not a typical characteristic
- Mild to moderate articulation disorders (omissions, distortions, and weak consonant productions); complicated by hypotonia and velopharyngeal insufficiency
- Initially slower but later somewhat accelerated language development; limited by the degree of intellectual disabilities
- Hypernasality and nasal air emission due mostly to hypotonia

Refsum Syndrome.   Genetic syndrome characterized by progressive sensorineural hearing loss, neurological deterioration, cerebellar ataxia, chronic Polyneuritis, and Retinitis Pigmentosa

Etiology

- Autosomal recessive inheritance
- Biochemical imbalance involving excessive storage of Phytanic Acid in tissue or plasma

Physical Symptoms

- Chronic inflammation of the peripheral nerves (Polyneuritis) and disturbed balance (cerebellar ataxia)
- Pigmentary degeneration of the retina and night blindness
- Heart diseases in about 50% of cases
- Skeletal abnormalities including Spondylitis and Kyphoscoliosis in about 75% of cases

Speech, Language, and Hearing

- Slowly progressive sensorineural hearing loss that begins during the second or third decade of life in 50% of cases
- Articulation disorders consistent with acquired hearing loss
- Dysarthria if the facial muscles are involved
- Harsh voice and variable pitch and loudness; hypernasality and nasal emission
- Prosodic problems (associated with dysarthria) include altered rate of speech and stress patterns

Stickler Syndrome.   Genetic syndrome characterized by facial deformities, ophthalmologic problems, musculoskeletal deficiencies, Pierre-Robin sequence including cleft palate or submucous cleft, and hearing impairment; normal intelligence.

Etiology

- Autosomal dominant inheritance
- Abnormalities on 12q13.11–11q13.2

Physical Symptoms

- Ophthalmologic problems include cataracts, retinal detachments, and severe myopia

- Musculoskeletal problems include joint diseases and juvenile rheumatoid arthritis; prominent ankle, knee, and wrist bones; long and thin legs and hands
- Craniofacial deviations include <u>Micrognathia</u>, midface <u>Hypoplasia</u>, cleft palate, submucous cleft or bifid uvula, round face, depressed nasal root, and epicanthal folds
- Upper airway obstruction
- Auricular malformations in 10% to 12% of cases

Speech, Language, and Hearing
- Feeding, sucking, and swallowing problems during infancy; complicated by upper airway obstructions
- Bilateral conductive hearing loss associated with cleft palate; sensorineural loss in some 15% of cases
- Language problems associated with hearing loss and cleft palate
- Hypernasality, nasal emission, and hyponasality
- Articulation disorders associated with cleft palate and micrognathia

Tourette's Syndrome. Genetic syndrome characterized by tics (rapid semivoluntary movements performed compulsively); patterned and stereotypical movements voluntarily suppressed for only a short duration; occurs in about 4 to 5 individuals per 10,000; more common in males than in females; may be associated with obsessive compulsive behavior, phobia, and hyperactivity.

Etiology
- No identified specific genetic abnormality; thought to be autosomal dominant
- Not due to neurological diseases or drug effects

Physical and Behavioral Symptoms
- Multiple motor tics (eye blinks, facial twitches, shoulder shrugging, grimaces)
- One or more vocal tics (throat clearing, grunting, humming, yelling, screaming, spitting, and making barking noises)
- Various behavioral problems, including depression, inattention, impulsivity, anxiety, sexual disorders, and aggressive behaviors

Speech, Language, and Hearing
- Vocal tics that may start as grunting and evolve into other forms as noted
- Coprolalia (compulsive swearing or utterance of obscenities)
- Palilalia (repetition of one's own utterances) and echolalia (repetition of what is heard)
- Higher than the typical incidence of stuttering
- Hyperkinetic dysarthria
- Self-talking and conversation assuming different roles or persons

S

Treacher Collins Syndrome. Rare genetic syndrome characterized by mandibulofacial <u>Dysostosis</u>, hearing impairment, cleft or velopharyngeal incompetence, dental problems, and external ear malformations; intellectual disabilities are uncommon; also known as *mandibulofacial dysostosis, Franceschetti-Klein syndrome,* and *Franceschetti-Zwahlen-Klein syndrome.*

Etiology
- Autosomal dominant inheritance
- Genetic abnormality on 5q32–q33 (called a TREACLE gene)
- Possibility of spontaneous mutation

Physical and Behavioral Symptoms
- Craniofacial anomalies, including a long face, beaklike nose, underdeveloped facial bones (mandibular Hypoplasia or small chin and malar Hypoplasia or underdeveloped cheeks); dental malocclusion and hypoplasia; downwardly slanted palpebral fissures; Coloboma of the lower eyelid; high hard palate; short or immobile soft palate; cleft palate in about 30% of cases; submucous cleft in some cases; cleft lip and palate in a few cases; pharyngeal hypoplasia (very small pharynx), hair growth on the cheeks, absence of lower eyelashes; strabismus
- Auditory abnormalities, including stenosis or atresia of the external auditory canal, malformations of the pinna, and preauricular ear tags; middle and inner ear malformations including a fixation of the footplate of the stapes
- Sucking and swallowing problems during infancy

Speech, Language, and Hearing
- Early feeding disorders because of cleft palate and airway obstruction
- Congenital, bilateral, and conductive hearing loss; sensorineural loss in a few cases
- Speech disorders; posterior carriage of the tongue due to micrognathia, causing misarticulation of anteriorly produced speech sounds; compensatory articulation associated with cleft palate
- Language disorders associated with hearing impairment; deficient syntactic and morphological skills
- Hypernasality, hyponasality, and nasal emission possibly due to cleft palate, velopharyngeal incompetence, and the narrow pharynx; muffled resonance because of the posterior tongue position

Turner Syndrome. Genetic syndrome characterized by defective gonadal differentiation; congenital edema (swelling) of neck, hands, or feet; webbing of the neck; low posterior hair line; intellectual disabilities in 10% of cases; occurs only in females because the cause is a missing X chromosome; a similar syndrome that occurs in both males and females is called *Noonan syndrome*; also known as *XO syndrome*, *Morgagni–Turner–Albright syndrome*, *Schereshevkii–Turner syndrome*, *Bonnevie-Ulrich syndrome*, and *Turner–Vamy syndrome*

Etiology
- Missing X chromosome; females with a single X chromosome (called monosomy X); severity of the syndrome is dependent on the extent to which the X monosomy is found in the body cells

Physical and Behavioral Symptoms
- Absence or underdevelopment of the secondary sexual characteristics; ovarian abnormality resulting in amenorrhea (absence of menstruation) and infertility

S

- Congenital swelling of the foot, neck, and hands; webbing of the neck (excess skin over the neck)
- Cardiac defects
- Broad chest with widely spaced nipples, hip dislocation, and skeletal dysplasia
- Dysplastic nails, low posterior hairline, and pigmented skin lesions
- Craniofacial anomalies include Micrognathia (abnormally small lower jaw), maxillary Hypoplasia (underdeveloped or very small maxilla), high arched and narrow palate, and cleft palate
- Anomalies of the auricle include low-set, elongated, and cup-shaped ears; thick earlobes
- Right hemisphere dysfunction in some cases
- Learning disabilities, although intellectual impairments are uncommon

Speech, Language, and Hearing

- Acquired sensorineural loss, noticed after the 10th year; with middle ear infections, mixed sensorineural and conductive loss
- Delayed speech development and articulation disorders consistent with hearing impairment and maxillary abnormality
- Delayed acquisition and disorders of language consistent with the level and type of hearing impairment
- Possible auditory processing, visual, spatial, and attentional problems

Usher Syndrome. Genetic syndrome characterized by Retinitis Pigmentosa and nonprogressive congenital hearing loss; disturbed gait; intellectual disabilities in some cases; 50% of individuals who are deaf and blind may have this syndrome; relatively common among people of French Canadian descent and Jewish descent in Berlin, Germany; also noted frequently in Nigerians and Argentineans of Spanish descent; four types (Usher types I through IV).

Etiology

- Autosomal recessive inheritance in Usher syndrome Types I, II, and III
- Suspected X-linked recessive trait in Usher syndrome Type IV

Physical and Behavioral Symptoms

- Type I associated with congenital sensorineural deafness, onset of night blindness before the age of 10, and limited and progressively worsening peripheral vision; eventual blindness
- Type II associated with congenital sensorineural deafness and visual field problems
- Type III associated with progressive hearing loss; not congenital; normal until puberty
- Type IV associated with hearing loss and vision impairments; has the lowest incidence of all four varieties; more frequent in males than females
- Cochlear abnormalities and ataxia in the different subtypes

Speech, Language, and Hearing

- Delayed speech acquisition due to hearing and vision impairments; impaired sign language acquisition due to visual impairments; minimal or no speech with congenital deafness and early-onset blindness

S

- Articulation disorders and impaired intelligibility consistent with hearing impairment
- Delayed language and language disorders consistent with hearing impairment and the time of onset of vision problems
- Hypernasality and nasal emission

van der Woude Syndrome. Genetic syndrome involving clefts; nearly 5% of clients with various forms and combinations of clefts may have van der Woude syndrome; mixing of the cleft types (incidence of cleft palate only, cleft lip only, and cleft palate and cleft lip among relatives) is a distinguishing characteristic.

Etiology
- Autosomal dominant inheritance associated with this syndrome
- Gene abnormality on 1q32

Physical Symptoms
- Craniofacial anomalies, the single most important characteristics
- Pits or cysts of the lower lip in all cases; cleft lip and cleft palate in many cases; ankyloglossia; missing premolars

Speech, Language, and Hearing
- Otitis media and conductive loss associated with cleft palate
- Early feeding difficulties in cases of cleft palate
- Normal speech onset; articulation disorders consistent with hearing loss and cleft palate; compensatory articulation associated with palatal clefts and velopharyngeal insufficiency
- Language disorders are not typical, but errors consistent with hearing loss (e.g., missing morphological features)
- Hypernasality and nasal emission is associated with cleft palate and velopharyngeal insufficiency; voice is generally normal

Velo-Cardio-Facial Syndrome (VCFS). Common genetic syndrome of numerous anomalies, with over 180 clinical features; associated with congenital heart disease, psychiatric problems, and communication disorders.

Etiology
- Autosomal dominant inheritance
- A deletion at the long arm of chromosome 22 (22q11.2)

Physical and Behavioral Symptoms
- Craniofacial and oral anomalies include a flat skull base, microcephaly, long and asymmetric face, small or missing teeth characterized by deficient enamel, occasional cleft lip, prominent nasal bride, narrow nostrils, upper airway obstruction, laryngeal web, deficient adenoids, arytenoid hyperplasia, thin pharyngeal muscle, and unilateral vocal cord paresis
- Auditory disorders include overfolded helix; small, protruded, asymmetric, and cup-shaped ears; and narrow external ear canal
- Optic anomalies include small eyes, strabismus, narrow palpebral fissure, iris nodules, and puffy eyelids

- Cardiovascular abnormalities include ventral and atrial septal defects, right-sided aorta, interrupted aorta, aortic valve anomalies, defective subclavian arteries, abnormal origin of the carotid artery, and structural abnormalities of the internal carotid and vertebral arteries
- Neurological disorders include seizures, hypotonia, cerebellar growth abnormalities, spina bifida, and enlarged sylvian fissure
- Skeletal abnormalities include small hands and feet, short fingers, polydactyly, and syndactyly
- Various digestive, respiratory, renal, endocrine, and genitourinary disorders
- Psychiatric problems include bipolar affective disorders, schizophrenia, obsessive compulsive disorders, anxiety, and phobia

Speech, Language, and Hearing
- Early feeding and swallowing problems due to airway obstruction
- More common conductive hearing loss; occasional sensorineural hearing loss; mild to severe; unilateral or bilateral
- Severe articulation disorders; error patterns consistent with severe velopharyngeal insufficiency
- Delayed early language acquisition; somewhat accelerated in later years; negative effects of hearing loss
- A high-pitched, hoarse, and breathy voice
- Severe hypernasality, associated with velopharyngeal insufficiency

Waardenburg Syndrome, Type I and Type II. Genetic syndrome subclassified into two types: Type I is characterized by wide bridge of the nose caused by lateral displacement of inner (nasal) canthi, pigmentary disturbances, and hearing impairment in about 25% of cases; Type II is characterized by cranial and facial anomalies, Brachydactyly, cleft palate, cardiac defects, and hearing impairment in about 50% of cases.

Etiology
- Autosomal dominant inheritance in Type I syndrome

Physical Symptoms, Type I
- Lateral displacement of the inner (nasal) Canthi, causing wide bridge of the nose, medial flare of eyebrows, and white eyelashes
- Pigmentary anomalies including white forelock, Heterochromia irides, and Vitiligo
- Cochlear anomalies

Physical Symptoms, Type II
- High-domed skull (Acrocephaly), orbital and facial deformities, and cleft palate
- Shortness of fingers (Brachydactyly), fusion (Syndactyly) of soft tissue, a variety of glaucoma (Hydrophthalmos), and cardiac malformations

Speech, Language, and Hearing
- Early feeding and swallowing problems consistent with cleft palate
- Mild to profound congenital unilateral or bilateral sensorineural loss, more common in Type II than in Type I

S

- Language disorders consistent with congenital hearing impairment; especially deficient syntactic and morphological features
- Hypernasality and nasal emission

Articulation disorders consistent with hearing impairment and compensatory articulatory gestures consistent with cleft palate.

Baraitser, M., & Winter, R. M. (1996). *Color atlas of congenital malformation syndromes.* London: Mosby-Wolfe.

Dorland's Illustrated Medical Dictionary (1994, 28th ed.). Philadelphia, PA: W. B. Saunders.

Jones, K. L. (2005). *Smith's recognizable patterns of human malformations* (6th ed.). Philadelphia, PA: W. B. Saunders.

Jung, J. H. (1989). *Genetic syndromes in communication disorders.* Austin, TX: Pro-Ed.

Kahn, A. (2000). *Craniofacial anomalies.* San Diego, CA: Singular Publishing Group.

Shprintzen, J. R. (2000). *Syndrome identification for speech-language pathology.* San Diego, CA: Singular Publishing Group.

Shprintzen, J. R. (1997). *Genetics, syndromes, and communication disorders.* San Diego, CA: Singular Publishing Group.

Wiedemann, H. R., & Kunze, J. (1997). *Clinical syndromes* (3rd ed.). London: Mosby-Wolfe.

Synostosis.   Fusion of bones that are normally separate; congenital; may be genetic.

Syntactic Component.   Aspect of language that includes rules for combining words into phrases and sentences and rules that help transform one form of sentence into another.

Syntax.   Collection of rules in any language that dictate how socially acceptable sentences and sentence varieties may be produced.

S

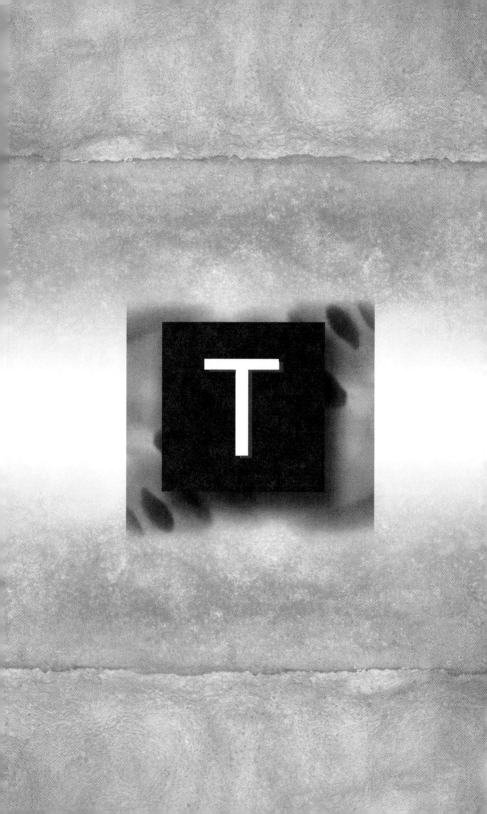

Tactile Agnosia. Neurological disorder associated with brain injury; clients cannot recognize objects they touch and feel but cannot see (as in darkness or when blindfolded); see Agnosia.

Taybi Syndrome. Same as Oto-Palatal-Digital syndrome (see Syndromes Associated With Communication Disorders).

Telegraphic Speech. Truncated speech devoid of certain grammatical elements; telegraphic in nature; a characteristic of children normally learning language, Language Disorders in Children, and people with nonfluent Aphasia.

Third Alexia. Same as frontal alexia; see Alexia.

Threshold of Hearing. An intensity level of an auditory stimulus that is faintly heard at least 50% of the time it is presented; a measure used in hearing testing.

Thrombosis. Disease process leading to blood clot formation in larger arteries of the body; due to accumulation of fat and other materials, arteries harden and restrict the movement of blood, encouraging clot formation; clots then cut off blood supply to areas beyond their location; unlike *emboli*, thrombotic clots remain at their point of origin; cerebral thrombosis is a frequent cause of stroke and resulting Aphasia.

Tongue Thrust. A deviant swallow in which the tongue is pushed forward against the central incisors; also known as *reverse swallow* or *infantile swallow*, but these are not preferred terms; part of Orofacial Myofunctional Disorders; controversially related to articulation disorders in the past; does not imply that the tongue is thrusting against the front teeth; characterized by:
- Forward (anterior) gesture of the tongue during swallow, which is typical of young children because of their relatively large tongue and smaller oral cavity; the tongue tip may be in contact with the lower lip
- Forward carriage of the tongue that results in the tip being in contact with the anterior teeth, with a slightly open mandible
- Fronting of the tongue during speech production; the tongue may be between or against the front teeth; again, the mandible may be slightly open
- Tongue thrust may be habitual or due to structural problems (e.g., enlarged adenoids or tonsils that partially block the posterior airway passage, thus forcing a more anterior tongue carriage)
- Articulation errors in some children and may include a lisp (distortions of /z/ and /l/) and a more anterior tongue position than normal in producing /ʃ/, /ʧ/, /ʤ/, /ʒ/, /t/, /d/, /l/, and /n/
- Forward (anterior) tongue resting position (between the anterior teeth at rest), more than tongue thrust alone during swallowing, may be associated with dental abnormalities or malocclusions

American Speech-Language Hearing Association (1991). The role of the speech-language pathologist in management of orofacial myofunctional disorders. *Asha, 33* (Suppl. 5)7.

American Speech-Language Hearing Association (1993). Orofacial myofunctional disorders: Knowledge and skills. *Asha, 35* (Suppl. 10), 21–23.

T

Topic Initiation. Pragmatic or conversational language skill to introduce new topics for conversation in a socially acceptable manner; may be impaired in persons with language disorders; abrupt introduction or introduction at wrong times constitute a topic initiation problem; see Language Disorders in Children.

Topic Maintenance. Talking on the same topic for an extended and socially acceptable duration; impaired when a speaker shifts a topic of conversation too soon or too abruptly; impaired topic maintenance is a feature of Language Disorders in Children.

Total Glossectomy. Surgical removal of the entire tongue, including its base in case of such incurable diseases as cancer.

Total Laryngectomy. Surgical removal of the entire larynx, including the cricoid and thyroid cartilages and the epiglottis in case of incurable cancer.

Tourette's Syndrome (Disorder). Genetic syndrome characterized by tics; see Syndromes Associated With Communication Disorders for details.

Tracheoesophageal Fistula. Pathological formation of a channel that allows food from the esophagus into the trachea; may be a congenital disorder, causing Dysphagia.

Transcortical Motor Aphasia. Variety of nonfluent aphasia, characterized by agrammatical, effortful, and telegraphic speech with good repetition skills; see Aphasia: Specific Types.

Transcortical Sensory Aphasia. A type of fluent aphasia; see Aphasia: Specific Types.

Transformational Generative Theory. Chomskyan theory of language in which grammar is the essence of languages; each child is born with the knowledge of a universal grammar, which helps generate varied forms of sentences; this innate knowledge helps each child acquire his or her native language; a theory that assigns little or no importance to environmental variables in learning language.

Chomsky, N. (1968). *Aspects of the theory of syntax.* Cambridge, MA: MIT Press.

Transient Ischemic Attacks. Minor strokes whose effects last a brief duration; may not produce any permanent effects; may be warning signs of more serious strokes that result in Aphasia and related symptoms.

Traumatic Brain Injury (TBI). An externally induced injury to the brain, also known as *craniocerebral trauma*; to be distinguished from injury to the brain caused by strokes and degenerative neurological diseases; may be Penetrating (Open-Head) Injury or Nonpenetrating (Closed-Head) Injury; in causing TBI, either the head moves and hits an object or an object moves and hits the head; third leading cause of death (cardiovascular diseases and cancer are 1 and 2); in more than two-thirds of individuals with TBI, the injuries are minor with no loss of consciousness; main symptoms of major TBI include restlessness, irritation, disorientation to time and place, and disorganized and inconsistent responses; impaired memory, attention, reasoning, drawing, naming, and repetition.

T

Epidemiology and Ethnocultural Variables
- TBI is the most common cause of death and disability among young people
- Causing an expensive medical emergency, TBI costs an estimated $25 billion a year for medical and rehabilitative services
- Each individual who sustains a serious TBI may incur a loss of up to $5 million in costs and lost wages
- Related but different concepts, head injury may not involve brain injury; brain injury almost always involves head injury
- Incidence of TBI varies across studies, but most sources suggest an incidence of about 150 to 200 per 100,000 persons in the U.S. general population; some reports suggest as high a rate as 367 per 100,000
- Annually, an estimated 1.4 million people sustain brain injury; about 54,000 people die of TBI before they reach a hospital; at least 350,000 people receive medical treatment and rehabilitative services after hospitalization; between 80,000 and 90,000 people with moderate to severe brain injury have long-term disability
- Prevalence rate is the highest for people in the age range of 15 to 24 years; young people in the age range of 15 to 19 years have 400 to 700 cases of TBI per 100,000 individuals; the prevalence picks up again for those who are 75 years or older, with a rate of 300 per 100,000 persons
- Males are more prone to TBI than females; three to five males for one female with TBI
- Higher TBI-related mortality rates for males than females
- Higher prevalence of TBI among people living in urban areas with a high population density
- People in the lower socioeconomic strata are more prone to TBI than those in the upper strata
- Limited ethnocultural data suggest a higher prevalence of TBI among African Americans and Hispanics than whites
- Head injuries due to gunshot wounds, assault, and other forms of violent behavior may be frequent among minority groups in lower socioeconomic strata living in poor neighborhoods, especially in inner cities
- Poor elderly living in inner cities are prone to TBI caused by violence

TBI: Two Main Varieties
- Penetrating brain injuries, also known as open-head injuries
  - Skull fractured or perforated
  - Meninges torn or lacerated
  - Some consider the injury penetrating when the skull is fractured but the meninges are intact; others require both to be involved to classify as a penetrating brain injury
  - Associated with a high mortality rate
- Nonpenetrating brain injuries, also known as closed-head injuries
  - Skull may or may not be fractured or lacerated
  - Meninges remain intact
  - Some consider the injury nonpenetrating only when the skull also is intact

T

Penetrating Brain Injury
Etiologic Factors
- Basic cause of penetrating brain injury is the piercing of the skull by an external object; the object may pass through the head
- Military weapons, rifles, and other automatic assault weapons produce high-velocity injuries
- Automobile accidents, blows to the head, and such other low-velocity forces when they produce a concentrated impact on a small area of the skull
- Arrow, nail gun, knife, and other projectile products produce low-velocity injuries; bullets shot from handguns also produce low-velocity injuries
- Falls and sports-related accidents
- Assaults (personal violence)

Neurophysiological Consequences
- Extent of brain injury depends on the projectile's entrance velocity; the greater the velocity, the more serious the injury
- The more zigzag the course of the object (called *yaw*) moving through the brain, the greater the extent of injury
- The higher the amount of fragmentation of the moving object within the brain (e.g., the bullets), the greater the damage
- The higher the number of wounds, the greater the extent of injury
- As the projectile travels through the brain, there might be injury to tissue on both sides of the projectile tract
- As the projectile hits the skull, it may be fractured or perforated
- Skull is more likely to be fractured (not perforated) with low-velocity impacts
- Foreign substance (hair, skin, and bone fragments) may be carried to the brain by the projectile
- Foreign materials that enter the brain may cause secondary infection
- Instant increase in intracranial pressure due to the impact and injury; pressure waves create a second round of increase in pressure within 2 to 5 minutes of impact
- Immediately after the impact, blood pressure drops, then rises, and drops again
- Flow of blood within the brain immediately drops and remains low for several hours; cerebral metabolic rate remains low
- Additional effects of brain injury include bleeding, infection, swelling, and hydrocephalus
- Injury causes a series of behavioral effects, including attentional deficits, memory, and speech and language problems (described later)
- Brain-penetrating objects may cause death; death rate is higher for those who sustain brainstem injuries than for those who sustain injuries to higher levels of the brain; death may be immediate in case of gunshot wounds; may be delayed in other cases

T

Nonpenetrating Brain Injury

Etiologic Factors

- Force is applied to a stationary head or the head hits a stationary object; head may move back-and-forth because of force applied to other parts of the body; mostly the same factors that cause penetrating brain injury also cause nonpenetrating injury, except that the meninges are not torn or lacerated
- Various kinds of industrial, domestic, or sports-related accidents that impact a stationary head (e.g., the collapse of an automobile on the head of a mechanic lying under the vehicle)
- Falls in which the head hits a stationary object
- Blows to the head with a blunt object, often a result of violence
- Automobile accidents in which the force is applied to a movable head, causing rapid back-and-forth movement of the brain inside the skull; the force also may be applied to other parts of the body (as in whiplash), setting the head in motion and causing movement of the brain inside the skull
- Abuse and interpersonal violence; Shaken Baby syndrome, for example, is a significant cause of nonpenetrating brain injury in children under 5 years of age; about 19% children subjected to this kind of brain injury die

Neurophysiological Consequences

- Nonpenetrating brain injuries are collectively called *acceleration/deceleration injuries* caused by the physical forces that strike the head or body and as a result, the head and the brain inside the skull rapidly move back and forth
- Acceleration may be linear or angular
- In linear acceleration, caused by force striking the head midline, the head moves in a straight line
- In angular acceleration, caused by force striking the head off-center, the head rotates; angular acceleration causes more serious brain injury than linear acceleration
- There is *impression (impact) trauma*, which is skull deformation at the point of impact; more common with linear acceleration; the impact will cause *coup injuries* to the brain (injuries at the point of impact)
- When the head is set into linear motion, the brain begins to move inside the skull; when the head movement decelerates, the brain continues to move for a few seconds; this movement then causes *contrecoup injuries*, which are injuries to the brain tissue on the opposite side of the impact
- Coup and contrecoup injuries cause focal damage to meninges, cortex, and subcortical structures; when the brain moves back-and-forth within the skull, the soft tissue on the underside of the brain, especially the basal portions of the temporal and frontal lobes, are damaged because of sharp bony projections over which the brain moves
- In angular acceleration, the head rotates away from the direction of the blow; the brain stays still for a few milliseconds when the head begins to move; this will cause *diffuse axonal injury* (twisting and shearing of

brain tissue); the brain eventually begins its angular movement, but when the head stops moving, the brain will continue its rotational movement for a few milliseconds, resulting in additional injury

- Nonacceleration brain injuries occur when there is no movement of the head or the brain inside the skull; an automobile crashing down on the head of a mechanic lying on a hard surface is an example of nonacceleration injury; generally, nonacceleration injuries occur less frequently and produce less severe effects than acceleration injuries

Primary Effects of TBI

- *Primary effects* are common to both penetrating and nonpenetrating injuries
- Fractures of the skull (a cause of fatality in 80% of individuals who sustain TBI)
- Diffuse axonal injury (torn nerve fibers in widespread areas of the brain); a direct effect of trauma, often due to angular acceleration; eventually causes small clusters of microglia (cell shapes that suggest neural damage); degeneration of long neuronal tracts, leading to severe disabilities or vegetative state
- Primary brainstem injury, causing coma
- Diffuse vascular injury (small and widespread ruptures in the brain's blood vessels), causing multiple hemorrhages in the brain
- Primary focal lesion (restricted, localized lesions in the brain); often due to linear acceleration
- Cranial nerve damage; speech impairments associated with injury to cranial nerves V, VII, X, and XII
- Altered consciousness; varied levels of consciousness depending on the extent and type of brain injury; the individual may be dazed, or in a state of stupor (not responsive except for pain and other strong stimuli) or coma (unconscious and unresponsive to most if not all external stimulation)
- Survival with no recovery of consciousness; individual lies in a vegetative state or persistent vegetative stage (beyond 30 days in this condition)
- Slow or sudden recovery from consciousness
- Brief loss of consciousness associated with concussion or minor head injury with quick regaining of consciousness followed by headache, neckache, backache, blurred vision, fatigue, and sleep disturbances; subtle but long-lasting physical and cognitive effects
- Interrupted respiration; lower blood pressure and heart rate
- Behavioral changes, especially in the acute stage, including restlessness and agitation, auditory hallucinations, confabulations, delusions, and depression

Secondary Effects of TBI

- Primary effects are followed by secondary effects
- Traumatic (intracranial) hematoma (accumulation of blood in the brain due to hemorrhage), often a result of automobile accidents
- Epidural hematoma (accumulation of blood between the dura matter and the skull), often in the temporal regions of the brain; also a typical result of automobile accidents
- Subdural hematoma (accumulation of blood between the dura and the arachnoid), a more frequent cause of death; frequently associated with sustained assaults and falls

- Intracerebral hematoma (accumulation of blood within the brain itself); a common occurrence in the temporal and frontal lobes, often due to diffuse axonal injury because of linear acceleration; a frequent cause of coma and death
- Increased intracranial pressure due (accumulation of blood, water, or cerebrospinal fluid); restricts blood flow to the brain tissue; may cause death if the pressure is extreme; leads to ventricular enlargement and edema
- Ischemic brain damage (injury to brain tissue due to oxygen deprivation), caused by reduced or interrupted blood supply due to breathing difficulties, hypotension, constricted cerebral blood vessels, and cerebral vasospasms (construction of the muscular layer surrounding blood vessels)
- Seizures associated with moderate to severe injury; vomiting or nausea, dilation of pupils, weakness or numbness of the extremities, and loss of coordination
- Infection of the head wound, meninges, or both
- Dysphagia (swallowing disorder), may be present in the early stage of TBI; frequently associated with intracranial bleeding, longer durations of coma, and brainstem injury

Initial Behavioral Symptoms of TBI
- Individuals who regain consciousness tend to be:
  - Inconsistent, disorganized, confused, and disoriented to time and place
  - Restless, irritated at minor issues, inattentive, and distractible
  - Amnesic (total loss of memory); amnesia without confusion or disorientation is often associated with damage to the medial temporal lobes and the hippocampus
  - Impaired memory; both pretraumatic memory loss (*retrograde amnesia*) and posttraumatic memory loss (*anterograde amnesia*) are more common than amnesia; impaired visual memory (difficulty recalling what is seen briefly)
  - Impaired judgment and abstract reasoning skills; unable to understand abstract language or interpret it literally
  - Impulsive and aggressive, with poor control over emotional responses
  - Anxious, paranoid, and depressed
  - Socially inappropriate
  - Slow in reacting to stimuli; distractibility a contributing factor
  - Aimless, lacking in purposeful behavior; unappreciative of his or her deficits; unconcerned about self-care; in need of constant care and supervision

Recovery From the Early Symptoms
- Symptoms of TBI improve gradually; in many cases the improvement may be stepwise (periods of little or no improvement alternated with rapid improvement); as physical conditions improve:
  - Confusion clears up
  - Orientation to space and time improves
  - Social awareness and awareness of the physical surroundings improve
  - Emotional responses become better controlled and more appropriate
  - Responses to simple questions become more appropriate and relevant

- o Self-care skills slowly re-emerge, although still needing assistance and supervision
- o General behavior becomes more purposeful
- o Behavior will be progressively more independent functioning in routine situations
- Some behavioral symptoms, though showing signs of abatement, may still be present:
  - o Irritability, restlessness, poor emotional control, aggressive tendencies, impulsivity, and slow reaction time
  - o Short attention span; impaired memory and judgment; impaired reasoning skills; failure to detect logical inconsistencies in statements, point out absurdities or missing elements in pictures, and generate reasoned responses

Communication Deficits. Clients with TBI have less pronounced communication deficits than attentional, cognitive, emotional, and general behavioral deficits; clients with mild brain injury may occasionally give irrelevant or inappropriate responses but otherwise may retain normal speech and language problems; some of their communication deficits may be a function of their behavioral and attentional deficits; other communication disorders (e.g., dysarthria or reduced word fluency) are due to brain injury that affects speech and language formulation and production; still other communication deficits may partly reflect the limited language skills the clients had before the brain injury; the more serious the brain injury, the higher the likelihood of speech and language problems; clients with severe brain injury exhibit serious and lasting communication deficits

- The varied communication disorders associated with TBI include:
  - o <u>Mutism</u> or <u>aphonia</u> in some extreme cases; mutism is likely in the acute stage of TBI
  - o Confused language in the initial stages of TBI, especially soon after regaining consciousness or coming out of mutism; unaffected grammar but incoherent, irrelevant, confabulatory, and circumlocutory verbal responses
  - o Bizarre, inappropriate, incoherent, and paraphasic language, especially if confusion persists
  - o <u>Anomia</u>, especially evident in confrontation naming, may partly be due to inattentiveness, distraction, and hasty responses; persistence of word-finding problems
  - o Preservation of verbal responses (inappropriate repetition of the same response)
  - o Reduced word fluency, especially rapid naming of as many as possible within a category (e.g., names of flowers or animals); fluency affected by naming difficulties
  - o Impaired pragmatic language skills; difficulty initiating conversation, taking appropriate turns in conversation, and maintaining topics during conversation; too brief or rambling speech; inappropriate shifts in topics; initiation of irrelevant topics
  - o Difficulty in narrative speech; lack of cohesion, contextual information; use of the pronoun *it* without specifying the referent

T

- o Imprecise speech; use of vague, general, and inaccurate terms
- o Impaired nonverbal communication; gestures and facial expressions are limited, nonexistent, or inappropriate
- o Impaired social interaction, in spite of good grammatical skills
- o Difficulty understanding proverbs and idioms; literal interpretation of abstract statements
- o Auditory comprehension deficits; difficulty understanding spoken speech, meaning of gestures and facial expressions of others, complex and abstract material, and speech spoken at a rapid rate
- o <u>Dysarthria</u> (motor speech disorder due to impaired control of speech muscles), especially when the brainstem or cerebrum are affected; occurs in 30% to 35% of people with TBI; symptoms include reduced breath support for speech, limited phrase length, hypernasality, impaired rate of speech, imprecise production of consonants, abnormal stress patterns, monotonous speech with limited pitch and loudness variations, prolonged intervals (pauses) in speech, reduced speech intelligibility, and harsh and hoarse voice quality; typically mild to moderate in severity; all symptoms not always present
- o Nearly normal or normal syntactic features in recovered clients; possibility of subtle grammatical problems
- o Reading problems; difficulty understanding what is read, especially complex or abstract material
- o Writing problems; rambling and incoherent writing; increased difficulty with longer passages; common and persistent spelling errors; partly due to impaired attention and concentration
- o Recovery of most communicative skills within the first two months; continued improvement for up to 1 year; residual pragmatic deficits and word-finding problems

Related Problems

- Brain injury produces several related problems, including:
  - o Sleep disturbances in 30% to 70% of people with a recent history of TBI; clinical insomnia in 30%; risk factors for persistent sleep problems include fatigue, depression, and pain
  - o Endocrine disorders including hypopituitarism, secondary hypoadrenalism, and hypothyroidism in a small but significant number of clients
  - o <u>Foreign Accent Syndrome</u>; speech pattern, especially the prosodic and phonological features, that are alien to the client's premorbid (native) speech
  - o Possibility of brain tumors later in life

Subsequent and More Persistent Symptoms

- Possibility of long-term or permanent disability; worsening of a few persistent symptoms; worsening of problems with abstract reasoning and conceptualization, inhibition, memory problems, agitation, lack of self-appraisal, lack of diminished initiative, and flattening of emotional experiences
- Persistent physical disabilities including limited or impaired use of hands and limbs; persistent visual or other sensory deficits

- Emotional and social problems; as the recovery continues, the individual may experience:
  o Depression after the initial recovery possibly due to an awareness of deficits; may be unrelated to the degree of impairment
  o Feelings of helplessness or hopelessness, depending on the degree of recovery
  o Social withdrawal, especially if emotional and communication deficits persist
  o Suicidal tendencies
  o Lower threshold of tolerance for noise
  o Impulsivity
- Cognitive deficits; more persistent and more or less subtle symptoms, including:
  o Poor judgment
  o Memory deficits (impaired recall of events prior to or subsequent to the trauma)
  o Problem-solving skills and abstract reasoning
  o Distractibility and attentional deficits
  o Slower reaction time
  o Problems in drawing figures or geometric shapes
  o Visual-spatial deficits
  o Construction impairment
- Communication problems
  o Depending on the severity of the brain injury, more or less subtle naming problems and difficulty with abstract language may persist

Beukelman, D. R., & Yorkston, K. M. (1991). *Communication disorders following traumatic brain injury: Management of cognitive, language, and motor impairments.* Austin, TX: Pro-Ed.

Bigler, E. D. (Ed.). (1990). *Traumatic brain injury.* Austin, TX: Pro-Ed.

Center for Disease Control (2006). Incidence rates of hospitalization related to traumatic brain injury—12 states, 2002. *Morbidity and Mortality Weekly Report,* March 3, 2006, 55(8), 201–204.

Cooper, P. R., & Golfinos, J. G. (2000). *Head injury* (4th ed.). New York: McGraw-Hill.

Gillis, R. J. (1996). *Traumatic brain injury: Rehabilitation for speech-language pathologists.* Boston, MA: Butterworth-Heinemann.

Hegde, M. N. (2006). *A coursebook on aphasia and other neurogenic language disorders* (3rd ed.). Clifton Park, NY: Thomson Delmar Learning.

High, W. M., Sander, A. M., Struchen, M. A., & Hart, K. A. (2006). *Rehabilitation for traumatic brain injury.* New York: Oxford University Press.

Murdoch, B. E., & Theodoros, D. G. (2000). *Traumatic brain injury: Associated speech, language, and swallowing disorders.* Clifton Park, NY: Thomson Delmar Learning.

Silver, J. M., McAllister, T. W., & Yudofsky, S. C. (Eds.) (2005). *Textbook of traumatic brain injury.* Arlington, VA: American Psychiatric Publishing Inc.

T

Treacher Collins Syndrome. See Syndromes Associated With Communication Disorders.

Tremor. Pattern of shaking, an involuntary rhythmical movement of small amplitude.

Trisomy-21. Genetic condition in which three free copies of chromosome 21 cause a type of intellectual disability called Down syndrome (see Syndromes Associated With Communication Disorders).

Tumors. Space-occupying lesions that cause swelling in, and increased pressure on, surrounding tissue; associated with neurogenic communication disorders, including Aphasia, Apraxia of Speech, Dysarthria, and Dementia.

Turn Taking. Appropriately taking the role of a listener and speaker in conversational exchanges; a pragmatic language skill; impairments include interrupting the speaker to take a turn to talk or failure to take a turn when the conversational partner yields and expects the listener to talk; impaired in Language Disorders in Children.

T

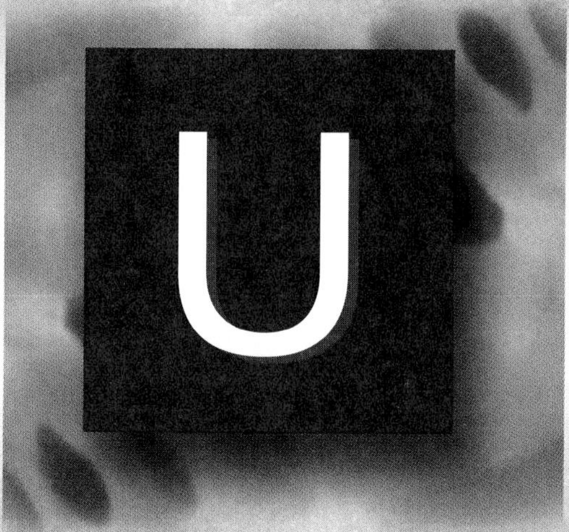
U

Underextensions. Word productions that are limited to restricted stimulus contexts; for instance, a child may say "car" only when the family car is seen, but not when other people's cars are seen; the production of words that are overly stimulus-selected with no generalization of the word meaning; normal unless they persist beyond age 3.

Unilateral Upper Motor Neuron Dysarthria. Motor speech disorder that includes problems of speech production; associated with lesions in the upper motor neurons (pyramidal and extrapyramidal tracts of motor control); a specific type of dysarthria; see Dysarthria and Dysarthria: Specific Types.

Unilingual. Person who speaks a single language.

Universal Grammar. A linguistic hypothesis that there are universal rules of grammar that apply to all languages; often presumed innately given in a child; part of the transformational generative theory of grammar.

Uremic Encephalopathy. Brain disorder caused by chronic kidney failure, resulting in a type of Dementia.

U

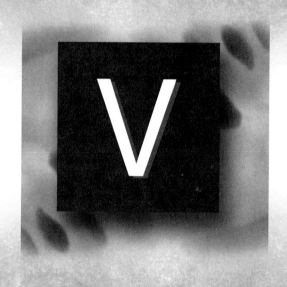

Valleculae.   Wedge-shaped space between the base of the tongue and the epiglottis; a space that food may fall into in cases of Dysphagia.

Variegated Babbling.   Infant-varying vocalizations of vowels, consonant-vowel combinations, and some consonant-vowel-consonant combinations; most children begin to show variegated babbling around 9 months; delay in variegated babbling or its persistence may be a sign of language disorder in a child.

Vascular Dementia.   Type of dementia caused by a variety of diseases that affect the cerebral vascular system; widespread and bilateral damage to the cortical and subcortical structures produce the second most common form of Dementia; vascular dementia is the second highest in frequency, dementia of the Alzheimer's type (DAT) being the highest; some experts believe Alzheimer's disease may be the underlying pathology of vascular dementia; vascular dementia is more common in men than in women; affects younger clients than does Alzheimer's disease; clients with vascular dementia die sooner than those with other types of neuropathology; vascular dementia is more common among African Americans than among whites; unlike other forms of dementia, vascular dementia has a sudden onset; three common types of vascular dementia have been identified: multi-infarct dementia, lacunar state, and Binswanger disease.

Multi-infarct Dementia.   Also known as *multiple bilateral cortical infarcts* (that lead to dementia); a form of mixed dementia because of both cortical and subcortical involvement; named *vascular dementia* in the DSM-IV; due to repeated strokes associated with a history of hypertension and arteriosclerosis; no familial pattern; varied symptom complex; younger age of onset compared to DAT; more frequent in men than in women; frequency may be just as high in nonwhite older women; may be more frequent in nonwhite populations because of their high frequency of vascular diseases.

Etiologic Factors
- Often a reported history of hypertension
- Vascular disorders with a history of arteriosclerosis, increasing the chances of repeated strokes
- Strokes due to large vessel occlusions in the major cerebral arteries (anterior, middle, posterior cerebral arteries), often producing focal damage

Neurological and Behavioral Symptoms
- Abrupt onset (versus insidious onset of other types of irreversible dementia); step-wise deterioration
- Early signs of cognitive impairment and confusion
- Inconsistent memory impairments (atypical of other forms of dementia); total inability to recall an event, followed by a sudden and total recovery
- Patchy distribution of impairment (coexistence of impaired and intact skills)
- Focal (specific and localized) neurological signs versus the more typical diffuse signs of dementia; include pseudobulbar palsy, gait abnormalities, and weakness of an extremity

V

- Progressive deterioration in memory and other cognitive skills, similar to other forms of dementia
- Impaired language (aphasia) and motor speech disorders
- Better preserved personality and behavior than those with other forms of dementia

Lacunar State. A kind of neuropathology characterized by a hollow space, cavity, or gap in the neural (or any other anatomic) structures; due to occlusion of small-end blood vessels deep with the brain; the resulting dementia is subcortical.

Etiologic Factors

- Occlusion of small-end arteries deep in the brain, causing ischemia
- Multiple, small, ischemic strokes in the basal ganglia, thalamus, midbrain, and brainstem
- Prolonged hypertension

Neurological and Behavioral Symptoms

- Initial stroke symptoms that improve
- Repeated infarcts that produce more persistent and serious problems, including rigidity, plasticity, pseudobulbar palsy, and limb weakness
- Dysarthria and dysphagia
- Nonspecific dementia symptoms in 70% to 80% of individuals, which become more severe in the late stage of the disease
- Language problems, only in the late stage
- Psychiatric symptoms, including apathy, disinhibition (inappropriate social behavior), and frequent mood swings

Binswanger's Disease. Also known as *subcortical arteriosclerotic encephalopathy;* associated with another form of vascular dementia; due to atrophy of the subcortical white matter; also may be due to multiple infarcts; lacunar states are also found in Binswanger's disease; mostly unaffected cortical structures.

Etiologic Factors

- Stroke risk factors (e.g., hypertension, vascular diseases)
- Multiple infarcts resulting in leukoareosis (atrophy of the subcortical white matter)
- Lacunar states in the basal ganglia and thalamus

Neurological and Behavioral Symptoms

- Symptoms are similar to those of lacunar states
- Acute strokes and a slow accumulation of focal neurological symptoms
- Motor symptoms similar to those associated with pseudobulbar palsy
- Intellectual deterioration and eventual dementia

American Psychiatric Association (1994). *Diagnostic and statistical manual of mental disorders* (4th ed.) Washington, DC: Author.

Clark, C. M., & Trojanowski, J. Q. (2001). *Neurodegenerative dementias.* New York: McGraw-Hill.

Hegde, M. N. (2006). *A coursebook on aphasia and other neurogenic language disorders* (3rd ed.). Clifton Park, NY: Thomson Delmar Learning.

Jagust, W. (2001). Understanding vascular dementia. *Lancet, 358,* 2097–2098.

Velo-Cardio-Facial Syndrome.   See <u>Syndromes Associated With Communication Disorders</u>.

Velopharyngeal Closure.   Approximation of the velum (the soft palate) and the pharyngeal sphincter to block the nasal resonance of phonated nonnasal sounds; needed for normal resonance of all oral (nonnasal) sounds; the mechanism may be congenitally incompetent or insufficient because of a lack of tissue mass; associated with such craniofacial anomalies as clefts, especially of the soft palate; also associated with <u>Dysarthria</u> and <u>Cerebral Palsy</u>; neuromuscular structures and actions involved in achieving velopharyngeal closure include:

- Muscles of the soft palate that help achieve normal velopharyngeal closure include the levator veli palatine, tesnsor veli palatine, muscular uvulus, salpingopharyngeus, superior pharyngeal constrictor, palatopharyngeus, and palatoglossus; palatal and upper pharyngeal muscles are mostly innervated by the cranial nerves glossopharyngeus, vagus, and accessory; trigeminal and facial nerves may be involved
- Levator veli palatine primarily elevates the soft palate during speech production and swallowing
- In achieving closure, the levator is moved upward and backward to make contact with the posterior pharyngeal wall; the contact is rarely firm and constant but remains flexible depending on the speech sound being produced; height varies during the production of different vowels
- Posterior pharyngeal wall moves anteriorly to meet the velum, and the lateral walls of the pharynx move medially to constrict the pharynx
- Combined actions of the soft palate movement and the pharyngeal wall movement and constrictions help achieve velopharyngeal closure; there are individual differences in the degree and force of the closure

Velopharyngeal Dysfunction.   A general term that suggests problems in velopharyngeal closure without specifying the causes; any kind of difficulty in achieving adequate velopharyngeal closure may be described as dysfunction; includes velopharyngeal inadequacy, velopharyngeal incompetence, velopharyngeal insufficiency, and velopharyngeal mislearning.

Velopharyngeal Inadequacy.   Most clinicians use this as a general term for problems in velopharyngeal closure, regardless of etiology, known or unknown; a variety of craniofacial structural and neurological problems may be responsible for inadequate velopharyngeal closure; inadequacy may be associated with adequate tissue mass; in most cases, insufficient tissue mass causes inadequate closure during oral speech sound production; problems resulting from velopharyngeal inadequacy include:

- Hypernasality: Excessive nasal resonance on oral sounds due to velopharyngeal insufficiency and incompetence; more pronounced on vowels; does not affect voiceless sounds

V

- Nasal Air Emission: Air escape through the nose during speech production that may be audible or inaudible (though measurable); often noticed on consonants; adds a hissing sound to speech only if audible; insufficiency, incompetence, and mislearning may all cause nasal emission; may be due to excessive effort to achieve velopharyngeal closure; other problems related to nasal emission include a *nasal rustle* (a friction-like noise when the air escapes through a partially constricted velopharyngeal valve), audible *nasal snort* (forceful air escape through the nose that results in a sneeze-like sound), and nasal grimace (contraction of facial muscles surrounding the nose); sometimes attributed to nasal air emission, *phoneme-specific nasal air emission* is not related to velopharyngeal dysfunction; it is an articulation disorder (substitution of posterior nasal fricatives for /s/)
- Weak consonant production: Results from the loss of air pressure in the oral cavity because of air loss through the nose; weak consonants (and hypernasality) are typically associated with Cleft Palate and several types of Dysarthria
- Reduced utterance length: Limited phrase length due to wastage of exhaled air available for speech; another feature of Dysarthria
- Compensatory articulation errors: Retaining the manner of sound production but displacing the place of production; sounds produced in the more anterior portions of the oral cavity may be produced more posteriorly; result is glottal stops (consonants produced at the glottis), pharyngeal stops (production of sounds with the back of tongue making contact with the pharyngeal wall), and pharyngeal fricatives (production of sounds with approximations of the base of the tongue and the pharyngeal wall; tongue is retracted to achieve this approximation)
- Dysphonias: Hyperfunctional voice disorders due to excessive efforts at closing the velopharyngeal valve; vocal nodules and resulting voice problems
- Hyponasality, denasality, or cul-de-sac resonance: Due to blocked nasal passages or surgical procedures designed to correct clefts, resulting in a more restricted nasopharynx

Velopharyngeal Incompetence. Deficient movement of the velopharyngeal mechanism, often due to a neuromotor or physiological disorder; *incompetence* refers to the actions, not to the structures; etiologic factors that cause insufficient movement of the velopharyngeal mechanism may vary across individuals; effects on speech production are similar to those described under velopharyngeal inadequacy; some of the factors that lead to incompetent movement include:

- Abnormal muscle insertion (e.g., levator veli palatini may be inserted into the hard palate, instead of the soft palate)
- Poor muscle function due to cleft palate surgery
- Poor lateral pharyngeal wall movement
- Lesions in the motor control systems (causing Dysarthria, Apraxia of Speech, and Hypernasality)

Velopharyngeal Insufficiency. Tissue deficiency in the velopharyngeal mechanism; varied etiologic factors making it physiologically impossible to achieve closure; effects on speech production are similar to those described under velopharyngeal inadequacy; common etiologic factors include:

- A short velum
- Deep pharynx that makes it difficult to achieve closure
- Deeper nasopharynx created by adenoidectomy, adenoid atrophy, irregular adenoids, jaw surgery, and surgical removal of oral tumors

Velopharyngeal Mislearning. Inadequate velopharyngeal closure presumably due to faulty learning; organic deficiencies do not explain the closure problem; mislearning is presumed when:

- Resonance and speech problems characteristic of velopharyngeal inadequacy persist in a child whose palatal clefts have been surgically closed
- Apparently adequate velopharyngeal mechanism yet inadequate closure, resulting in hypernasality
- Compensatory articulation that may have been learned before the surgical closure of the cleft (e.g., substituting posterior nasal fricatives for /s/ and /z/), causing nasality and audible nasal air emission
- Significant hearing loss with little or no auditory feedback

Kummer, A. W. (2001). *Cleft palate and craniofacial anomalies.* Clifton Park, NY: Thomson Delmar Learning.

Peterson-Falzone, S. J., Hardin-Jones, M. A., & Karnell, M. P. (2001). *Cleft palate speech* (3rd ed.). St. Louis, MO: Mosby.

Ventricular Dysphonia. Voice disorder resulting from the use of the ventricular (false) vocal folds for phonation; possibly because the true folds have some pathology; sometimes associated with enlarged ventricular folds; ventricular folds overlap the true folds, thus dampening their vibrations; characterized by low pitch, monotone, decreased loudness, harshness, and arrhythmic voicing.

Verbal Aphasia. The same as Broca's aphasia (see <u>Aphasia: Specific Types</u>).

Verbal Apraxia. See <u>Apraxia of Speech</u>.

Verbal Behavior. An alternative view of language conceptualized by behavioral scientists, especially B. F. Skinner; contrasts with the linguistic view of language as a mental system; defined as a form of social behavior maintained by a verbal community; does not include structural components (e.g., phonologic, morphologic, semantic, and syntactic); classified on the basis of causes that lead to behaviors, not on the basis of their structures; includes the following functional or cause-effect classes of behavior:

- Mands: A class of verbal behaviors caused by states of motivation or deprivation; they specify what will reinforce them (e.g., *may I have a glass of water* is uttered when the person is deprived of water, and the response specifies its own reinforcer: a glass of water); reinforcers are typically primary or biological, of survival value (e.g., food, water, procreation, and avoidance of harm); includes what are called commands, demands, and requests; often impaired in children with language impairment; impairment may lead to undesirable or aggressive behaviors to seek what is needed; teaching mands may eliminate such undesirable behaviors

- Tacts: Verbal behaviors that are caused by environmental objects and events; not based on states of motivation (deprivation) like the mands; hence, "disinterested" verbal behavior in a certain sense; reinforced socially, with agreement, praise, and so forth (e.g., a speaker's statement, *It is raining heavily*, may be reinforced by someone who agrees); verbal behavior consists mostly of tacts (e.g., descriptions, narratives, and comments)
- Echoics: Verbal behaviors that match the acoustic properties of a model; behavior that duplicates its own stimulus; reinforced by one or more persons on the basis of the similarity between the stimulus (the model) and the echoic response; the greater the similarity, the higher the chances of reinforcement; also known as *imitation*; not limited to children, and not posited as the main means of language acquisition; adults, too, echo experts when they try to learn something.
- Intraverbals: Verbal behaviors that are caused by speaker's own prior verbal behaviors or prompted by one's own utterances; most of connected speech is intraverbal behavior; what a speaker says one moment may be stimulus for what he or she says next; fluency of speech is possibly a function of intraverbal control; when a speaker speaks continuously on a topic, intraverbals are emitted because, putting it colloquially, "one thing leads to another" (e.g., *that reminds me of . . .* followed by additional continuous verbal behavior).
- Autoclitics: Verbal behaviors that comment upon or point to the causes of other verbal behaviors of the same person; account for grammar in the behavioral view of human communication; the speaker who says "I see two cups, not one cup," is pointing out the numerical property of the stimulus event (two, not single) that causes the verbal behavior; a speaker who says, "I read in the newspaper that global warming is a reality," is essentially telling why he or she is indeed saying what is being said.
- Textuals: Verbal behaviors whose causes are printed material; includes reading and writing, both involving printed material as their controlling stimuli; in learning to write, the child has to match the printed stimulus of letters to his or her own motoric responses (writing); in learning to read, the child has to literally name the sounds in the form of printed letters.

B. F. Skinner (1957). *Verbal behavior.* New York: Appleton-Century-Crofts.

Visual Agnosia.   Failure to grasp the meaning of objects seen normally; a rare neurological disorder; see <u>Agnosia</u>.

Vitiligo.   Anomaly of skin pigmentation resulting in white patches surrounded by hyperpigmented border; part of some genetic syndromes; see <u>Waardenburg Syndrome</u> under <u>Syndromes Associated With Communication Disorders</u>.

Vocal Fold Paralysis.   Laryngeal pathology resulting from damage to the branches of the vagus (cranial nerve X) nerve; unilateral or bilateral paralysis of the vocal folds; one or both folds may be fixated; may be unilateral (more common) adductor paralysis, which is inability to close the folds, often due to trauma or accidental cutting of the recurrent laryngeal nerve during surgery; bilateral abductor paralysis, often caused by a brainstem lesion, associated with dysarthrias; results in aphonia or dysphonia; see <u>Voice Disorders</u>.

317

Vocal Hyperfunction. Speaking with excessive muscular effort and force; vocal abuse or misuse; a frequent cause of voice disorders associated with such structural changes as vocal nodules; see Voice Disorders.

Vocal Nodules. Form of laryngeal pathology associated with vocally abusive behaviors; benign lesions of the vocal folds; generally bilateral; found at the junction of the anterior one-third and posterior two-thirds of the true vocal folds; symptoms may include hoarseness, harshness, periodic aphonia, frequent throat clearing, hard glottal attacks, tension, and a dry vocal tract; see Voice Disorders.

Voice Disorders. Various disorders of communication related to faulty, abnormal, or inappropriate loudness, pitch, quality, and resonance of voice; voice that does not help meet the social and occupational demands of communication; voice that deviates from expectations based on age, culture, or gender; may be associated with tension or a sense of discomfort in some cases; many descriptive terms of voice disorders lack objective definitions; classification varies across experts; many classifications confuse voice disorders (deviations of loudness, pitch, quality, and resonance) with their immediate or more or less remote causes (nodules, vocal abuse, cancer, papilloma); causes include vocally abusive behaviors resulting in laryngeal structural changes, physical trauma to the laryngeal mechanism, problems in neural control of the laryngeal mechanism due to central nervous system pathology, various physical diseases including cancer, reaction to stressful life situations (psychogenic), and no apparent cause (idiopathic) leading to the inference of faulty learning (functional disorder); may be the first and only sign of a serious laryngeal pathology; those associated with nodules are the most common; those associated with edema, polyps, carcinoma, and no known laryngeal pathology occur with decreasing frequency; those associated with carcinoma and vocal fold paralysis are most common in the elderly; nodules are most common in males under 14 years of age and females in the age range of 25 to 45 years; people who talk excessively or those who are professional voice users are more prone to voice disorders.

Epidemiology and Ethnocultural Variables

- Reliable and replicated evidence on the prevalence of voice disorders in the general population is limited; there are studies on the prevalence in specific populations (e.g., teachers or singers); estimates in the general population vary across sources
- Most if not all children and adults may have an episode or two of voice problems in their lifetime; episode may not last long or require medical or voice treatment; nonetheless, the lifetime incidence of voice disorders (at least one episode in a lifetime) is high
- Up to 10% of school-age children may have voice problems at any one time they are examined; about 7% of school-age children may have a more persistent voice problem; it is unlikely, however, that 7% of school-age children are enrolled in clinical voice services in public schools
- Perhaps 3% of adults have persistent voice disorders that may need medical or voice assessment and treatment; in telephone interviews of nonteachers, 6% reported voice problems (Roy et al., 2004)

V

- Prevalence of voice disorders may be higher in particular groups than in the general population; those who regularly use their voice in their occupational settings have a higher risk of developing voice disorders; for instance:
  - Among teachers, the prevalence may be as high as 20% or as low as 11% (Roy et al., 2004; Smith et al., 1997); either estimate is higher than that for the general population, which varies from less than 1% to 15%; some recent sources suggest between 3% and 6% for the general population; up to 58% of teachers may report a lifetime incidence of voice disorders compared with 28% of nonteachers; however, only 14% of those who report a voice problem may have actually consulted a physician or speech-language pathologist, compared to 5.5% of nonteachers
  - More females than males, especially female teachers, report voice problems; voice problems in female teachers may be more chronic than those in male teachers
  - Teachers in the age range of 40 and 59 years with 16 or more years of education may be more likely to have voice disorders than are others in the general population
  - Family history of voice disorders is a risk factor; this may be a function of genetic vulnerability as well as environmental (behavioral) variables
  - People who experience frequent episodes of allergies, asthma, colds, sinus infection, and postnasal drip have a high risk for voice disorders
  - Cheerleaders are another vulnerable group; up to 75% of cheerleaders may experience voice problems soon after a game
  - Preachers, sportscasters, disk jockeys, auctioneers, and others who regularly talk for extended durations on their job have a high risk for voice disorders
- Prevalence of voice disorders in different ethnic groups has not been studied adequately; available data are about medical conditions that cause voice disorders; variations in the prevalence of diseases of the mouth, larynx, pharynx, and esophagus can cause differential prevalence of voice disorders in different ethnocultural groups:
  - Prevalence of laryngeal cancer, a major disease that causes voice problems, is highest among African Americans and lowest among American Indians; the prevalence is progressively lower among Hawaiians, Hispanics, Japanese, Chinese, Filipinos, and Native Americans
  - Prevalence of oral cancer alone (no laryngeal or pharyngeal involvement), from the highest to lowest, is found in African Americans (the highest), Native Americans in Alaska, Chinese, Hawaiians, Filipinos, Mexicans, and Japanese and American Indians (the same lowest rate)
  - Prevalence of oral and pharyngeal cancer is highest in African American males, followed by white males and Chinese who may be especially predisposed to nasopharyngeal cancer
  - The highest to lowest incidence of esophageal cancer is found in African Americans (the highest), Hawaiians, Filipinos, Chinese, Japanese and American Indians (roughly the same rate), and Hispanics (the lowest rate)
  - Thyroid deficiencies that can cause voice disorders are more common in whites than in African Americans

319

o Incidence of cleft palate, which often causes resonance disorders, is, per 1000, 4 among the Chinese, 3 among American Indians, 2.5 among the Japanese, 2 among Hispanics, and slightly less than 1 among whites

o Vocal nodules are more prevalent in white males than in white females; they are more common in African American females than in African American males

• Most prevalence data are for voice disorders due to heavy vocal use or vocal abuse; prevalence data on other kinds of voice disorders are inadequate; in addition to various kinds of cancers, neurological diseases also can cause voice problems; several forms of dysarthria are associated with hyponasality, hypernasality, monopitch, monoloudness, and harshhoarse voice; no specific prevalence data are available on neurogenic voice disorders

• Abnormalities in the oral structures and muscles of respiration may contribute to voice disorders; abnormal function of the laryngeal and the velopharyngeal mechanism contributes to most voice and resonance problems; voice disorders refer to deviations in pitch, loudness, and quality of voice; resonance disorders refer to an improper distribution of phonated air between the oral and nasal cavities; all voice disorders, except for aphonia, may be classified as dysphonias; in dysphonia, voice is present but is impaired in one or more of its dimensions; in aphonia, the voice is absent

Classification of Voice Disorders. Voice disorders are traditionally classified as functional, organic, and neurological:

• Functional voice disorders: caused by faulty vocal behaviors of the speaking persons (e.g., misuse or abuse of voice), not by any organic conditions

• Organic voice disorders: caused by tissue changes that are due to disease processes (e.g., cancer of the larynx or hyperkeratosis)

• Neurological voice problems: caused by neurological diseases that affect the regulation of the vocal folds and other speech-related structures (e.g., the velopharyngeal mechanism)

• This classification is problematic because the immediate or proximal causes of many so-called *functional voice disorders* are indeed tissue changes that are due to abuse or misuse; it is the cause of tissue change that is functional (not due to disease, but abuse), but the voice disorder itself is caused by organic changes in most functional voice disorders; very few voice disorders (e.g., aphonia without an organic basis, too high or too low pitch, and too loud or too soft voice in some cases) are truly functional

Functional Aphonia. Loss of voice; technically, aphonia of any kind is a complete absence of voice; an inability to produce phonation (sound) for speech; complete and constant absence of phonation is unusual, and is called muteness; phonation may be heard during coughing, laughing, or throat clearing; problem may be constant or intermittent; most clients who have aphonia communicate effectively with whispers, gestures, and facial expressions; some clients may speak with a faint voice with breathiness or with a weak shrill voice; aphonia with a sudden onset is classified as

V

functional if no organic causes are found for the lack of voice; associated factors include:

- Psychological or behavioral factors are thought to play a causative role in functional aphonia
  - Sometimes described as an hysterical reaction (conversion reaction); a psychoanalytic (Freudian) term that means that unconsciously, some other problem (e.g., repressed sexual impulses) has been transformed (converted) into aphonia
  - Reaction to difficult life situations involving acute or prolonged stress (e.g., a person may become suddenly aphonic during a courtroom testimony); this description avoids the psychoanalytic connotations of conversion reaction; loss of voice, often temporary, may have some reinforcing consequences that maintain the disorder (e.g., escape from the stressful witness stand)
- Reaction to physical diseases
  - Onset of aphonia in some cases may be preceded by the flu, upper respiratory illness, meningitis, or other physical illnesses
  - Possibly, temporary loss of voice due to organic causes which cease to operate but aphonia persists
- Following laryngeal surgery
  - Following laryngeal surgery, the client who was ordered complete voice rest for a period of time may fail to regain voice and remain aphonic even though the vocal folds are intact

Voice Disorders of Loudness (Intensity). Socially inappropriate vocal loudness; include the following:
- Excessively loud voice: Voice that is judged too loud from the standpoint of social situations; associated factors include:
  - Habitual vocal hyperfunction (voice produced with excessive force); the speaker may be accustomed to speaking in a loud voice and thus the disorder may be purely functional (no organic cause or tissue change)
  - Neurological factors that affect vocal fold activities; loudness variations may include excessive loudness; Dysarthria is associated with loudness problems, although too soft voice may be more common than too loud voice
  - Hearing loss may be associated with loudness problems; inability to monitor one's own speech and voice adequately, a person with a hearing loss may speak too loudly (or too softly)
- Excessively soft voice: Voice that is too soft to meet the social and occupational demands of communication; associated factors include:
  - Neurological diseases; various neurological diseases (e.g., amyotrophic lateral sclerosis, Parkinson's disease) may reduce vocal loudness, resulting in excessively soft voice
  - Laryngeal pathologies; various structural laryngeal pathologies (regardless of their origin) may affect vocal loudness; these include vocal nodules and paralysis that may reduce vocal loudness because of loss of air pressure

      o Cultural or personal variables; these are poorly understood, but some individuals speak too softly because of their family or general cultural practices; loud speech is considered too impolite, and their soft speech may be too soft in a different cultural context

- Shimmer; this is intensity (loudness) perturbations; a cycle-to-cycle variation that exceeds 1 dB is called shimmer; may be described as a voice quality disorder; associated factors include:
  - o Possible neurological factors
  - o Various organic factors, including vocal nodules

Voice Disorders of Pitch (Frequency). Voice characterized by various deviations in pitch that may be unacceptable for age and gender; include the following:

- Inappropriate pitch: Inappropriate in relation to the speaker's age and gender; includes falsetto or puberphonia: very high pitch in postpubertal males and females; associated factors include:
  - o Faulty learning; failure to learn the new voice pattern with lower pitch
  - o Persistence of prepubertal vocal pattern with its high pitch
- Pitch breaks: A high-pitched voice may break lower; a low-pitched voice may break higher; may be described as a quality disorder; associated factors include:
  - o Developmental changes in the laryngeal mechanisms in adolescents
  - o Speaking at inappropriate pitch levels; consequently, voice may break an octave or two up or down in children and adults
  - o Vocal fatigue due to prolonged voice use
- Lack of pitch variations: Monopitch; associated factors include:
  - o Vocal fold paralysis
  - o Neurological diseases (e.g., Parkinson's disease)
  - o Faulty learning (functional)
- Diplophonia: Production of double pitch; associated factors include:
  - o Vocal folds vibrating at different rates because of differences in mass between the two
  - o Vocal fold paralysis, laryngeal web, ventricular fold vibration, and aryepiglotic vibration
  - o Faulty learning (functional)
- Jitter: Frequency perturbations; cycle-to-cycle variations in vocal intensity that exceed 1%; may be described as a voice quality disorder; associated factors include:
  - o Possible neurological factors
  - o Vocal fold structural anomalies, including nodules
  - o Faulty learning (functional)

Voice Disorders of Quality. Voice characterized by undesirable vocal qualities due primarily to faulty approximation of the vocal folds; include the following:

- Breathiness: Excessive and audible air leakage associated with phonation; primary and immediate cause is a failure to achieve optimum approximation of the vocal folds; associated factors include:
  - o Various organic factors including nodules and polyps; paralysis of vocal cords
  - o Faulty learning (functional)

V

- Harshness: Unpleasant, strident, or rough voice; aperiodicity of laryngeal vibration; associated factors include:
  o Excessive vocal effort, hard glottal attacks, and abrupt initiation of voice
  o Vocal tract constriction
  o Possible neurological problems
  o Laryngeal structural problems
  o Vocal abuse and faulty learning (functional)
- Hoarseness: A grating or husky voice quality that includes voice breaks, diplophonia, low pitch, harshness, and breathiness; the most commonly observed voice disorder; dry hoarseness (because of lack of sufficient lubrication of the folds) or wet hoarseness (because of excessive mucous secretions on the vocal folds); associated factors include:
  o Various laryngeal structural alterations including nodules, polyps, cysts, papilloma, and cancer
  o Laryngitis and upper respiratory infections
  o Vocal abuse and misuse
- Glottal or vocal fry: Popcorn popping or bubbling kind of voice occurring toward the lower end of the pitch range; a slight hoarseness may be heard; not necessarily a disorder of voice because glottal fry is a normal voice characteristic; too frequent production may constitute a clinical problem; the major associated factor is the following:
  o Contact between the vocal folds and ventricular folds
- Tense voice: Voice produced with excessive adduction and medial compression of the folds; voice sounds tensed; associated factors include:
  o Various organic conditions that promote compensation resulting in hyperadduction
  o Faulty learning (functional)
- Spastic voice: Spasticity in voice production; intermittent stoppage of voice because of an extreme degree of tensed vocal fold approximation; a symptom of spasmodic dysphonia; associated factors include:
  o Neurological problems
  o Faulty learning (functional)

Voice Disorders of Resonance. Voice characterized by inappropriate resonance; may also be described as voice quality disorders; include the following:

- Hypernasality: Excessive nasal resonance because of the open velopharyngeal port; associated factors include:
  o Craniofacial anomalies including cleft soft palate
  o Structural problems unrelated to clefts including short hard palate, short velum, partial submucous cleft palate, and deep pharynx
  o Tonsillectomy and adenoidectomy resulting in reduced tissue mass
  o Neurological diseases that cause problems in motor control of the velopharyngeal mechanism (as in dysarthrias)
- Hyponasality: Too little nasal resonance because of limited resonance of the nasal cavity; almost all associated factors are organic:
  o Pharyngitis and tonsillitis
  o Diseases of the nasal cavity

- o Allergies and upper respiratory disorders
- o Nasal polyps and papillomas
- o Foreign bodies in the nasal cavity
- o Nasal neoplasm (growth in the nasal cavity)
- o Deafness
- Cul-de-sac nasality: "Bottom of the sac" or hollow-sounding nasality; associated factors include:
  - o Excessively posterior carriage of the tongue
  - o Anterior nasal obstruction with posterior opening
  - o Faulty learning (functional)
- Assimilative nasality: Nasal resonance in the production of oral sounds that are adjacent to nasal sounds; associated factors include:
  - o Recent tonsillectomy and adenoidectomy
  - o Premature opening of the velopharyngeal port (nasality prior to nasal sounds)
  - o Failure to promptly close the velopharyngeal port (nasality after nasal sounds)

Etiologic Factors Associated with Voice Disorders

- Well established interaction between laryngeal pathologies and behavioral patterns; some of the behavioral patterns induce laryngeal pathology; all laryngeal pathologies are described in this section, including those that have behavioral origins

Laryngeal pathologies. Various pathologies involve structural changes in the laryngeal mechanism; pathological changes may have physical or behavioral causes; the deviations in voice parameters are directly related to those pathological structural changes, regardless of the origin of those changes.

- Cancer: Carcinoma of the laryngeal structures; may affect the vocal folds (glottal), supraglottal structures, subglottal structures, or a combination of these; causes and consequences include:
  - o Potential causes include damaging behaviors including smoking, excessive drinking, and a combination of the two which is thought to produce the most negative consequences; genetic predisposition because most cancers seem to be due to an interaction between genetic and behavioral/environmental variables
  - o Voice problems related to cancer include hoarseness of voice
  - o Related problems include pain, bleeding, respiratory problems, and swallowing difficulties
- Contact ulcers: Lesions mostly on the posterior third of the vocal folds that cause voice problems; entire approximating margins of the vocal folds may be granulated; some inflammation may be evident; a relatively infrequent cause of voice disorders; causes and consequences include:
  - o Excessive slamming of the folds (behavioral) with a low-pitched voice, excessively loud voice, and frequent throat clearing and coughing may be the behavioral causes of contact ulcers; perhaps only a few clients have this as the primary cause of contact ulcers

V

- o Gastric reflux (medical); stomach acids may migrate upward, causing irritation of the laryngeal areas; this factor may account for a substantial number of cases
- o Intubation; intubation pre- or post-surgery may cause contact ulcers
- o Voice problems due to contact ulcers include vocal fatigue and hoarseness or roughness of voice
- o Pain in the throat, frequent throat clearing
- Cysts: Whitish oval-shaped nodule-like lesions under the surface of vocal folds; possibly traumatic lesions; submucosal; may be confused with nodules; some, but not all, may be fluid filled; typically unilateral, but may be bilateral or multiples; typical site is the Reinke's space; most are benign; causes and consequences include:
  - o Congenital or acquired
  - o Consequence of surgery for nodules
  - o Dysphonia
- Endocrine abnormalities: Disorders of the endocrine system that typically affect a still-growing larynges; several glandular abnormalities may lead to voice problems: causes and consequences include:
  - o Pituitary gland abnormalities may delay laryngeal growth and prevent voice change in pubescent children (high-pitched voice in males may continue)
  - o Hypofunction of the adrenal gland may lead to a continuation of high-pitched voice in boys
  - o Hypothyroidism, which increases vocal fold thickness and causes a low-pitched voice
  - o Virilization of the female voice, associated with birth control medication or menstrual periods
- Granuloma: Firm, granulated, sac-like, vascular growth on the vocal process of the arytenoid process (posterior larynx); causes and consequences include:
  - o Vocal abuse and misuse
  - o Surgical intubation, a traumatic cause; women and children, because of their smaller airway passage, are more prone to it than men
  - o Gastric reflux is a medical condition; perhaps the most frequently encountered factor
  - o Limited pitch range, hoarseness, and breathiness are the main voice characteristics associated with granuloma
  - o Vocal fatigue, throat pain, and frequent throat clearing are related problems
- Hemangiomas: Soft, blood-filled sacs on the posterior larynx; similar to granulomas except hemangiomas are softer; causes and consequences include:
  - o Vocal hyperfunction (vocal abuse)
  - o Hyperacidity and intubation-induced trauma
  - o Voice problems associated with hemangiomas are similar to those found in granulomas: hoarseness, breathiness, low pitch or limited pitch range

- o Related problems include vocal fatigue, pain in the throat, and frequent throat clearing
- Hemorrhage: Vocal fold hemorrhage that may resolve by itself or produce a chronic condition of fibrous and scarred vocal folds; causes and consequences include:
  - o Main cause is trauma to the vocal folds
  - o Main vocal characteristic is hoarse voice
- Hyperkeratosis: Pinkish rough growth; leaf-shaped keratinized (horny) cell growth on the folds or inner glottal margins; unilateral or bilateral; may be premalignant (transforming later into cancerous growth); may be found under the tongue and the arytenoid prominence; causes and consequences include:
  - o Causes not clearly established, although excessive drinking and smoking and exposure to smoke-filled environments are clinically linked to hyperkeratosis
  - o Vocal hoarseness
- Increased vocal fold mass: May be only a slight thickening of the vocal folds; sometimes temporary; thicker folds vibrate more slowly and may not approximate; causes and consequences include:
  - o Hypothyroidism is an endocrine disorder that can increase vocal fold mass; may be relatively permanent if the endocrine problem is not treated
  - o Lowered estrogen and progesterone in women during menstruation can cause thickening of the folds; temporary condition
  - o Lower pitch and hoarseness
- Infectious laryngitis: A general term, laryngitis means inflammation of the larynx, often associated with dryness and soreness of the throat, affecting the voice; causes and consequences include:
  - o Viral infection due to a cold is more common than bacterial infection; infectious laryngitis is likely in individuals with fever and cold
  - o Hoarseness; low pitch in some cases
- Leukoplakia: Patchy, white lesions on the vocal folds and under the tongue; not always malignant, but may be precancerous in some cases, leading eventually to squamous cell carcinoma; hard to distinguish from cancer by visual examination; causes and consequences include:
  - o Excessive and prolonged smoking
  - o Hoarseness, diplophonia, and reduced vocal intensity
- Papilloma: Mulberry- or wart-like growth on the vocal folds and related structures; may obstruct the airway; may be life-threatening; tend to recur in younger and older children, requiring repeated surgical removal; causes and consequences include:
  - o Papillomas are caused by the human papilloma virus
  - o Shortness of breath because of airway obstruction
  - o Frequent hoarseness and infrequent aphonia
- Polyps: Typically unilateral, soft, fluid-filled growth on the anterior and middle third portion of vocal fold edges (the same typical site of vocal nodules); may be broad-based *sessile* or narrowly based *pedunculated;* the latter type of polyp may look more like a small balloon with a narrow

V

stem; larger pedunculated polyps may hang down and obstruct the airway; causes and consequences include:

- o Vocal abuse and misuse; acute onset because unlike nodules, polyps may develop as a result of a single episode of vocal abuse
- o Severe voice problems; may include hoarseness and breathiness (partly due to inadequate glottal approximation and asynchronous vibration because of vocal fold mass differences)
- o Frequent throat clearing; this may exacerbate the problem

- Reinke's edema: Type of vocal fold thickening; may be considered a mild form of polypoid degeneration; an accumulation of fluid under the vocal fold cover in the Reinke's space (hence the name); causes and consequences include:
  - o Smoking and vocal abuse
  - o Hoarseness and low pitch

- Laryngeal growth problems: Larynx may fail to attain normal size; this will affect voice production; causes and consequences include:
  - o Endocrine disorders, especially pituitary disorders in women
  - o Pitch disorders

- Sulcus vocalis: Bilateral development of a groove along the vocal fold edges; the glottal opening may have a long oval shape; voice problems may be the early and presenting symptoms; causes and consequences include:
  - o Congenital or acquired condition whose etiology is not well understood
  - o Trauma and vocal abuse
  - o Decreased vocal intensity, breathiness, and hoarseness

- Traumatic laryngitis: Also known as functional laryngitis; characterized by vocal fold swelling; the glottal edges are swollen and thickened; irritated, blood-accumulated vocal folds alter phonation; causes and consequences include:
  - o Vocal abuse as seen in overly enthusiastic sports fans
  - o Hoarse and low-pitched voice

- Vocal fold thickening: Anterior two-thirds of the glottal margins (the vibrating portion) may be thickened, sometimes as a precursor to nodules or polyps; may be more extensive in some cases; causes and consequences include:
  - o Chronic abuse or misuse (e.g., loud talk, frequent screaming and yelling) is a behavioral cause of vocal fold thickening
  - o Genetic predisposition to vocal fold thickening
  - o Persistent upper respiratory problems
  - o Laryngeal postsurgical reaction; hoarseness (with low pitch), harshness, and possibly breathiness

- Vocal nodules: Typically bilateral, whitish, benign, callous-like growths on the edges of the vocal folds; often at the midpoint of the folds (anterior and middle third portion) but the site of growth may vary; multiple nodules in some cases; causes and consequences include:
  - o Vocal abuse and misuse (including frequent yelling and screaming, hard glottal attacks, excessive talking, and singing in abusive ways) over a period of time

- o An "aggressive personality" and excessive arguing with others
- o Alcohol abuse
- o Prevents optimal approximation of the folds, causing breathiness, lower pitch, hoarseness, and voice that sounds to lack proper resonance; vocal fatigue toward the end of the day
- o Jitters and shimmers and reduced maximum phonation duration and (possibly) abnormal s/z ratio
- o Frequent throat clearing, causing additional abusive effects on the folds
- Webbing: Thin and web-like tissue growth across the vocal folds; may be small or large; typical site of growth is the anterior commissure where the two folds come together; causes and consequences include:
  - o Congenital (observed at the time of birth) in some individuals; may be due to an abnormality during the embryonic period when the membranes of the two vocal folds normally separate but fail to
  - o Acquired in other individuals; trauma to the medial edges of the folds may cause a web to grow across them; traumatized tissue (e.g., infected larynges) come together and tend to grow into each other
  - o Severe Dysphonia
  - o Respiratory distress (shortness of breath)

Laryngeal Trauma. Externally induced injury to laryngeal structures that result in voice problems, often requiring immediate medical or surgical treatment; variety of conditions may induce laryngeal trauma, although they may be conveniently grouped into three major categories:

- Injury to larynx: Various conditions can cause laryngeal injury that may be mild to severe (involving the crushing of the laryngeal structures); causes and consequences include:
  - o Automobile accidents that crush or damage laryngeal structures
  - o Injury due to assault and gunshot wounds to the throat; attempted strangulation
  - o Accidental penetration of the laryngeal area by sharp objects
  - o Voice problems are less urgent than the surgical repair of the damaged laryngeal structures; postsurgically, various kinds voice problems may be evident
- Burning of the laryngeal area: Burning of the laryngeal area results in severe damage because of the delicate nature of the vocal folds; causes and consequences include:
  - o Smoke damage because of burning buildings or crashed automobiles in which people get trapped
  - o Gas inhalation; automobile exhaust inhalation when trapped in a closed space
  - o Harmful chemical ingestion in industrial accidents or during an attempted suicide
  - o Varied voice disorders
- Surgical sequelae: Consequences of certain surgical procedures that induce trauma to the vocal folds; causes and consequences include:
  - o Tracheostomy and endotracheal intubation may irritate the vocal folds

- o Long-term use of nasogastric tube for various reasons may cause more severe or persistent damage to the vocal folds
- o Vocal fold irritation, edema, webbing, granuloma, and vocal fold paralysis may be among the consequences
- o Various kinds of voice disorders, depending on the nature and extent of the injury

Neurological Pathologies. Voice disorders are associated with various neurological disorders; neuropathologies may affect the structure or function of the vocal folds; basic cause is disordered neural control of the laryngeal mechanism, often due to central nervous system involvement.

- Bilateral vocal fold paralysis: Paralysis of both the vocal folds, affecting phonation; causes and consequences include:
  - o Various diseases and trauma that damage the brainstem and descending motor tracts
  - o Airway may remain open, resulting in serious swallowing problems
  - o Weakness or paralysis of oral structures (including the tongue, pharynx, or velum); Dysarthria is associated with such weakness or paralysis
- Unilateral vocal fold paralysis: Paralysis of one fold due to various factors; associated with voice problems; causes and consequences include:
  - o Damage to the superior or recurrent branch of the vagus (cranial nerve X) due to trauma, penetrating gunshot or stab wounds, neurological diseases, or surgical accidents (including thoracic surgical accidents)
  - o Laryngeal adductor muscles, especially the lateral cricoarytenoid muscle, may be unable to help achieve vocal fold approximations, although at the anterior commissure, the folds may approximate as well as vibrate
  - o Breathiness, hoarseness, and monotone; infrequent association of aphonia
  - o Cranial nerve damage, including that of the vagus nerve, is associated with flaccid dysarthria with hypernasality and audible nasal emission
- Bilateral upper motor neuron lesions: Affect both the direct and indirect motor pathways; causes and consequences include:
  - o Variety of factors including vascular and degenerative diseases, tumors, and trauma cause bilateral upper motor neuron lesions
  - o Spastic dysarthria is associated with bilateral upper motor neuron lesions
  - o Strained-strangled voice, pitch breaks, low pitch, harshness, monoloudness, and hypernasality
- Cerebellar lesions: Lesions to the cerebellum (which coordinates movement) affect speech and voice production; causes and consequences include:
  - o Variety of factors including degenerative and vascular diseases and demyelinating diseases
  - o Ataxic dysarthria
  - o Harshness, monopitch, monoloudness, and occasional voice tremors

- Lesions of the basal ganglia: Structures of the basal ganglia are involved in motor control; causes and consequences include:
  o Variety of factors including such degenerative diseases as Parkinson's disease and vascular disorders
  o Hypokinetic dysarthria
  o Monopitch, monoloudness, harshness, breathiness, hypernasality, weak phonation, and low pitch
- Amyotrophic Lateral Sclerosis (ALS): Degenerative motor neuron disease that affects bulbar, limb, and respiratory muscles; causes and consequences include:
  o Upper- and lower motor neuron lesions
  o Associated with mixed dysarthria (spastic-flaccid)
  o Hypernasality, harshness, monopitch, monoloudness, strained or strangled voice, breathiness, and nasal emission
- Multiple Sclerosis (MS): Demyelinating disease of the central nervous system that affects speech and voice production; causes and consequences include:
  o Demyelination of various brain structures, especially the white matter and periventricular areas of the brain; damage may be widespread
  o Associated with dysarthria (flaccid and spastic-ataxic)
  o Loudness control problems, harshness, impaired pitch control, breathiness, hypernasality, and inappropriate pitch
- Spasmodic dysphonia: Although not a neuropathology in itself, Spasmodic Dysphonia is a special category of voice disorders of suspected neuropathology; may be of the adductor type, which is more common, or abductor type, which is not only less common but controversial; causes and consequences include:
  o Uncertain etiology, although presumed to be of neurological origin; currently considered a form of dystonia (a movement disorder)
  o Uncertain brain lesion sites; not convincingly documented
  o Possibly other unknown causes
  o Strained, struggled, effortful voice production; jerky voice onset; intermittent voice breaks; vocal tremor (adductor type); breathy spasms, failure to maintain voice; worsening symptoms with voiceless sounds (abductor type)

Behavioral Patterns. Many behavioral patterns are associated with voice disorders; some behavioral patterns lead to tissue changes in the vocal folds and related structures (e.g., vocal nodules that are related to vocal abuse); other behavioral patterns, listed here, are not associated with pathological changes in the larynx; these disorders are truly *functional* (versus the voice disorders due to nodules, which are also classified as *functional,* but are really due to organic changes).

- Speaking at the upper end of the normal pitch range; this may be a habitual response with no organic basis; causes and consequences include:
  o Causes are mostly unknown
  o Failure to shift to a lower voice or a failure to learn to speak with appropriate pitch and pitch variations

V

o Downward pitch breaks
- Vocal reaction to stressful situations; voice disorders that are hard to explain because of a lack of physical bases are described as *psychogenic*; but the term does not explain anything, and often obscures potential observable environmental events; causes and consequences include:
  o Potential negative reinforcement (e.g., an otherwise unexplainable aphonia may offer a chance to escape from certain speaking situations; avoiding aversive situations is *negatively reinforcing* to the individual)
  o Conversion reaction is a Freudian explanation of behavioral problems—including certain voice disorders—with no known organic etiology (e.g., such hysterical reactions as functional blindness, deafness, or paralysis); however, the Freudian theory of behavioral disorders lacks experimental evidence
  o Combination of stress and organic pathology that disappears (e.g., laryngitis that led to complete rest); when the pathology recedes, the voice problem associated with it or imposed as a consequence may persist (see <u>Functional Aphonia</u> at the beginning of this entry)
- Persistence of childhood vocal pitch or use of even higher pitch beyond puberty; also called puberphonia or mutational falsetto (a high-pitched breathy voice in the postpubertal male); causes and consequences include:
  o Inadequate response to pubertal changes in the larynx
  o Concern about pitch breaks and the social reaction to them (embarrassment about pitch breaks at puberty that helps maintain the high pitch)
  o Suggested causes are mostly speculative
- Participation of ventricular folds in voice production; in some cases, the ventricular folds may be the primary or only source of phonation; causes and consequences include:
  o Loading of the ventricular folds on the true folds, resulting in some vibration of the ventricular folds as well
  o Disease of the true folds may force the use of ventricular folds
  o Effect is described as ventricular dysphonia, characterized by low-pitched, monotonous, and hoarse voice

Andrews, M. L. (2006). *Manual of voice treatment: Pediatrics through geriatrics* (2nd ed.). Clifton Park, NY: Thomson Delmar Learning.

Boone, D. R., McFarlane, S. C., & Von Berg, S. L. (2005). *The voice and voice therapy* (7th ed.). Boston, MA: Allyn and Bacon.

Case, J. L. (2002). *Clinical management of voice disorders* (4th ed.). Austin, TX: Pro-Ed.

Roy, N., Merrill, R. M., Thibeault, S., Parsa, R. A., Gray, S. D., & Smith, E. M. (2004). Prevalence of voice disorders in teachers and general population. *Journal of Speech, Language, and Hearing Research, 47,* 281–293.

Sataloff, R. T. (2005). *Clinical assessment of voice.* San Diego, CA: Plural Publishing.

Smith, E., Gray, S., Dive, H., Kirchner, L., & Heras, H. (1997). Frequency and effects of teachers' voice problems. *Journal of Voice, 11*(1), 81–87.

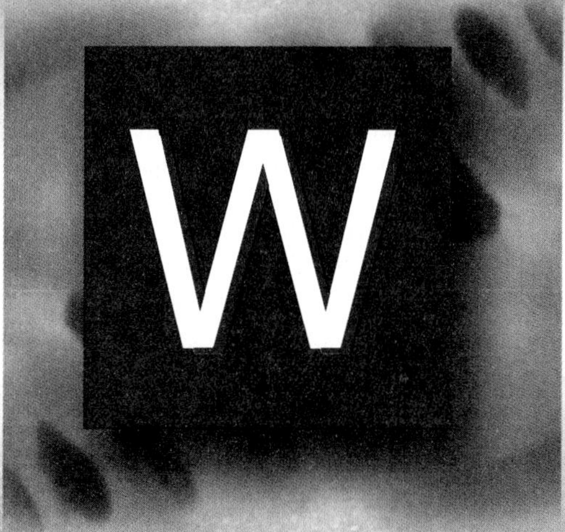
W

Watershed Area.   Region of the brain supplied by small end-branches (terminal branches) of the anterior, middle, and posterior cerebral arteries, receiving marginal amount of blood; disruption in blood supply to the watershed area of the brain is often associated with transcortical motor and transcortical sensory aphasias; see Aphasia: Specific Types.

Wernicke's Aphasia.   Type of fluent aphasia caused by damage to Wernicke's area; see Aphasia: Specific Types.

Wernicke's Area.   Posterior two-thirds of the superior temporal gyrus in the left or dominant hemisphere; responsible for comprehension and formulation of speech; damage to this area is associated with Wernicke's aphasia; see Aphasia: Specific Types.

Wilson's Disease.   Inherited, autosomal, progressive neurological disease with gradual onset; affects metabolism of dietary copper; toxic amounts of copper may be deposited in the corneas of the eyes, kidneys, liver, basal ganglia, and other parts of the brain; also known as *hepatolenticular degeneration* or *progressive lenticular degeneration*; associated with degeneration of the lenticular nuclei of the basal ganglia; late adolescent or early adult onset; tremor in the outstretched arms; slow movement; rigidity and bradykinesia of muscles; psychiatric symptoms including depression, mania, schizophrenic-like behaviors, and emotional lability; drooling; ataxia; dysphagia; hypokinetic, hyperkinetic, spastic, ataxic, and mixed dysarthrias, and subcortical dementia in some cases; effectively treated in early stages to prevent the onset of advanced symptoms; untreated, death occurs due to liver failure in about 3 years postonset.

Word Deafness.   Profound auditory comprehension deficit for spoken words; less commonly used name for Wernicke's aphasia; see Aphasia: Specific Types.

Word Fluency.   Fluency in rapidly producing words that start with a particular sound or words that belong to a certain category (e.g., animals or flowers); skill impaired in clients with Aphasia and Dementia.

Word Retrieval Problems.   Difficulty in recalling specific words during speech production, including conversation and picture naming (confrontation naming); often marked difficulty recalling nouns; may lead to paraphasic speech; symptom of Aphasia and Dementia.

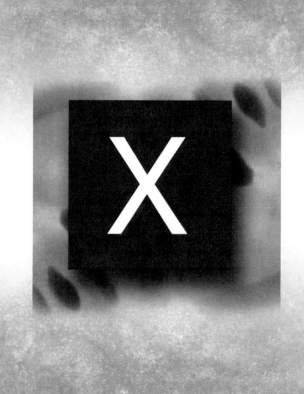

X

X-linked. Related to genes on the X chrome; inheritance of a trait related to the X chromosome(sex-linked), although the term *sex-linked* should include both X-linked and Y-linked conditions.

Xenophobia. Abnormal fear of strangers.

Xerostomia. Dry mouth; various medications, diseases, and radiological treatment may impair salivary glad secretion.

XO Syndrome. Same as Turner syndrome (see Syndromes Associated With Communication Disorders).

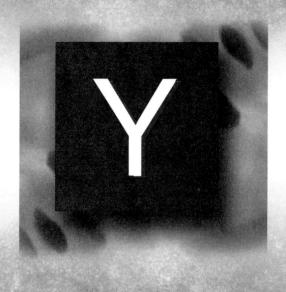

Y-linkage.   Related to genes on the Y chromosome; analogous to X-linkage.

Yaw.   Tendency of moving objects to change course; relevant to Traumatic Brain Injury; objects that penetrate the skull and change course as they move inside the brain; causes severe brain injury.

Z

Zenker's Diverticulum. Formation of a herniated pouch in the mucous membrane of the esophagus; collection of food within it may cause esophageal Dysphagia.

Z